MANIA

JOHNS HOPKINS BIOGRAPHIES OF DISEASE
Charles E. Rosenberg, Series Editor

Randall M. Packard, *The Making of a Tropical Disease: A Short History of Malaria*

Steven J. Peitzman, *Dropsy, Dialysis, Transplant: A Short History of Kidney Disease*

David Healy, *Mania: A Short History of Bipolar Disorder*

MANIA

❀ ❀ ❀

A Short History of Bipolar Disorder

David Healy

THE JOHNS HOPKINS UNIVERSITY PRESS
Baltimore

Johns Hopkins Paperback edition, 2011
2 4 6 8 9 7 5 3 1

The Johns Hopkins University Press
2715 North Charles Street
Baltimore, Maryland 21218-4363
www.press.jhu.edu

The excerpt from "Route" by George Oppen which appears on
page v is from *Collected Poems,* copyright © 1968 by George Oppen.
Reprinted by permission of New Directions Publishing Corp.

*The Library of Congress has catalogued the hardcover edition of
this book as follows:*

Healy, David, FRC Psych.
Mania : a short history of bipolar disorder / David Healy.
p. ; cm. — (Johns Hopkins biographies of disease)
Includes bibliographical references and index.
ISBN-13: 978-0-8018-8822-9 (hardcover : alk. paper)
ISBN-10: 0-8018-8822-0 (hardcover : alk. paper)
1. Manic-depressive illness—History. I. Title. II. Series.
[DNLM: 1. Bipolar Disorder—history. 2. History, 19th Century.
3. History, 20th Century. WM 11.1 H434m 2008]
RC516.H43 2008
616.89′5—dc22   2007036100

A catalog record for this book is available from the British Library.

ISBN-13: 978-1-4214-0397-7
ISBN-10: 1-4214-0397-8

*Special discounts are available for bulk purchases of this book.
For more information, please contact Special Sales at 410-516-6936 or
specialsales@press.jhu.edu.*

For Sarah, Justin, Helen, and Rita
Not as short as Crusoe we say was rescued
but with myths and Greeks

Tell the beads of the chromosomes like a rosary,
Love in the genes, if it fails
We will produce no sane man again

I have seen too many young people become adults, young
friends become old people, all that is not ours,

The sources
And the crude bone
        -we say
Took place
. . .

I think we try rather to understand
We try to stay together

From "Route," by George Oppen

CONTENTS

Disease is a fundamental aspect of the human condition. Ancient bones tell us that pathological processes are older than humankind's written records, and sickness still confounds our generation's technological pride. We have not banished pain, disability, or the fear of death, even if we die on the average at older ages, of chronic and not acute ills, in hospital or hospice beds, and not in our own homes. Disease is something men and women feel. It is experienced in our bodies—but also in our minds. Disease demands explanation; we think about it and we think with it. Why have I become ill? And why now? How is my body different in sickness from its quiet and unobtrusive functioning in health? Why in times of epidemic has a whole community been scourged?

Answers to such timeless questions necessarily mirror and incorporate available ideas and assumptions. In this sense, disease has always been a social and linguistic as well as biological entity. In the Hippocratic era, physicians—and we have always had them with us—were limited to the evidence of their senses in diagnosing a fever, an abnormal discharge, or seizures. Classical notions of the somatic basis for such alarming symptoms necessarily reflected and incorporated contemporary philosophical and physiological notions, a speculative world of disordered humors, "breath," and pathogenic local environments. Today we can call for understanding upon a variety of scientific insights and an armory of diagnostic and therapeutic practices—tools that allow us to diagnose ailments unfelt by patients and imperceptible to the doctor's senses. In the past century disease has become increasingly a bureaucratic phenomenon, as well, as sickness has been defined and in that sense constituted by formal disease classifications, treatment protocols, and laboratory thresholds.

Sickness is also linked to climatic and geographic factors. How and where we live and how we distribute our resources all contribute to time- and place-specific incidence of disease. For example, ailments such as typhus fever, plague, malaria, dengue, and yellow fever reflect specific environments that we have shared with our insect contemporaries. But humankind's physical circumstances are determined in part by culture—and especially agricultural practice in the millennia before the growth of cities and industry. Environment, demography, ideas, and applied medical knowledge all interact to create particular distributions of disease at particular moments in time. The contemporary ecology of sickness in the developed world is marked, for example, by the dominance of chronic and degenerative illness—ailments of the cardiovascular system and the kidneys and cancer. These are ailments not easily explained and evaded, nor are they easily managed.

Disease is thus historically as well as ecologically and biologically specific. Or perhaps I should say that every disease has a unique past. Once discerned and named, every disease claims its own history. At one level biology creates that idiosyncratic identity. Symptoms and epidemiology as well as generation-specific cultural values and scientific understanding shape responses to illness. Some writers may have romanticized tuberculosis—think of Greta Garbo as Camille—but, as the distinguished medical historian Owsei Temkin noted dryly, no one had ever thought to romanticize dysentery. Tuberculosis was pervasive in nineteenth-century Europe and North America and killed far more people than cholera did, but it never mobilized the same widespread and policy-shifting anxiety. Unlike tuberculosis, cholera killed quickly and dramatically and was never accepted as a condition of life in Europe and North America. Its episodic visits were anticipated with fear. Sporadic cases of influenza are normally invisible, indistinguishable among a variety of respiratory infections; waves of epidemic flu are all too visible. Syphilis and other sexually transmitted diseases, to cite another example, have had a peculiar and morally inflected attitudinal history. Some diseases such as smallpox or malaria have a long history, others like AIDS a rather short one. Some have flourished under modern conditions; others seem to reflect the realities of an earlier and less economically developed world.

These arguments constitute the logic motivating and underlying the Johns Hopkins Biographies of Disease. Biography implies a coherent identity, a chronology, and a narrative—a movement in and through time. Once inscribed by name in our collective understanding of medicine, each disease entity becomes a part of that collective understanding and, thus, inevitably shapes the way in which individual men and women think about their own felt symptoms and prospects for future health. Each historically visible entity—each disease—has a distinct history, even if that history is not always defined in terms familiar to twenty-first-century physicians. Dropsy and Bright's Disease are no longer terms of everyday clinical practice, but they are an integral part of the history of chronic kidney disease. Nor do we speak of essential, continued, and remittent fevers as categories in our classifications of disease, even though they played an important role in the history of medical ideas.

Melancholy and mania have a similarly lengthy pedigree. Since classical antiquity, physicians have described disturbing and sometimes incapacitating levels of affect—men and women unnaturally depressed and others morbidly if often episodically exhilarated. Our contemporary notion of bipolar disease is in some ways conceptually novel, yet its defining aspects are as old as medicine itself. In his biography of bipolar disease, David Healy traces the persistent yet shifting and elusive historical fortunes of this aspect of human experience. He doubts neither the felt reality of these clinical phenomena nor the fact that each era perceives and manages them in a historically specific way. It is in this sense that bipolar disease is a social entity—constituted by a time- and place-specific configuration of ideas, practices, and institutions.

That conceptual entity—and thus lived reality—we call bipolar disease today is peculiarly a product of our world. It is a world in which reductionist notions of disease have come to dominate our way of thinking about sickness. It is a world of bureaucratic categories and psychopharmaceutical practice. It is a world created in part by the laboratory's accomplishments, but it is also a social world shaped in part by mass media and advertising, by corporate strategies and government policies. And, as is illustrated by highly visible contemporary debates over the problematic increase of bi-

polar diagnoses in children, it is shaped as well by the public con-
testation of such clinical judgments—decisions that are in theory
individual, private, and objective.

It is in this multidimensional sense that the subject of David
Healy's biography exists outside the bodies and emotions of any
particular man, woman, or child. But these aggregated social, cultural, and institutional realities can and do intrude into very real
bodies and minds. Healy never lets us forget the men, women,
and children who feel emotional pain and incapacity no matter
how much such disquieting experience is modified by drugs and
ideology, by business plans and bureaucratic rationalities, by professional strategies and rewards. His subject is both timeless and
timely, situated in social and cultural space, yet anchored implaca-
bly in the idiosyncratic circumstantiality of particular lives.

Charles E. Rosenberg

Stories about Mania

❊ ❊ ❊

Meet Alex. Alex could be anyone's partner, parent, child, brother, or sister. He or she has a nervous problem of some sort. Many of us do. Throughout human history, we have struggled to understand just what might be involved when we have a nervous problem. Do we have a disease or are we stressed because we are caught in a crisis or does our malaise have a spiritual origin? In order to get by, we need answers or at least hypotheses.

The challenge for a history is to show in some sense that this struggle for meaning has always been with us and that people have been no less rational and no less insightful at different times, even if the answers they have offered now seem strange or odd. The job is to suggest that in one sense nothing ever really changes, no matter how bizarre certain practices or hypotheses may now seem. We who now find these views odd would have come to similar views placed in the same times and circumstances. This would be fine if at the same time the historian didn't also have a brief to convey how radically strange the past can be. Often it seems that just going back three or four years into the past propels us into another country, where we are the foreigners.

So the job becomes one of simultaneously conveying how alien the past was and at the same time how familiar it is. This task has become layered with further complexities for anyone who wants to tackle nervous problems today, when diseases or problems of the self have come so much to center stage as a focus for our existential concerns. The complexity is particularly apparent for the kind of nervous problem that Alex had, which was finally diagnosed as manic-depressive illness or bipolar disorder.

The landscape of bipolar disorder is changing from month to month, never mind from decade to decade. If we want some insight on the forces that shape the answers we can give to the question of what is wrong with us, a disease like bipolar disorder, which offers such a rapidly changing tapestry, can give insights on what might be going on in a way not easily gained elsewhere.

Mania is a curious beast in that the term crops up in antiquity, whereas schizophrenia and depression do not. As part of recent efforts to educate clinicians and the public about bipolar disorder, pharmaceutical companies and academics have commonly cited the lineage of this disorder, stressing that it goes back to the Greeks and that many famous figures through history have had the illness. But does having mania or being bipolar now mean the same thing as it meant to have mania in Athens in 400 BC or during the Renaissance or in Paris in the 1850s, when the concept of bipolar disorder first came into being?

Alex's story is a modern one. The time spent in treatment with psychotropic drugs occupied 75 percent of his or her life. This simple fact dates the story to the 1960s or later. That a clinician settled on a diagnosis of bipolar disorder after trying and rejecting a number of other possibilities dates the story somewhere closer to the 1990s. While being treated with one of the antipsychotics released since 1996, Alex dropped dead. She died aged two years old.[1] This last detail dates the story to the early years of the twenty-first century, and immediately makes it clear that no Greek, no European from the Renaissance, and no nineteenth-century Parisian ever had anything like what Alex had.

Alex's story feeds into the overall narrative in this book, not because it indicates we have now entered a new period and can add one further bead to a necklace of dates and epochs, but rather for the shaft of light it throws into the dark caverns of how we grapple with ourselves. This history is not a chronology, although it will progress from ancient Greece through the Renaissance to the present and will include many dates and names—indicating who discovered what and when. Rather, it aims to outline how the ways in which we have gone about trying to understand ourselves in the face of morbidity can shed light on the question of who are we.

Although the book includes material from ancient through recent to modern times, the use of the modern is not aimed at adding a final block to the edifice, an indication of the goal toward which progress was heading all the time. It is geared much more toward using a period of history where the processes of disease making (with the consequent effects on how we understand ourselves) have been speeded up, perhaps allowing us to pick out some of the key factors in these processes.

My assumption for the most part is that variations on these same processes have in fact applied through history but perhaps have never been deployed before with the same industrial efficiency. The disease mongering, chicanery, and deployment of the latest jargon to foster the interests of an establishment are ever the same. They can be seen in close up in the present but must be assumed to apply to some extent in other epochs.

The story could almost have been written backwards, but, backwards or forwards, this is a story. It is about the ultimate stories we tell our children or the most profound issues that friends help friends with. It is about the fact that parents have always had to share profundities with children to help them cope with the uncertainty of this world. Among the first things I can remember is my father recounting Greek myths to me and reciting a poem—Robert Louis Stevenson's "Where Go the Boats." Both the myths and this poem curiously work for 4-year-olds and 104-year-olds, although the sonority and timbre of my father's voice perhaps made the poem in particular stick for me. Many physicians and scientists would be happy at the notion that history is little more than stories told at bedtime. But if the answers we hand on fail to work, society has a crisis. If the answers work, this will be a part of ourselves that lives on in our children or friends.

Why, a scientist might ask, do you not hand on the truths of science? We can imagine some "Victorian" parents did just this at bedtime. With the emergence of science, there was a sense in the West that a new Truth had been born. The perception was that scientific discoveries built on previous discoveries and the resulting edifice managed to become ever more stable while inching slowly toward the heavens. At the same time the builders seemed to be moving toward a common and universal language. History was almost unnecessary. All that needed to be done was to chronicle progress. The first histories of medicine and science did just this.[2]

Science and medicine were often written with the initials of its authors missing. As late as the mid-1960s, George Carraz, one of the key figures in this story, references himself and coauthors by surname only—Carraz, followed by the name and page numbers of a journal. Later articles appear with an apologetic initial in brackets—Carraz (G). Emil Kraepelin, the central figure of the book, in his memoirs notes as something of an afterthought the death of his children. He names neither his wife nor surviving children. From the point of view of science, the personal details of these people were unimportant. The history of science and medicine needed people only insofar as a story of progress needed convenient heroes to celebrate. Diseases were important primarily in order to demonstrate their eradication. Heroes and victories were what would entice children into the field.

By the start of the twentieth century, however, the knowledge that science appeared to offer became ever less certain. Science began to be viewed not so much as an engine of social progress but as an engine powering into goodness-knows-what future. The history of science also changed character, offering a vision of recurring revolutions rather than steady progress.[3]

More recently, the history of science and medicine has come to seem almost the most important branch of history. History is in some sense about the things that change our understandings of ourselves. Once upon a time, these shifts in understanding were occasioned by battles or politicians, and they occurred over decades or longer. But with the emergence of modern science in the sixteenth and seventeenth centuries, these shifts increasingly followed events that had taken place in scientific laboratories and clinical practice. In recent years drugs like Prozac, Valium, Viagra, and chlorpromazine, technologies such as cloning, and diseases like bipolar disorder have all changed how we view ourselves, and these changes now occur within years or sometimes within months of each other.[4]

In these domains the struggle to formulate what has been happening to us is revealed, and within this struggle the history of health and disease reveals our most intimate secrets. Histories can be and are written about sex and gender, but Viagra and conflicts about whether homosexuality is a disease are the moving points in this story. Developments in health now feature on the front pages of our leading newspapers or as the first item on the television news, often trumping what would formerly have been seen as significant political events. In another twist to the story, if the development involves a drug, even though the news is trivial, some public relations agency will ensure front-page coverage.

If this is the furnace in which we are being tempered, how do we guarantee the truth-value of the tales that some may bring back from the furnace? To return to the bugbear of science, a story has protagonists and a plot, and how can you know whether I might have been duped by some of the recent protagonists to tell their story rather than their competitors' story or, in the case of historical figures, whether I have simply picked convenient aspects of their careers for the sake of the story or inserted twists into the plot because good stories need twists? Furnaces, after all, are places where things are forged.

These are problems for all histories, but there are additional problems with this one. An anonymous reviewer of the proposal for this book, while welcoming the book overall, cautioned that the author is a player in the events he proposes to tackle. It is only fair to pass on this health warning. In addition to being critical of many current trends and of the figures linked to those trends, I have done research in some of these areas. How is the reader to know that I am not bringing difficulties in other domains of my work inappropriately into this account?

Another reviewer of an earlier book of mine put his issues like this: "For some time now, critics of David Healy have been suggesting he has lost the plot. My own situation is distinctly worse in that despite two readings of *The Creation of Psychopharmacology* I am not sure I have got the plot at all. . . . The intoxication of the argument gets the better of the facts. . . . Healy appears to have a good memory of the 1960s, which means, I imagine, that he was not there."[5] This is taking Mark Twain's adage—that the older he got, the better he remembered things that had never happened— one step further to suggest I am endowed with an even better memory of things that I could never have been present at. If this is true for the 1960s, how much more true is it likely to be for events from centuries ago? But more to the point, in the face of hostility like this, how is the reader to know whether I have written this reviewer out of the script in revenge?

On the topic of passion, who would not be passionate about a topic that involves two-year-olds dropping dead on drugs? Although passion may cloud judgment, by some alchemy it is also often what is needed for us to reach beyond ourselves. Perhaps we should not hope that this history can be objective. It certainly won't suit everyone. The value lies in whether it is picked up and—as with scientific ideas, and with boats—set afloating.

But behind the protests of critics who themselves have been players in the story where readers may think, "Well, they would say that, wouldn't they?" and protests that may stem from sibling rivalry or other dynamic factors, readers should also listen for the failure of scientists. Science is supposed to be an ever-questioning enterprise, ever open to revision, and in this lies its strength. From this point of view, history, which opens up new perspectives on established truths, should be one of science's greatest allies. Where science supposedly progresses by embracing the inconvenient observations that current experiments present, history can stimulate by outlining a series of inconvenient but forgotten observations.

Far from welcoming this, scientists all too often view the efforts of history as a force making for nihilism when it suggests that the truths of science are not eternal. When they rail against history, scientists often reveal that, while the process of science may be open, the mind-sets of individual scientists are closed and they cling to beliefs as rigidly as any fundamentalist does.

This story then is not a mirror held up to the world but an addition to that world, written by a creature of flesh and blood who winces in response to hostile reviews. It will become a contested element in the mental health world. There is one message that both those who agree and those who disagree with the details of the story offered here might want to consider. Francis Fukuyama recently suggested that, with the triumph of liberal capitalism, history as we are used to it was over. It seems clear that in the sense he meant it, this idea was wrong.

But there is another way in which history could end. In chapter 8, this book suggests that the most potent cultural forces in our world today are the marketing departments of pharmaceutical corporations. They have been able to suck into their ambit the academics who were supposed to act as a counterweight to industry, as well as the apparatus that was supposed to regulate companies, and have in addition transformed those in the media, who distrust every politician once their lips move, into the bearers of the good tidings of salvation through pharmaceuticals. There is no reason to think they won't also move in on the history of medicine and science and, if they do, that might be the end of history.

It often seems the bottom line for marketing departments is that a boring message or no message is better than a message with a spin that the marketers cannot control. It is when there is agreement about a Stepford history that it will be time to get worried, not when critics dispute elements of a book like this.

ACKNOWLEDGMENTS

Carbon neutrality is the order of the day. The only way to get airborne and remain carbon neutral is in a glider or parapent. But gliding or paragliding leaves you so much at the mercy of the elements that if this was the only way to get from A to B, many reasonable people might opt to stay at A forever.

If someone else abducts your ideas for their trip from A to B, reading the results might feel not unlike being an unwilling traveler on a glider. Those who may be feeling queasy in this case include Tom Ban, Ned Shorter, Kal Applbaum, Barbara Marshall, Steve Lanes, Annemarie Mol, Ray Moynihan, many of whose ideas I have commandeered, as well as German Berrios and Charles Rosenberg, who have played a part in kindling my interest in gliding. Margaret Harris, Joanna Le Noury, Richard Tranter, Stefanie Tschinkel, Fiona Farquhar, Di Bell, Dinah Cattell, and David Linden have been co-workers on projects central to some of the ideas and data presented here. Ross Baldessarini, Nassir Ghaemi, Joel Braslow, and Peter Parry have been involved in related work on bipolar disorders. Charles Medawar, Shelley Jofre, Sarah Boseley, Cindy Hall, Dee Mangin, Vera Sharav, Karen Menzies, Carl Elliott, Trudo Lemmens, Andrea Tone, Emily Martin, Elizabeth Lunbeck, Max Fink, Andy Vickery, Nancy Olivieiri, Osamu Tajima, Peter Rosenthal, and Jim Turk have been party to some of my previous efforts to get off the ground on this and related ventures.

A number of organizations have facilitated my absorption in these issues, particularly the North West Wales Trust and its mental health directorate, which could have legitimately required me to give more time to other things.

CHAPTER ONE

Frenzy and Stupor

❁ ❁ ❁

In lectures, articles, or textbooks tackling bipolar disorder, or manic-depressive illness, distinguished professors of psychiatry and other academics repeatedly, indeed almost universally, start by claiming the Greeks and Romans recognized this disorder.[1] But while the terms *mania, melancholia, insanity, dysphoria, dysthymia, paranoia, frenzy,* and *lunacy* all go back to the Greeks and Romans, manic-depressive disease does not and indeed could not.

Ten years ago, it might have been possible to write off 2,000 years of history and start instead at the end of the nineteenth century when the German psychiatrist Emil Kraepelin established manic-depressive illness in its modern form.[2] From 1899, even though the illness is more likely to be called bipolar disorder now, we have a history that can be researched as solidly as anything in biological psychiatry. Claims about events from the end of the nineteenth century onward can be supported by solid banks of evidence or challenged by an appeal to other evidence. It should be possible to establish areas of consensus about the history of mood disorders and move on to collect evidence on areas of continuing uncertainty just as science does.

But the launch of mood-stabilizing drugs for bipolar disorder in the mid-1990s means that we cannot write off these 2,000 years, because since then contemporary biological psychiatrists have invoked the past repeatedly. Their invocations suggest that modern manic-depressive illness is not set on solid ground and that claiming Greek precedents stems from a hope that the antiquity of such authorities will confer legitimacy on contemporary therapeutic and research endeavors. Almost every artist, composer, or author of note in the eighteenth and nineteenth centuries, as we shall see in chapters 5 and 6, has been similarly invoked as a prior sufferer from this illness.

If my argument that the disease was not and could not have been recognized before the nineteenth century is right, then this is a case of the present colonizing the past. If present powers seek to rewrite the past in this way, we need to see whether the edifice of manic-depressive illness we are faced with today is quite as stable if the props marked *history* are knocked out from under it.

But there are further reasons for not ignoring the past. The first is that this book is not just a history of one disease. It is also about how we understand ourselves, about how we fit ourselves into our bodies or fit our minds into our brains. We have had great difficulties in embodying the mind and in understanding how a "mind" can be diseased, and these difficulties played a key role in blocking recognition of manic-depressive disorder. If this is the case, then conversely current conceptions of this disorder (and perhaps this disorder more than any other) and the embodiment such conceptions imply must have implications for how we understand ourselves now.

Second, the difficulties in establishing the existence of a mood disorder tell us something about how clinicians make diagnoses. For the Greeks, visible signs made it reasonable to locate the problem in the body of the sick person. For us, diagnoses depend on what people say (chapter 7). As a result, we have moved into a world in which illnesses are negotiated, the consequences of which will be considered through the book. We have moved into a world in which, in the absence of visible pathology, we have no way of being certain whether it is the individual or society that is sick.

Third, whether a disease entity was recognized before the nineteenth century or not, "dis-ease" has provided a living for physicians and the suppliers of medications for more than 2,000 years. The commerce driven by dis-ease is an important factor underpinning or inhibiting the recognition of disorders. Within this commercial domain, advocates of specific treatments and advocates of cocktail treatments have struggled in a dynamic that can be traced back over centuries, and this dynamic is one of the most profound cultural forces in our world today, as we shall see in chapters 4 and 8.

THE MANIA OF HIPPOCRATES

Hippocrates was the first to put mania and melancholia on our cultural radar.[3] Our story opens at Meliboea where "a young man who had been running a temperature for a long time as a result of drinking and sexual indulgence took to his bed. His symptoms were shivering, insomnia, nausea, and lack of thirst." He is then described as being beside himself (πάρέκρουσεν) on the tenth day. "On the 14th day his symptoms generally became more pronounced and he was beside himself and raving. On the 20th day he went mad. There was much tossing about. On the 24th day he died. This was a case of frenzy[4] [φρενῖτις]."[5]

A host of other such vignettes appear in Hippocrates, some diagnosed as frenzy and others as mania (μανία). But this mania is clearly different from the mania that typifies manic-depressive illness. And it is against this background that we need to interpret the case of the woman at Thasos, whose story (at least the unbracketed parts of the following translation) psychiatrists today cite more than any other from antiquity.

A sensitive [δυσάνιος][6] woman became unwell, having been sad [λύπης] after a loss, and although she did not take to her bed, she suffered from insomnia, loss of appetite, thirst, and nausea. . . . [Early on the night of the first day,] she became frightened [φόβος], began to rave and became dysthymic [δυσθυμία][7] [and had a slight fever. In the morning she had many spasms (σπασ-μοί);[8] when the spasms had passed,] she talked incoherently. [She developed a series of severe pains. On the second day, she was much the same, unable to sleep and with a more marked fever].

[On the third day, the spasms ceased but she became sleepy and obtunded, followed by a return to consciousness, when] she leapt up and could not be restrained. She began raving [and showed a high fever. That night she sweated profusely all over with warm sweat. She lost her fever and] slept well, becoming collected and lucid and reaching the crisis. [On the third day her urine was black with substances floating in it. At the time of the crisis, she had a copious menstrual flow].⁹

Is this an early case of manic-depressive illness? Today's clinicians argue that manic-depressive illness and schizophrenia are more likely to cause symptoms at certain times of the year such as spring and autumn, and Hippocrates notes that mania and melancholy were more likely in spring and autumn, along with epilepsy, hemorrhages, sore throats, catarrh, hoarseness, coughs, leprosy, vitiligo, ulcerative eruptions, tumors, and arthritis. Fevers, heat spots, vomiting, diarrhea, and gangrene of the genitalia predominated in summer.¹⁰

But to argue that Hippocrates describes manic-depression here involves a careful selection of the facts and a gross selection of text. Lecturers today literally omit the translated material in brackets in this passage. Depending on text selection and the translation of key words, the case of the woman of Thasos can be made to look like manic-depressive illness. Indeed, it is even claimed that Hippocrates is describing the mixed states outlined by Kraepelin more than two millennia later. But this can happen only because stripped-down versions of this case circulate like a virus in manic-depressive circles, and no one goes back to place this woman in context. She had a mania that, like that of the youth at Meliboea, could be influenced by the airs, waters, and spices in the environment. When talking about these cases, Hippocrates makes constant references to risks, such as that of drinking standing water, which at certain times of the year might lead to quartan fever.¹¹ The cases invariably involved fever and often resulted in death.

There are similarities and differences between Hippocratic and modern views on health—ones that do not always work in favor of modernity—but the similarities do not involve manic-depressive illness. Although the guiding humoral spirit behind the Hippocratic and modern complementary health care systems appears similar in important respects, the Hippocratic system had a feature that distinguishes it from other premodern views and contemporary complementary views. Unlike Yin and Yang, the dhosas, and even the serotonin of popular culture, the four Hippocratic humors were visible. *Blood,* the liquor of vitality, made the body hot and wet. *Choler,* bile or gastric juice, made the body hot and dry. *Phlegm* was all colorless secretions, as in sweat and tears and the thickened concentrated form that appeared in illness at the nose and mouth; it made the body cold and wet. It was also found in the brain, where one of its roles was to cool the ardor of the blood. *Black bile,* or melancholy, was the one hidden humor, seen only insofar as it led to the darkening of other fluids, such as blood and stools; it made the body cold and dry. The spleen was the leading candidate location for this somewhat more mysterious humor. But the fact that the humors were visible and could even be quantified left the Hippocratic system open to revision and development.[12]

These humors had corresponding elements, which were also visible and potentially testable. Blood was linked to fire, choler to air, phlegm to water, and melancholy to earth. The humors were in balance with the seasons, so that, for instance, blood was linked to summer and phlegm to winter.

The humors were not simply blood, bile, and phlegm, as we know them now, but vital forces as exemplified by blood and bile. As forces or influences, they penetrated the fabric of the body to "color" individuals and peoples. In the case of blood, this might literally color an individual to make him ruddy but also lead to a sanguine or lively, energetic, and robust temperament. The choleric person was bilious in nature. The term *distemper* was originally used to indicate a disposition that was out of balance or a crisis that stemmed from dispositional factors rather than from acute disturbances of the more visible humors—something we might now talk of in terms of personality problems rather than acute breakdowns. Hippocrates, in fact, uses μελαγχολικός (melancholic) more often to describe a disposition than a disease.

These latter ideas about dispositions have correspondences in modern neuroscience. Neurohumors such as serotonin and norepinephrine occur in the body to a much greater extent than they occur in the brain. Even within the brain, there is better evidence that different configurations of norepinephrine and serotonin influence our personalities than evidence that disturbances of these humors provide a chemical basis for any nervous or mood disorder.[13]

The text of Hippocrates makes it difficult to avoid the impression that these physicians were interested in more than treating disease. As the following passages suggest, they appeared keen to understand why we behave the way we do:

> Those of a bilious constitution are liable to shout and cry out during the night when the brain is suddenly heated. . . . Warming of the brain also takes place when a plethora of blood finds its way to the brain and boils. It courses along the blood vessels in great quantity when a man is having a nightmare and is in a state of terror. He reacts in sleep in the same way that he would if he were awake; his face burns, his eyes are bloodshot and he is as scared as when the mind is intent upon the commission of a crime.
>
> The brain may be attacked by both phlegm and bile and the resulting disorder can be distinguished thus; those whose mania results from phlegm are quiet and neither shout nor make a disturbance; those whose mania results from bile show frenzy and will not keep still, and are always up to some mischief. Such are the causes of continued mania, but fears and frenzy may be caused by changes in the brain.[14]

Hippocrates was unusual in allocating to the brain a role in behavior, in contrast to Aristotle and others who located the drivers of behavior in the heart or elsewhere.

> It is the brain too which is the seat of madness and delirium, with the fears and frights which assail us often by night but sometimes even by day; it is there where lies the cause of insomnia and sleep walking, of thoughts that will not come, forgotten duties and eccentricities. All such things result from an unhealthy condition of the brain. . . . when the brain is abnormal in moisture it is necessarily agitated, and this agitation prevents sight or hearing being steady. Because of this, varying visual and acoustic sensations are produced, while the tongue can only describe things as

they appear and sound. So long as the brain is still, a man is in his right mind.[15]

But this is to some extent a trick of translation. This was not the brain as we understand it. It took no clearer form than the encephalon—that which is within the skull. The image put forward of an excess of hot bile flooding into the brain or a deficient production of cooling phlegm causing mania made sense of some of the key clinical observations that were visible in the *face* and *head*. For Hippocrates, the foreheads of maniacs and melancholics would commonly have literally felt hot with the fevers that gave rise to delirious or frenzied states.

Mania was essentially delirium. Those afflicted were maniacs rather than manics. On a probabilistic basis, it could not have been anything else. Before the antibiotics, high fevers gave rise to agitated and raving states far more commonly than any "mental" disorder did. The word *frenzy*, stemming from the Greek φρένες, points to how things must have been. The same frenzy is at the heart of the word *schizophrenia*. But far from meaning a brain, φρένες can describe midriff, breast, soul, mind, heart, sense, understanding, and reason.[16]

The contrast with frenzy or mania was not melancholia, as that term might now be used, but rather stupor. Stupor happened when the phlegm in the brain became overly cool, bringing behavior to a full stop. On a probabilistic basis, the most common causes of melancholia or stupor in this sense must also have been infective or states of postinfective lethargy, although conditions now known to be Parkinsonism or hypothyroidism may also have contributed. Infections, which gave rise to delirium and later lethargy, would have led to the perception that mania might be preceded by or followed by melancholia.

The argument that it is not possible to make links between Hippocrates' use of the word mania and modern bipolar disorder is not the same as saying that Hippocrates was unable to distinguish modern diseases. Modern psychiatry is making an even bigger mistake than that. Delirium, epilepsy, impotence, leprosy, and a variety of vesical, menstrual, respiratory, digestive, and neurological syndromes can be picked out with confidence in Hippocrates' writings. Other classical authors, such as Aretaeus, described glycosuria, and Galen gives very clear descriptions of cataplectic stupor or catatonia, while both Galen and Hippocrates describe hysteria.

Among the forty-two cases in books I and III of Hippocrates' "Epidemics," sixteen involve women. Of the female cases, nine stem from the postpartum period, making postpartum problems the single biggest corpus of disorders discussed in his writings. Clearly, Hippocrates was medically correct to identify the postpartum period as a time of risk. Consider now another of his women from Thasos, who, after giving birth to a daughter, had loss of appetite, despondency (ἄθυμος), insomnia, anger, dysphoria (δυσφορίαι),[17] and a mental state (γνώμην) that was melancholic (μελαγχολικά). On the basis of these symptoms, she meets modern criteria for an affective disorder. The problem is that these symptoms all occur against a background of retained lochia and in the midst of an eighty-day clinical saga dominated by fevers, rigors, delirium, coma, pain, and ultimately death.[18] Only 5 percent of the vignette contains material that we might now think refers to a mood disorder.

These postpartum manias, as they were called for the following 2,000 years, would now be termed postpartum fevers or infections. Not until the early nineteenth century, as we will see in chapter 5, did physicians begin to distinguish between the insanities of the postpartum period that were accompanied by fevers and the quite comparable but much less common states without fever.[19] Furthermore, classic mental illnesses such as general paralysis of the insane have since been identified as infective disorders without a fever, while in recent years it has become clear that ulcers, tumors, and other disorders may stem from infections that do not cause fevers.

Hippocrates' postpartum cases make it clear his focus was on what we would now recognize as infections. He and his medical successors through to the nineteenth century were faced with the desperate facts of contagion and wondered about air, water, and other sources of transmission of disease. Against a background of terrifying and lethal epidemics, what is now called manic-depressive illness was almost an irrelevance. It was a rare disorder.

In contrast, the landscape we look out on now contains much fewer apparently infective disorders but is dominated by mushrooming epidemics of attention deficit hyperactivity disorder (ADHD) and bipolar disorder, raising questions about how these contagions spread. Our modern, supposedly scientific treatments seem about as effective in containing these new epidemics as blood-letting once was for the Greeks.

Finally, another Greek text that brings mania into play with a slightly different meaning is Plato's *Phaedrus*.[20] In this dialogue, Plato anticipates Shakespeare's lines from *A Midsummer Night's Dream* that poets whose eyes in a fine frenzy roll from earth to heaven and back again have much in common with lovers, madmen (μανίαν), and seers whose seething brains and shaping fantasies apprehend more than cool reason ever comprehends. This use of mania has little link to mental illness. It comes closer to enthusiasm or the use later found in the Netherlands' tulip mania of the seventeenth century that hints at the delusions of crowds. This mania, as we shall see in chapter 7, can lead to putting infants on potent psychoactive medication.

FROM DIAGNOSES TO TREATMENTS

In distinguishing between delirium or frenzy involving fever and other manias that might not, Soranus of Ephesus brought closer the possibility that a Greek or Roman physician might recognize manic-depressive disease. Soranus also noted connections between melancholy and mania, but not as two poles of one disorder. Mania was a state of overactivity, in which hallucinations and delusions were common. Patients with melancholia showed "mental anguish and distress, dejection, silence and animosity towards members of the household, sometimes a desire to live and at other times a longing for death, suspicion when a plot is being hatched against them, weeping without reason, meaningless muttering and again occasional joviality."[21]

This melancholia was seen as part of the developing picture of a chronic form of insanity without fever that was commonly focused on a fixed obsession. The problem was thought to begin with the pooling of black bile in the hypochondrium. This led to an awareness of bodily symptoms and complaints, which developed into melancholia, a prodrome of mania (insanity) rather than an opposing pole to mania. Cases of melancholia that got worse might topple over into mania. On a probabilistic basis, if not describing physical illnesses here, Soranus might have been describing schizophrenia or psychotic depressions that typically show fluctuating levels of agitation and delusions, both of which are much commoner than the swings between mania and depression found in manic-depression.

The theme of melancholy developing into mania recurs with Aretaeus of Cappadocia, who in addition was one of the first to describe the glycosuria that is a concomitant of diabetes. In addition to citing the woman from Thasos, modern biological psychiatrists regularly cite Aretaeus to claim that manic-depressive illness was recognized in antiquity just as diabetes was and to imply thereby that it is as real a disease as diabetes is.[22]

Aretaeus offered the standard descriptions of melancholia as a state of "low spirits stemming from a single phantasy, a state without fever, where the understanding is turned to sorrow and despondency only. Those affected with melancholy may not all be identically affected, but they either are suspicious of poisoning, or flee to the desert from misanthropy, or turn superstitious, or end up with a hatred of life."

Melancholia, he noted, starts with patients becoming dull, strained, dejected, and unreasonably torpid, without any manifest cause. They also become peevish, dispirited, and sleepless and begin to start up from a disturbed sleep. They become prey to anxieties, as the disease worsens, when their dreams become true, terrifying, and clear. Whatever they have an aversion to when awake rushes in upon their vision in sleep.

In the course of their illness, these patients are prone to change their mind readily, switching from being base, mean-spirited, and illiberal to a short time later being simple, extravagant, and munificent; this does not happen from any virtue of the soul, but rather simply from the changeableness of the disease. But if the illness becomes more urgent, the patients develop hatreds, avoid others, and begin to lament and complain about life, desiring to die.[23] If read one way, this can be taken as a description of a disposition. Alternately, suggestions like these of overactivity can fit into any developing psychosis, including psychotic depression.

This view that an insanity or mania might appear as a development of an initially melancholic state is widely found in Roman writers.[24] The usual connection was in terms of melancholia being an earlier stage or mild form of madness with mania being the term used for the later and more severe stages. But these terms were almost completely nonspecific, and little meaning would be lost from the original texts if the terms underactive and overactive insanity were substituted for melancholia and mania.

The key issue for these physicians was the visible presentations of their patients. Take, for example, this celebrated description from Galen of Pergamon, the key figure after Hippocrates. He describes a student "who had worn himself out by steady application to this studies, was seized by this disease and lay as if he were wood, stretched out stiff and unbending. He gave the impression that with his eyes open he was looking at us; he did not even blink, but nonetheless he did not say anything to us. He said [later] that he heard us at the time we were speaking, not always clearly, but there were things, which he recalled. He said that he saw everyone who was present so that he was able to describe some of their actions which he had observed, but he could neither speak nor move any member."[25]

In this description, the features of an extraordinary condition come through with great freshness across almost 2,000 years. Greek, Roman, and later medieval physicians practicing in Latin called this state *catalepsy*. This was the ultimate underactive insanity. A person might remain mute, immobile, and stuporous for weeks or months. When vernacular languages took over in medicine, in the English-speaking world the dominant word for this condition was stupor, until Karl Kahlbaum in the nineteenth century coined a new term—catatonia (chapter 3).[26]

Catalepsy was readily reconciled with a humoral model. Whereas frenzy involved an excess of bile in the brain or a deficiency of phlegm, stupor was explained in terms of an excess of thickened phlegm. Giving too much opium or giving it at the wrong time was the kind of thing that physicians at the time thought might lead to phlegm congealing.

The texts of Galen and Hippocrates make clear that physicians in antiquity often described diseases, and even mental disorders, that can be recognized today, but they did so on the basis of the visible appearances of the disorder—the swelling, heat, and redness of a tumor, the smell of urine, the mute rigidity of stupor, the frenzy of delirium. These were not diseases based on what the affected subject reported about some inner mental state. Galen also described cases of hysteria, but for his time, and for almost two millennia afterward, the commonest presentation of hysteria was in the very visible form of convulsions.

With Galen, however, a new dynamic comes into play. Shortly after the Hippocratic school established an empirical form of medicine, Aristotle elaborated his philosophy and, in particular, his system of logic that was dominated by the syllogism. This system put a premium on correct reasoning rather than careful observation. Galen effected a synthesis between Aristotelian and Hippocratic systems, in the process creating a corpus of work that remained almost unquestioned for 1,500 years.

The Galenic systematization of the humoral framework led to treatments that were increasingly based on the prescriptions of a model rather than the presentation of the patient. The logical and theoretical aspects of Galenic medicine are now seen as inimical to the development by observation and experiment that medicine needs. Galenism is cited as a force against which Vesalius, Paracelsus, and other medical pioneers of the Renaissance had to struggle. What is much less often noted is the role of the commercial opportunities that the new synthesis presented.

The step after diagnosis is treatment. Within the humoral framework, various "drug" treatments were developed of which the most famous—Theriac—was later closely linked to Galen. Roman and Greek remedies were drawn from herbs, some of which were recognized to contain a sole active principle (the simples), whereas others were thought to contain a number of active principles. Based on the patient's predicament, the physician would take (thus Rx, the abbreviation for the Latin *recipe*, meaning "take") a variety of active principles and mix them. The principles were aimed at stimulating certain bodily functions or opposing others. Theriac was the most celebrated of the resulting compounds. Many versions of Theriac contained up to 100 supposedly active ingredients. For 1,500 years, this was the preeminent treatment for nervousness—in twenty-first-century terms, the ultimate brand.[27]

Although Theriac seems almost the exact opposite of a modern medicine, which aims to have a single potent ingredient, appearances and rhetoric can deceive. Unless the modern medicine contains a single replacement ingredient like iron, the chances are it is a compound medicine not unlike Theriac. This is particularly true for drugs that act on the brain, which act on a multiplicity of brain systems and receptors and are better thought of as cocktail compounds rather than thought of as specific "magic bullets," as they are commonly portrayed.

Theriac had another similarity to modern medicines in that it and related compounds were significant factors in the trade and commerce of Western states, such as Venice. The survival of Galenism may have owed a good deal to this commercial dominance. There is little reason to believe that the merchant classes of the late Roman period or the Middle Ages would have welcomed a new science of disease any more readily than the makers of H-2 blocking antihistamines in the 1980s welcomed news that ulcers, then the most lucrative area of therapeutics, might be completely eliminated by antibiotics.

COMMERCE AND SCIENCE

In the Middle Ages, humoral frameworks became very elaborate, and a number of health handbooks were developed offering advice on the correct foods to eat at particular times of the year and correct times for certain activities in order to counterbalance environmental influences. These handbooks contained beautiful and masterly depictions of the health economy or health landscape of the Middle Ages. One of the most famous of these books was the *Tacuinum Sanitatis*.[28] Some of the best art of the medieval period went into the *Tacuinum* to illustrate combinations of seasons, herbs, and dispositions, with instructions for optimal health. Thus, an industry in health and well-being was flourishing at a time when the explicitly medical management of serious disease was relatively impotent to effect much meaningful difference in peoples' lives.

A turning point came with the scientific revolutions of the Renaissance. The Galenic system was faced with a challenge from anatomists like Vesalius and later Willis (see chapter 2), as well as from Paracelsus and the chemical doctors who followed him. Basel was the epicenter of change. Vesalius's *Anatomy* was first published there. In 1526 Paracelsus was appointed the professor of medicine in Basel but was stripped of the title two years later, after he famously burned the books of Galen and other ancient authorities and instructed his pupils that "proofs derive from my own experience and my own reasoning and not from reference to authorities."[29]

Paracelsus railed against the Galenic system and argued for a more empirical medicine. But his main point of attack had to do more with the remedies in use than with the theoretical framework. "What sense would it make for a physician if he discovered the origin of diseases but could not cure or alleviate them?"[30] Paracelsus had two problems with Galenic remedies. He advocated the use of purified remedies, such as metals, rather than Galenic compound medicines like Theriac, and he introduced the notion that for each specific illness there might be a specific remedy (although his notions of specificity were a long way from ours). A further objection was that physicians had handed over the compounding of remedies to apothecaries and, as a result, were less familiar with what their remedies contained and their treatment effects.[31] In modern terms, Paracelsus appears to have been asking for a greater awareness by physicians of the functional changes they wished to bring about and a deployment of therapies aimed at producing such changes rather than using a potent, multipurpose compound like Theriac.

The legacy of Galen was not readily overthrown. New drugs like quinine and mercury, which seemed to contradict humoral predictions, were accommodated within establishment thinking. Through the seventeenth century, medical treatises, except for a few exceptional cases such as works by Willis in Oxford, continued to refer primarily to authorities such as Galen rather than to actual cases physicians may have been seeing.

What we get with Paracelsus and his successors—the chemical doctors—though, is a new form of attack on medicine. From the sixteenth century onward, there is a growing use of new treatments such as metals and other purified chemicals that were not based on and could not readily be explained in terms of humoral frameworks. As they were adopted, medicine slowly became responsive once more to observations and data.[32] Medicine did so because ultimately it followed the money. In boxing parlance, this was the equivalent of hitting the body to get the head to fall. Change the practice, and the thinking will follow. It has ever been thus, although medical history has almost exclusively focused on the scientific head and rarely on the commercial body.[33]

The clinical theses of the sixteenth and seventeenth centuries dealing with psychiatric issues continued to stress health themes from Hippocrates and Galen onward—physical factors such as food, air, and water. Despite this emphasis on the physical, this approach cannot be seen as a biological medicine or orientation, in that biology as we know it had not been born at the time. But slowly from the mid-1700s onward two developments begin to shape thinking. The first development, an awareness of the course of disorders, became a key issue in the evolution of modern psychiatry after the opening of the asylums in the early 1800s offered the chance to observe the course of a patient's illness systematically over time (chapters 2 and 3). Second, understanding behaviors from nostalgia through to alcoholism, rape, insane love, and homicide, all of which require some exploration of the inner life of the subject, began to come within medical purview (chapter 2).

There was also a slow shift to a discussion of actual cases. Dissertations began to describe new cases of melancholia, epilepsy, catalepsy, somnambulism, and other behavioral disorders. Some of the ideas that these cases prompted can sound remarkably modern. For instance, William Thoner from Basel described the onset of melancholy in 1590 as involving wakefulness, disturbed sleep, sluggishness, and fatigue. He emphasized that there may be no obvious triggers—it can just happen.[34] This sounds very much like descriptions of endogenous depression from the mid-twentieth century.

Henningus Unverzagt, whose dissertation was lodged in Helmstadt in 1614, talks about primary melancholy as having "as its subject the brain only. The disorder in this case would arise from

actual imbalance in the brain itself, or from causes, which generate melancholic matters in the brain e.g., worry, fear, frighten-
ing sights, violent imagination, and wakefulness."[35] With a bit of
updating of its language, this description could be slotted into a
line-up of various formulations of the amine/serotonin theories
of depression and not be picked out as anomalous—which might
give readers worries about the epistemological character of some
of the most cherished notions of modern psychiatry.

When they began to focus on their own cases, physicians found
themselves pushed into almost open revolt against the dominant
Galenic ideas. As Christian Vater of Wittenberg in 1680 noted,
"melancholia often passes into mania and vice versa. The melancholics themselves now laugh, now are saddened, now express
numberless other absurd gestures and forms of behaviour. . . .
It is vain to look to humors, or spirits for an explanation of this
[change]."[36] Vater's mockery of the older humoral models arguably deals as much of a setback to modern notions on the biology
of mood disorders or emotional change. While it is easy to relate
the invariant rigidity of Parkinson's disease to lowered dopamine
in the brain, it is not clear what it is about the multiform presentations of depression, both between individuals and even within
the one subject, that could conceivably correspond to a lowering
of serotonin.

Perhaps the most compelling case was one described by
Thomas Sydenham in 1681, that of a woman who "shrieks irregularly, and inarticulately, and strikes her breast and has to be held
down by the united efforts of the bystanders." Sydenham went
on to outline what would now be considered the dynamics behind the syndrome from which this woman and others suffered.
"The patients [with this condition] feel dejected. The mind sick-
ens more than the body. An incurable despair is so thoroughly
the nature of this disease, that the very slightest word of hope creates anger. . . . They have melancholy fore-bodings. They brood
over trifles, cherishing them in their anxious and unquiet bo-
soms. Fear, anger, jealousy, suspicion, and the worst passions of
the mind arise without cause. . . . there is no moderation. All is
caprice. They love without measure those whom they will soon
hate."[37]

Here is a description of a syndrome characterized by such variability that Vater would have said, "It is vain to look to humors, or spirits for an explanation of this [change]." Sydenham's description coincided with Thomas Willis's contemporary groundbreaking research on the anatomy of the brain outlined in chapter 2. But Sydenham held little hope that brain research would help in cases like this: "[Anatomy] will be no more able to direct a physician how to cure a disease than how to make a man."[38] It must be doubtful that Sydenham would have found his description any more readily reconciled with modern brain theories of mood disorders than he would have found it explained by the humoral models criticized by Vater, or the brain research of Willis.

Sydenham's description of this patient and his formulation of the dynamics of cases like this pose even bigger problems than a mere threat to the amine theories of mood disorders. The condition he outlined maps beautifully onto modern criteria for borderline personality disorder. And borderline personality disorder is just the kind of disorder that enthusiasts for bipolar disorder, as will become clear, would now regard as part of the bipolar spectrum (chapters 5 and 6). Borderline disorders typically display a rapidly alternating euphoria that the modern clinician might see as mania or hypomania and dysphoria that the modern clinician might see as depression.

But Sydenham called this condition hysteria. Hysteria is, of course, the disorder that gave rise to modern dynamic psychology just when Emil Kraepelin was formulating the concept of manic-depressive disease. Without hysteria, it is unlikely we would have had Freud and all the changes to modern and Western sensibility that he brought about. Whereas the Greeks had souls and bodies, we, as a result of the struggles of Freud and Janet with the protean manifestations of hysteria, have minds and psyches and bodies.[39]

Sydenham's formulation makes it clear that looking back through the historical record to the Greeks, who first described hysteria, can produce cases with alternating phases of mania and melancholia, or overactivity and underactivity, that are clearly psychiatric but not so clearly manic-depressive. In the case of Galen's catalepsy, it is now recognized that this condition also swings from pole to pole (chapters 3 and 5). Unless every clinical state that shows variability is deemed bipolar, this evidence would seem to fatally undermine our abilities to state with confidence what was happening in the Greco-Roman cases extant in the literature, other than when these involved gross cases of frenzy or stupor.

With hysteria and the birth of dynamic psychiatry at the end of the nineteenth century, diagnosis within psychiatry changed radically. Whereas the Greeks had made their diagnoses based on the visible presentations of disorders, psychiatrists began to turn to words and reports of internal mental states. This trend culminated in the United States in the 1950s when an older system of diagnosis was overthrown in favor of a new dynamic psychiatry, in which even the visible signs of physical disorders, such as ulcers or the immobility of Parkinson's disease, were liable to be interpreted as manifestations of psychopathology.[40]

The psychoanalytic heyday was a brief one that ended in 1980 with publication of the third edition of the American Psychiatric Association's *Diagnostic and Statistical Manual of Mental Disorders*. The *DSM-III* superficially appeared to reject a diagnosis based on hidden inner forces in favor of more obvious disturbances of behavior that met operational criteria. One of the new disorders for which operational criteria were provided was bipolar disorder (chapter 5).

Yet, far from being a radical break with analysis and a return of psychiatry to mainstream medicine, or to what many described as its Kraepelinian bedrock (see chapter 5), the new diagnoses were still based for the most part on what people said. Despite claiming to be biological, modern psychiatrists listen to words rather than look at patients. But even though words are their métier, these clinicians have rejected the range of linguistic and hermeneutic tools developed during the middle years of the twentieth century to manage words and are arguably like a musician attempting to realize a symphony with one instrument only.

Based on words, twenty-first-century psychiatrists diagnose a range of disorders from compulsive shopping disorder to social phobia that physicians before the 1980s had never heard of. These diagnoses are made in the absence of diagnostic tests to point to the validity of these conditions. In the case of ADHD and mania in one- and two-year-old children, the diagnoses are based on the words of third parties (see chapter 7). This new use of mania may mean that continuity will soon be lost between how the word is being used in the twenty-first century and how it was used in the twentieth century. Ironically, the twenty-first-century use may end up closer to the Greek use, where it connoted overactivity.

While words reign in this way, repeated surveys have shown that the most visible of psychiatric disorders, catatonia, still occurs in up to 10 percent of patients, but that it goes unseen and undiagnosed.[41] The panoply of neuropsychiatric signs on which psychiatrists like Kraepelin depended almost certainly go equally undetected. Psychiatry is in a muddle, and there would seem to be scope to get things badly wrong.

ACROSS TIME

The key point to take from this selective sweep through twenty-five centuries of the usage of the words mania and melancholia is that modern authorities on manic-depressive disorder make a gross error when they try to effect a link between modern presentations of a disease they call bipolar disorder and ancient precedents. There is little excuse for this mistake, in that the pit into which modern commentators fall was clearly signposted a quarter of a century ago.

In 1981, in an article on the history of mania, Edward Hare put forward the view that a difference between schizophrenia and manic-depressive illness had appeared only very recently.[42] Hare's work engaged Andrew Scull, who disputed the suggestion that there was anything recent about schizophrenia. Scull's response made everyone more aware of the role that the interests of the medical profession and the power of institutions might play in the history of a disease. The controversy between Hare and Scull did a great deal to put the history of psychiatry on the map.

But another important response came from German Berrios who made it clear that Hare's argument was based on a complete misreading of the word mania.[43] Modern psychiatrists, Berrios made clear, could not assume mania has always meant what it means to them. It is not clear that many psychiatrists have heard or understood this yet.

This is not just an arcane problem. As we shall see, there were few if any patients in the Western world described as having manic-depressive disorder before the 1920s. In the United States, few patients had this disease before the 1960s. Invoking Greek precedents therefore both misreads the older literature and makes it difficult to understand where manic-depressive disease went for two millennia.

Few would doubt that there were individuals in antiquity affected with core features that might lead to a diagnosis of manic-depressive illness now. But, as we shall see in chapter 3, this condition until recently occurred in a severity that was likely to impinge on the radars of physicians at an annual rate of ten new cases per million. Given that there were not many millions of people in Rome or any major population centers until quite recently, it was just not likely that manic-depressive illness would be picked up and certainly not widely recognized.

The primary concern of physicians up to the time of Kraepelin at the end of the nineteenth century was with epidemics. The appearance and explosive increase in these lethal conditions was a problem that threatened everyone. Against these epidemics, physicians from Hippocrates through Willis and on to Esquirol and Kraepelin, who feature in chapters 2 and 3, watched essentially powerless as these diseases took away their wives, children, friends, and colleagues. Kraepelin in his memoirs written after the First World War described as a matter of routine the deaths of several of his children through the 1880s and 1890s and near deaths of others. Epidemics removed governments and destroyed empires.[44] How much of what was happening was down to biological forces or to social arrangements or individual failings? What were the vectors of transmission? These were the key questions. Medicine for these physicians was a desperate and passionate calling rather than a dry and sterile matter, but it was all too easy to see why the overwhelming nature of these hostile forces might encourage a retreat to sterile formulae.

In contrast, comparatively few of the physicians in the generations between Willis in the 1640s and Kraepelin in the 1890s will have had relatives affected by mental illness. Now, however, we seem subject to new epidemics of behavioral disorders that come from nowhere and seize our children and relatives. Are the vectors of transmission biological, social, or individual? In the face of these new threats, we seem to have no more ideas as to the mode of contagion than Hippocrates and Willis had in their days. This point of continuity with the past, this grappling of individual physicians and others involved in health with the fact that the new disorders may blight the lives of their families, is at least as important an aspect of disease and its impact on all of us as is the question of whether there is a continuity of particular disease entities.

Insofar as having a disease depends on the expectations that go with a specific diagnosis, then even though there is a continuity to the disease, the experience of modern and ancient sufferers might be entirely different. Having tuberculosis now is entirely different from the mid-nineteenth-century experience of having consumption. But one ground that can unite older and modern experiences lies in the expectations that stem from the availability or nonavailability of treatments that are thought to make a difference. This is the ground on which commerce as well as hope and despair flourish—a ground that can leave many physicians in Africa today in the same position vis-à-vis infective epidemics such as AIDS as physicians from Hippocrates through to Kraepelin were, while at the same time making it seem to physicians in the West as though manic-depressive disease is one of the most pressing scourges facing humanity.

A final point of continuity with the past lies in the dialectical opposition between empirical and theoretical orientations. An empirical orientation as found in Hippocrates, Paracelsus, and, later, Willis and Kraepelin, commonly leads to breakthroughs, while a theoretical orientation as found in Galen and Freud attempts to integrate developments into a worldview against which people can make sense of what might be happening to them. These latter worldviews provide commercial opportunities because they typically have implications for health and well-being and not just simply for the management of acute disease. But these theories also risk becoming sterile formulae, and the risk for all of us faced with threatening realities is that the formulae to which we turn will be sterile. If these formulae provide commercial opportunities, there is an added risk, namely, that the thera-

peutic establishment may hinder our efforts to come to grips with
new problems. This is the issue that will face us in chapter 8.

The medical establishment in Greco-Roman times was organized in schools linked to protoclinics. Later, during the Middle
Ages and Enlightenment, except in some notable European centers, medicine was largely outside of or loosely linked to universities like Oxford or Cambridge, which were institutions in the first
instance devoted to the disciplines of theology and philosophy.[45]
Medicine during this period and indeed until the mid-twentieth
century often seemed to academicians too pragmatic and empirical to be considered a university discipline. It was only with the
commercial opportunities created by research linked to biology
and the pharmaceutical industry in the second half of the twentieth century that the university systems in America and Britain
fully embraced medicine.

The flowering of academic medicine witnessed in the middle
of the twentieth century may turn out to have been a relatively
brief bloom. When the psychopharmaceutical events that sit at
the heart of this book began to unfold from 1949 onward, professors of medicine or psychiatry from Harvard, Oxford, or Paris
would barely have known the names of pharmaceutical companies in the field. It was unlikely that even the most senior company figures would have been invited into the inner academic
sanctums. But now the biggest university names in the field are
likely to be found vying for the attentions of company personnel,
and the establishment arguably now sits in company boardrooms
rather than in universities.

Whereas in the 1960s physicians carried out the research on
the host of new compounds that formed potent weapons in a new
medical armory, by the end of the century research had passed
out of medical hands to clinical trial organizations, key publications were for the most part ghostwritten, and the rate at which
new breakthroughs were being made had slowed to a trickle. In
the face of this, what would a Paracelsus make of modern physicians, whose prescribing, as we shall see in chapters 7 and 8, is
constrained by guidelines rather than by their own experience?
What would Hippocrates or Kraepelin have made of a world in
which companies market diseases, and people with little true dis-

ability and certainly little risk of death, appear to catch fashionable diseases?

What, indeed, will we make of the brave new medical world that is brought into view so well by considering the fortunes of bipolar disorder? While there are continuities and discontinuities of importance to us when considering this story that stretches back to the Greeks, a specifically modern story starts in seventeenth-century England, when Thomas Willis brought the brain as we now know it into view for the first time, and Thomas Sydenham began classifying diseases. Soon afterward, lunacy came into view in a new way as the building of the asylums exposed physicians to madness in all its guises. These developments led in 1854 in Paris to descriptions of an apparently rare new illness, *folie circulaire*, which was subsumed by Karl Kahlbaum and Emil Kraepelin into bipolar disorder and manic-depressive illness. The new disorder remained rare until a controversy arose in the 1960s about whether it might respond to treatment with lithium. This dispute in which the protagonists were both concerned to rein in the pharmaceutical industry paradoxically laid the basis for an astonishing pharmaceutical company gold rush into bipolar disorders in the 1990s that has en passant transformed the way we understand ourselves and the way our physicians approach the practice of medicine, and has also raised profound questions about the intersection between science and commerce.

CHAPTER TWO

Circling the Brain

❀ ❀ ❀

The emergence of psychiatry in the early nineteenth century finally eclipsed humoral models of mental disorders. The same forces that laid the basis for the new discipline remade our world but brought in their train secularism and concerns about a biological reductionism of behavior.

Among these forces was the confluence of elements that gave rise to the revolution in the natural sciences that began in Europe in the seventeenth century. Although it gave rise to the work of Galileo, Newton, Descartes, Harvey, Boyle, Leibniz, and others, this was also a period of profound social dislocation that led on to the Enlightenment, in which science came to be seen as the best hope for social progress and as offering humanity some control over the forces of nature. More recently, doubts have emerged about the capacity of science to effect meaningful social reform and concerns that our control of nature may lead to environmental catastrophe, and these doubts and concerns have fueled critiques that have portrayed science as simply a manifestation of capitalism. This interplay between scientific progress and social dynamics will follow us to the end of the book.

While the birth of physics and chemistry in the mid-seventeenth century has been celebrated, a new science of the brain, born at the same time, has received much less attention. Thomas Willis was one of the central figures in creating this science of the brain, a science that meant we had to find new ways to fit ourselves into our bodies and into society. Compared with physics and chemistry, the new neuroscience was initially an all-but-dormant volcano, but its slow emergence was marked by a growing rumble of secularism. A second set of social forces in the early nineteenth century led to the creation of asylums to house the insane. The asylums called forth a new cadre of physicians, the alienists, who offered medical input to the care of inmates confined in these institutions. Confronted with insanity in all its guises, it was inevitable that, in the hands of these alienists, not only would our views of madness change, but the process would eventually affect how we view ourselves.

A third group of forces stemmed from attempts to devise an explicit set of rules to determine when individuals should be held accountable for their actions. Late eighteenth- and early nineteenth-century legal cases forced society to grapple with the issues thrown up in cases of murder in which the defendant appeared to be insane. Who, if anyone, might be spared execution on the grounds of illness? The problem called for a new expertise, one that blended the legal and medical fields.

THE NEW BRAIN

Nowadays images of the brain are ubiquitous. In magazines and on television screens, we see the grays and blacks of computed tomographic (CT) and magnetic resonance imaging (MRI) scans. In drug advertisements, we often see different regions of the brain lit up in the colors of positron emission tomography (PET) scans. These images were introduced in the mid-1980s and became common in medical settings only in the mid- to late 1990s, the decade of the brain. They seeped into popular consciousness at the start of the twenty-first century as Internet sites flourished, offering new services promising the ability to maximize our potential through a proper utilization of our brains.[1]

Until the late 1980s, the bones of the skull stood out on X-rays in solid relief, but within the bony surrounds of the skull there was a vacuum where the brain should be. In the mid-1970s movie *The Exorcist,* for instance, psychiatrists investigating the brain did so using angiograms that outlined the arteries snaking around the brain, making it visible in the way a sprinkle of dust made *The Invisible Man* semivisible.

Pneumoencephalograms were also used in which bubbles of air within the ventricles of the brain allowed clinicians to guess— "to make inferences"—based on disturbances in the shapes of the ventricles as to the existence and nature of any pathology in the surrounding lobes of the brain. This was a neurological version of "blindman's bluff."

The astonishing transformation in the visibility of the brain in the last decades of the twentieth century parallel a transformation that took place in the visualization of the brain in the mid seventeenth century, with the work of Thomas Willis in Oxford.

With the Renaissance and the early phases of the scientific revolution, there was a growing emphasis on experiment, epitomized by Paracelsus's chemical therapeutics and by Andreas Vesalius's dissections of human corpses. Vesalius's dissections directly contradicted Galen on a number of key points. The publication in Basel in 1543 of his *On the Structure of the Human Body* fueled the emerging questioning of Galenic concepts of how the human body functioned.[2] A host of related anatomical discoveries outlining features, such as the refractory properties of the lens of the eye, emphasized continuities between animals and even machines and man. The most dramatic result of this new approach came in 1628 when William Harvey published his findings in *On the Motion of the Heart and Blood in Animals,* demonstrating that the heart functioned as a muscular pump, pushing blood through the arteries, which delivered it around the body, for it to be returned to the heart by the veins before being circulated through the lungs and redistributed again through the body.

Prior to Harvey's publication, the heart had been considered a mysterious organ in the human body, quite possibly the seat of the soul. It was the part of the body that most clearly responded to the influence of the emotions. The presumed involvement of the heart in thinking is still found in a number of everyday phrases, such as learning it "by heart."

One of the first efforts to incorporate the nascent biological sciences into a new vision of what it means to be human came in the work of René Descartes. In response to the new anatomy and physiology, Descartes produced a radical view of man as a mechanical being inhabited by a soul. In the process, he famously left unresolved the issue of where the soul took up its residence within the body. In the *Passions of the Soul*,[3] the soul appears coterminous with the entire body, but in Descartes' *Treatise on Man*, the residence of the soul is placed in the pineal gland.[4]

Localizing the soul in the pineal gland seemed plausible. It is the one single organ in the brain. Everything else comes in duplicates, one on the left and one on the right. The pineal is also in the midline of the brain. Most crucially, the pineal hangs down into the cerebral ventricles through which the animal or nervous spirits inhabiting the brain were thought to travel, and on their travels they could be imagined subtly influencing this gland or being influenced by it.

For most of the previous two millennia insofar as anyone had seen the brain, the ventricles, or chambers of the brain, were the features of greatest interest. More than any other areas of the brain, the ventricles had been seen as a possible hall of residence for a spirit. Hippocrates clearly considers the possibility that the diaphragm was the organ of thinking, but he rejects it in favor of the brain because the diaphragm "has no cavity into which it might receive anything good or bad that comes upon it."[5] The cerebral ventricles were, moreover, filled with a liquor or humor that was essential for humoral models of human functioning. This fluid, which was variously termed animal spirits or a subtle fluid, could be conceived as distributing itself down through the channels of the nerves to various parts of the body to animate them. The white cords emanating from the brain, now called nerves, had been observed by Galen as early as the second century AD.

The remainder of the brain surrounding the ventricles, which we now see as a solid mass that conceivably could house the cerebral computer that we imagine directs physical and psychological functions, did not look so solid to the Greeks or Romans or during the dissections of the Renaissance. When heads were split open in battle, the brain contents literally leaked out. By the time postmortems or the dissections of corpses took place, particularly in hotter climates, the brain had little more shape than a mass of pudding would have. Within this mass, the ventricles at least had some shape, and as a result representations of the brain often featured an organ inside the head in which the ventricles occupied, even in Descartes' work, much more space than in fact they do, with the rest of the brain having no distinctive features.

The new Cartesian view was still an essentially ancient view of the brain, in which the ventricles and the fluid that they contained were critical and open to outside influences from God or the environment. It could still be affected by the wind or *pneuma,* which was the dominant metaphor for the presence of God in the world. Hippocrates had put this beautifully: "Everything contains moisture to a greater or lesser degree and thus all things feel the effect of the south wind and become dark instead of bright, warm instead of cold, and moist instead of dry. Jars in the house or in the cellars which contain wine or any other liquid are influenced by the south wind and change their appearance."[6]

Beautiful though this was, this view did nothing to force people to examine what might be happening within their brains when they contemplated the meaning of life, or they fell in love, or they had to tell their children about what it meant to be human.

There were many reasons to continue to think that the heart and the blood were the seat of the soul and the seat of life. The blood was clearly warm to the touch. Under the influence of Paracelsus, it came to be seen as a site of fermentation processes, which might deliver heat and energy to various parts of the body, including the brain. The brain, in contrast, appeared to be a cold organ.

It was the genius of Thomas Willis and his colleagues in Oxford to revisit the brain (introducing the use of preservatives) and give it its modern shape.[7] Working in Oxford at a time of Civil War in England, Willis moved in the group of early scientists that established the first scientific society—the Royal Society. This Oxford circle included Robert Boyle, Robert Hooke, Christopher Wren, Richard Lower, and others. Willis was heavily influenced by Harvey, who spent his final years in Oxford, and by William Petty, another anatomist.

The ferment of experimentation these early scientists stimulated, despite the war, led in 1664 to Willis's breakthrough work, *Anatomy of the Brain.* In this volume, the anatomical drawings of the brain were radically different from anything that had gone before. The most famous featured the undersurface of the brain with its folds and fissures and a plethora of discrete features, such as the brain stem, the pons, the medulla, and the circle of arteries surrounding the base of the brain that have ever since been known as the Circle of Willis. Other views showed the corrugated infolding of the cerebellum and the cerebral cortex. There was little emphasis on the ventricles. This was a new solid brain. For the first time, clinical and scientific attention was directed to what we now call the brain.[8]

The representation of the brain as a solid organ made it possible to start thinking systematically about how this might be the organ of thought. Prior to Willis's time, the cerebral ventricles, as containers of fluids, were assumed to be in some way open to the influence of environmental and other pressures, whether from the promptings of God through the pineal gland, or though the influence of the seasons or other contagious factors on the humors circulating through the ventricles. The new brain as envisaged by Willis appeared to be a closed organ, which, if it were open to outside influence, would be so through the medium of active subjects learning by using their senses in order to make judgments as to what was happening in their world.

Dissection made it clear the new brain had different strata— cerebral cortex, cerebellum, and then midbrain structures. This pointed to the possibility of a new mental economy where different systems would have different functions not unlike the way different parts of society cooperated under the direction of a monarch. The new vision of the brain called for two new sciences—neurology and psychology. Willis himself coined the term *neurology,* and his new discipline laid the basis for the ultimate localization of ancient disorders such as epilepsy and apoplexy.

John Locke, one of Willis's students, taking seriously his teacher's ideas of brain function, argued that human beings began life with a tabula rasa, a blank slate, and, through sensory inputs from outside, built up their personalities and thinking styles through impressions and associations laid down within the matter of the brain.[9] This led to his seminal work of modern philosophy, *An Essay Concerning Human Understanding.* Locke coined the term *psychology* in the 1680s to deal with the new learning.[10]

Besides its philosophical implications, the new work pointed to ways in which we might live that are now seen as characteristic of the Enlightenment. While good example had always been seen as important, if a person were not primarily influenced by the *pneuma,* but rather by the impressions and associations laid down from birth, pedagogy became of compelling importance and a correct education became an increasingly significant religious and political tool.[11]

Locke's interest in the implications of the new brain contrasted to the views of another contemporary. The physician Thomas Sydenham abjured brain anatomy as a fruitless exercise, likely to yield little of value for either the therapeutics of disease or our understanding of how to live. In common with Willis, however, Sydenham also put a renewed emphasis on clinical observation.[12] He was one of the first to raise the possibility that there might be disease entities—that is, something that ran a characteristic course regardless of who was affected. The traditional Galenic approach to illness involved treating the individual rather than treating a disease. If there were disease entities, Sydenham recognized they would need to be classified, just as the botanists were classifying plants.[13] This led him to establish one of the first classifications of the disorders encountered in medical practice—a first stab at what would later become the *Diagnostic and Statistical Manual* (*DSM*) system in psychiatry and International Classification of Diseases (ICD) for medicine in general.

The new thinking had implications for what would now be called the emotions but were then termed the passions. The word *passion* stems from the Greek *pathos,* which implies the experience of having one's body being acted upon, as in suffering. People suffered powerful impulses. This idea took shape in a context that assumed that the body was porous and open to outside influences but that the control of the passions was the duty of a rational individual. Such control could be exercised through the notion of moderation in particular, and this notion of moderation was bound up with a humoral model that strove for balance. In terms of managing or not unduly disturbing the humors, moderation was seen as a virtue when it came to diet, activity, and sexual activity.

Between 1700 and 1800 the term passion began to be replaced by the new term *emotion*. In contrast to the passions, the emotions were seen as stemming from within the individual and therefore potentially, rather than being subversive influences from outside, were guides from within that might steer an individual along the right path. Where before there was no question but that the rational faculty should subdue all others, a world began opening up in which there might be competing sources of wisdom with much less certainty that "conventional rationality" was the supreme virtue.[14] The notion that one might opt to be guided by one's feelings emerged. This innate knowledge stood in contrast to Locke's tabula rasa.

All of these ideas were dangerous. Willis's work took place against a background of great uncertainty. The Civil War had turned the English world upside down.[15] While much of the political ferment was driven forward by radical religious sects, a new phenomenon began to appear for the first time—the possibility of a lack of belief in any overarching god or cosmic principle. It had previously been almost impossible to conceive of a desacralized or mechanical world.[16]

This science raised new questions. What did one tell one's children about what our purpose in life was, or about how the human body might shape human behavior? Even though almost all scientists at the time studied the book of Nature as another path to God,[17] Descartes left his *Treatise on Man* unpublished, and the constant risk that Willis and his colleagues ran was of being accused of laying a basis for atheism and materialism. Their political skill lay in pushing forward the boundaries of science while at the same time persuading a variety of political masters that their new discoveries were consistent with traditional values and with the maintenance of order in society. This new knowledge was no less dangerous if not contained within a moral framework than twentieth-century nuclear knowledge would later be.

THE NEW BRAIN AND ITS "NERVES"

Both Sydenham and Willis regarded hysteria as a convulsive disorder. In referring to it as the "*so-called* uterine disease," Willis made one of the first breaks with traditional views on this disorder. He claimed instead that its etiology lay in an alteration of the nerves and brain, invoking a mechanism that could be regarded as a prototype of the modern reflex.[18] By means of the nervous system, he wrote, "are revealed the true and genuine reasons for very many actions and passions that take place in our body that would otherwise seem most difficult to explain: and from this fountain, no less than the hidden causes of diseases and symptoms, which are commonly ascribed to the incantations of witches, may be discovered."[19]

In 1682 Sydenham classified hysteria as the commonest chronic nervous disease. It took almost a further 100 years for hysteria to become more clearly established as a disorder of the nerves—a neurosis. The term *neurosis* was formally introduced by the Edinburgh physician William Cullen in 1785, although the idea that general lassitude or suboptimal behavior of obscure origin could be attributed to "nerves" had probably been put forward as early as 1765 by another Edinburgh physician, Robert Whytt.[20] Cullen defined the neuroses as disorders that involved disturbances of nervous functioning, without any obvious lesion or inflammation of the nerves (neuritis) being apparent at postmortem. In much the same way, the word *nephrosis* had been coined to categorize functional kidney disorders in the absence of demonstrable abnormality or inflammation (as in nephritis). For Cullen, who was a medical classifier like Sydenham, hysteria was one subdivision of the spasmodic neuroses—all of which involved abnormal movement of muscles or muscle fibers. The neuroses also included tetanus, epilepsy, colic, diabetes, palpitations, and whooping cough. This classification system survived for more than a century. As late as 1899, Kraepelin still classified epilepsy, chorea, tetanus, and migraine along with hysteria as neuroses.[21]

The recognition of nerve cells and the idea that nerve fibers conducted impulses between nerve cells lay 100 years in the future, so it is not clear what Cullen meant by neurosis. It seems likely that he saw the neuroses as malfunctions of the system as a whole, with no one definite, localized disturbance. These generalized disturbances of function displayed themselves in symptoms of pain, increased or decreased sensitivity to internal or external stimuli, spasms and general disorders of muscular movement, and weakness.

This was a nervous system still permeated in some way by an immaterial spirit. Philippe Pinel, the first of the great French alienists, who had Cullen's work translated into French, for example, could still see the neuroses as caused by the passions of the soul. With Cullen and Pinel, the notion of a neurosis became fashionable, and there was a huge expansion in the number of diseases that were considered neurotic.

Shortly afterward, however, one of the so-called neuroses, apoplexy (stroke), was discovered to have a very real and demonstrable cause in loss of brain tissue. By 1840 it was clear that many of the disorders that Pinel and Cullen had described as neuroses had been demonstrated either to have a localizable basis in nervous destruction or, indeed, to have nothing to do with nerves. For the remainder, who had "neurotic" behavior in the absence of a localizable lesion, a new explanatory notion emerged—the reflex.

When Descartes suggested that men and animals might function in many respects like automata, he postulated that physical and mental operations might take place by means of tugs and pulls, using some equivalent of ropes and pulleys and springs, or by a hydraulic process involving fluid and valves.[22] The obvious candidates for such threads or pipes were the nerves. Descartes suggested that on stimulation by pain, for example, delicate threads lying in the nerve bundles are moved, which open valves within the brain and release animal spirits (sensitive and irritable substances), which then lead to muscular movement. However, he did not envisage this as an automatic and unconscious reaction, of the kind that we now mean when we use the term *reflex*.

For example, he meant that the physical sight of fire would be associated with a mental image of flames. Animal spirits in the brain on catching a glimpse of such an image would be reflected in fright toward the muscles disposing them for flight. Until about 1830, the primary meaning of the term reflex connoted some form of reflection in the sense of judgment. Although some actions may seemingly occur beneath the level of awareness, as in mechanically removing one's foot from a flame that one is not looking at or in knee jerks, these did not happen without the reflection of the soul. Such acts were, after all, invariably wise.

Robert Whytt, 100 years after Descartes, argued that a lower faculty of the soul might govern some acts. The case of anencephalic infants, who were nevertheless capable of movements, pointed to the possibility of an unconscious agency—deeply troubling for those who believed that all human acts had to be governed by some wisdom of the soul.[23] Also disturbing were experiments on removing the brains of animals, which did not necessarily lead to complete passivity of the animal. These findings troubled many scientists and philosophers, for whom the nervous system was still primarily seen as a whole piece—without subdivisions.

In 1810 the Austrian physician Franz Gall postulated a nervous system organized in layers as part of his new science of phrenology.[24] The potential autonomy of the different layers in this system pointed to the possibility that things could happen outside the control of the soul. The disturbing implications of this view forced Gall to move from Vienna to Paris.

The unified nervous system was fractured by the work of François Magendie and Charles Bell, who separately in 1823 provided the physiological basis for Marshall Hall's demonstration in 1832 that the spinal column was not just a system for carrying messages from the brain but one that contained reflex systems that could operate independently of the brain.[25] This discovery made it possible to conceive of actions being automatic and unconscious. But in introducing the term *reflex* for such automatic and unconscious acts, Hall stood the original notion of a reflex on its head.

Hall envisaged reflexes as playing a part in the functioning of the spinal cord. He did not envisage their extension to the central nervous system. But progressively over the following thirty years, the German alienists Wilhelm Griesinger and Karl Wernicke (chapter 5), the British neurologists Thomas Laycock and Hughlings Jackson, and others postulated higher and higher reflexes to account for increasingly more complex behaviors.

The view of man that was taking shape was radically different from anything conceived by previous generations. Clearly some idea of an unconscious had been around since the Greeks, but essentially earlier ideas of unconsciousness took the form that the soul had depths, some of which might be effectively impenetrable. The reflex laid the basis for mechanical operations that could function without either a soul or consciousness. As Laycock put it, "many will consider it dangerous to concede that apparently pure mental acts are only the results of vital machinery excited into action by physical agencies."[26] "Researches of this kind," he argued, "whether instituted on the insane, the somnambulist, the dreamer, or the delirious must be considered like researches in analytical chemistry. The reagent is the impression made on the brain; the molecular changes following the application of the reagent are made known to us as ideas."[27]

The notion of a reflex gave substance to an idea postulated by Willis that the nervous system might become disturbed in sympathy with disturbances in other organs such as the kidneys, teeth, or uterus by a reflex mechanism operating outside consciousness. For example inflamed kidneys might lead to spinal irritation and thereby to a disturbance of other organs or a generalized nervous irritability. This possibility was not just an armchair theory of the neuroses. It led to the removal of kidneys and teeth in patients, who far from having renal or dental problems, had presented with complaints of being generally unwell. Where hysteria was concerned, the notion of a reflex overcame the difficulties that resulted from an exclusive reliance on a uterine pathology. Rather than have the uterus migrate, it was now possible to have nervous impulses from the uterus diffuse upward bringing abnormal sensations to other areas of the body. One obvious treatment for such a condition was a hysterectomy. These ideas still had a potent appeal in America in the 1920s, where they laid the basis for the extraordinary program of organ extraction from psychiatric patients overseen by Henry Cotton in New Jersey.[28]

The political and social implications of the new science were profound. Much of the speculation about cerebral reflexes was made possible by demonstrations of hypnotic "reflexes." And the earliest form of hypnosis, mesmerism, was closely linked to the revolutionary foment that overthrew the French monarchy in the 1790s. As a direct consequence of this revolution, hypnosis was banned by the medical establishment for almost a century and by the Catholic Church for almost two centuries.[29]

Later in the nineteenth century, the new neurophysiology was allied with evolutionary theory, which was widely regarded as another push toward atheism and materialism. The automatic and unconscious nature of reflexes raised the possibility that consciousness might be an unimportant spectator of human activity rather than its guiding focus. Thomas Huxley dramatically put forward this point of view in defense of Darwin, suggesting that consciousness was no more important to human functioning than the whistle of a locomotive was to the running of a train or that conscious awareness was akin to the mist or steam that hovers over machines while they work.

Not everyone saw the new biology as giving rise to a reductionist materialism. For Charles Sherrington, the new brain was an enchanted loom. Another successor of Willis, another neurologist, was Sigmund Freud. Ever one to incorporate the latest biology into his theories, in 1895, just when his studies of hysteria were leading to the birth of the modern psyche, and Kraepelin was outlining manic-depressive insanity, Freud wrote the "Project for a Scientific Psychology."[30] This unpublished text postulated that individual memories might reside in the then just discovered nerve cells, and a reflex linking of memories might be responsible for complexes and for repression and might in addition provide a scientific basis for therapy.

Freud abandoned this idea, deciding that this was not the way that minds fit into brains. Instead, in turning to the idea that character formation hinged on how we handle our biology, our instincts and impulses, he created psychoanalysis, a mode of viewing man that, with its emphasis on handling our passions, has clear continuities with earlier humoral views.

Although Freud was deeply suspect in many quarters, given his framing of religious belief as neurotic, the vision of the brain that he opened up was one that seemed much more compatible to many with notions of meaning in human life than the apparently even more materialistic behaviorism with its conditioned reflexes that appeared soon after. In many Catholic countries, for example, the depth psychologies were acceptable where behavior-ism was not.[31]

THE BRAIN IN THE ASYLUM

The impetus to the creation of asylums has generated great dis-putes that go to the heart of what psychiatry is. Did the asylum originate as an agent of social control,[32] or was it as much a branch of medicine as any other?[33] I take the expressed humanitarian wishes of the early advocates of asylums at face value (see chap-ter 3). The dictates of humoral medicine mandated an orderly environment with good food, regular exercise, and appropriate discipline as a means to restore wits to the witless. However, there are issues of social cohesion and control involved in managing maniacs, and this issue will return with all its bloody wounds still gaping at the end of the chapter.

Whatever the impetus to their creation, with the opening of the asylums in the early nineteenth century an emerging group of physicians, the alienists, was faced with the first assemblage of mentally disordered patients. Before the asylums, it was simply not possible for physicians or others who might comment on the human condition to have seen sufficient numbers of patients and a full range of types of insanity to be able to offer views of insan-ity that were likely to endure. Perceptive observations of idiosyn-cratic features or occasional syndromes were all that could be ex-pected. But when larger numbers of the insane were collected in the same place for the first time, it became inescapably clear that not all raving madmen had the same condition. This recognition prompted the first specifically psychiatric attempts to classify the various manias.

The name firmly linked to the first widely influential clas-sification in psychiatry was Jean-Étienne Dominique Esquirol. Born in Toulouse in 1772, Esquirol went to Paris and took up medicine relatively late. He joined the most famous of the early French alienists, Philippe Pinel, and after working with Pinel at the Salpêtrière for many years, he took charge of Charenton hos-pital on the outskirts of Paris. Pinel's public profile in liberating the insane from their chains has in the public mind eclipsed the reputations of subsequent nineteenth-century alienists, including that of Esquirol, but in terms of enduring contributions to psychiatry, Esquirol's achievement was the greater.

Faced with hundreds of patients in the Salpêtrière and later at Charenton, institutions that he was responsible for redesignating as asylums rather than hospitals, Esquirol distinguished monomanias from mania proper. Others grappling with these issues in Germany and England came up with the term partial insanity. This notion had been up to that point literally inconceivable. But now the concept seemed all but demanded by many of the new inmates of the asylum who could appear almost normal in every respect until one touched upon the point at which their belief systems became fixed. Esquirol argued that rather than being entirely manic or insane, these patients had a disturbance of one of their faculties only, and this disturbance led to their particular monomania or partial insanity.[34]

Standing in the way of views like this was one of the dominating notions of Western civilization—the soul. Traditional definitions of the soul concurred that it was indivisible. Everyone agreed that the soul was the rational center of a human being. If a person's behavior became irrational, mad, or deranged, it followed that a bit of the soul could not be mad or deranged but that the entire person had to be deranged. This led observers to expect to see madmen as wholly deranged or raving. And, as the majority of madmen were probably delirious or frenzied, the appearances of madness supported rather than refuted this.

This backdrop meant that clinicians or anyone else interested in the issue of madness would have great difficulty with the notion of a periodic or recurrent disorder. It was difficult if not impossible to conceive of a soul being somewhat restored to sanity only to relapse again. It was easier to maintain the belief that once insane, always insane. Apparent well-being in between episodes was more likely to be interpreted as a lucid interval rather than a restoration of sanity.

Toward the end of the eighteenth century, the emergence of faculty psychology in Edinburgh with Thomas Reid, the philosophy of the Scottish enlightenment, and the neurophysiology of Whytt and Cullen helped provide a model that overcame some of the difficulties. While not denying the unity of the soul, these authors introduced the operational notion of faculties, arguing for faculties of cognition, emotion, and volition. The introduction of faculties took place in just the same way that models of neurotransmitter receptors were adopted in the 1960s. In both cases, there was a backdrop of orthodox hostility, and the proponents of the new thinking did not argue for the reality of either faculties in the 1780s or receptors in the 1960s but rather for the utility of a convenient fiction. This new model of the soul made it possible to think that one or another of the faculties of the soul might be disordered without the rest of the brain or mind being disturbed. This conceptual breakthrough, married to a growing awareness that not all mad patients appeared the same, underpinned Esquirol's proposal that there might be monomanias distinct from full-blown mania.

> Writers since the time of Hippocrates have denominated that form of delirium which is characterized by moroseness, fear, and prolonged sadness, Melancholy. . . . Some moderns have given a more extended signification to the word melancholy, and have called melancholic, every form of partial delirium, when chronic, and unattended by fever. It is certain that the word melancholy . . . often presents to the mind a false idea. This . . . has caused me to propose the word monomania, a term that expresses the essential character of that form of insanity in which the delirium is partial. . . . Monomania expresses an abnormal condition of the physical or mental sensibility with a circumscribed and fixed delirium.[35]

It became possible, for example, to think that there might be disorders of an emotional or mood faculty that did not involve an intellectual disorder. Esquirol proposed intellectual, affective, and instinctive monomanias. One of these monomanias was lypemania. Derived from the Greek λύπης, which refers to sorrow, pain, and distress and was used to describe the woman of Thasos, lypemania was painted as a state in which individuals were excessively sad and miserable but typically without other features of traditional insanity: "a cerebral malady characterized by partial, chronic delirium, without fever and sustained by a passion

of a sad, debilitating or oppressive character."[36] Benjamin Rush
a few years before had described much the same condition and
given it the name *tristimania*. In the mid-twentieth century this
state would have been called endogenous depression. This new
disorder, depression, as it was later called, was seen as a different
disorder from melancholia, because the latter involved delusional
beliefs, whereas the former did not. Melancholia was a subdivision of mania, whereas lypemania or depression was not.

In addition to lypemania, Esquirol described volitional monomanias, such as obsessive-compulsive disorder, graphomania,
nymphomania, kleptomania, dipsomania, homicidal monomania, and other syndromes, some of which are still recognized. Esquirol's resulting classification system had similarities to *DSM-IV*,
which has a tendency to regard almost every prominent symptom
as a new illness in its own right. There are distinct echoes of kleptomania or graphomania in modern disorders like compulsive
shopping disorder.

This explosion of different syndromes paralleled developments in faculty psychology where the three primary faculties
multiplied up to forty different faculties. These putative faculties
underpinned Franz Gall's development of phrenology, according
to which different parts of the brain were the presumed seat of
different faculties and the relative developments of these faculties led to different bumps and protuberances on the skull, which
"scientists or skilled practitioners" could use to measure the abilities or character of the person.

The idea of monomania or partial insanity took root across
France, England, Germany, and Italy. Esquirol's role was more
one of offering a formula that captured these changes rather than
as the sole instigator of such changes. James Prichard and Forbes
Winslow in England, for instance, described conditions that
equally appeared to involve behavioral disturbances without intellectual disturbances.

In 1833 Prichard outlined the notion of moral insanity:[37] "This
form of mental derangement has been described as consisting in
a morbid perversion of the feelings, affections, and active powers, without any illusion or erroneous conviction impressed upon
the understanding."[38] Prichard's moral insanity has typically been

taken for the past fifty years or more to be a forerunner of the modern concept of psychopathy, but it could not have indicated any such connection. Patients with what would now be termed personality disorders simply did not get into the asylums. Asylum physicians were quick to distinguish between fools and the occasional knave who came their way, and they discharged the knaves. The knaves moreover had little to gain from asylum admission.

Prichard's morally insane, like Esquirol's lypemanics, had a disorder of their behavior in the absence of any defect of intellectual functioning, in contrast to the vast majority of patients entering the asylum, who were frankly deluded. Having a derangement of intelligence had been the essence of madness. It took time to realize that there were other patients confined to the asylum because of grossly impaired functioning who were simply not deluded. And this realization depended on and in turn supported notions that there might be emotional and volitional faculties that were distinct from an intellectual faculty.

Despite these changes in the perceptions of brain function and madness, there was little change when it came to making links between mania and melancholia. English, Dutch, and German physicians continued to see mania and melancholia as stages on the path to insanity.[39] Thus, John Haslam, the superintendent of the Bethlem Hospital in 1798, points to the common ground between mania and melancholia: "I would strongly oppose to them being considered opposite diseases. In both, the association of ideas is equally incorrect, and they appear to differ only, from the different passions, which accompany them. On dissection, the state of the brain does not show any appearances peculiar to melancholy, nor is the treatment which I have observed more successful, different from that which employed in mania. . . . we see everyday the most furious maniacs suddenly sink into a profound melancholy; and the most depressed and miserable objects become violent and raving."[40]

Alexander Crichton in Edinburgh noted cases of melancholia "terminating, or at least alternating, with the state of furious delirium, having all the true character of mania."[41] These ideas if anything may have become even stronger under the influence of Esquirol's notions of partial insanity. It was even easier to see mania as the progression from partial to complete insanity rather than a swing from one pole to another. On this issue, Esquirol himself in 1835 wrote:

> I have already mentioned that all the species of insanity may be variously combined, and frequently interchange one with another. It may be proper further to note that the same patients sometimes go through several kinds of insanity—which may be reckoned in such places as so many degrees of stages—during the course of the same illness. Of these combinations, and changes, there is an almost endless variety. One remarkable, and not uncommon transition of insanity, is from great dejection, and distress, to ease and cheerfulness and sometimes to an uncommon flow of spirits.[42]

Two developments were to change this perspective. One was an astonishing scientific breakthrough, the like of which would transform any future *DSM* as completely as it challenged Esquirol's new edifice. Using postmortem samples, Auguste Bayle demonstrated that one of the disorders that appeared in the asylum, general paralysis of the insane, was a distinct illness, showing distinctive postmortem brain changes not found in other manias.[43] The significance of this discovery was that it became clear that general paralysis of the insane or tertiary syphilis, involved a multipolar clinical picture in which patients might at one point be elated and grandiose but at others depressed and paranoid and toward the end might have dementia. Bayle's discoveries put a premium on following the clinical development of a disorder and argued against viewing symptoms or even dramatic syndromes as discrete illnesses in their own right.

The greater appreciation of disease entities stemming from Bayle posed problems for Esquirol's notion of monomanias that Jean-Pierre Falret, one of Esquirol's pupils, brought out.[44] First, the idea of monomania made it difficult to distinguish between normality and insanity. If an intensely passionate fixation on an unattainable individual was to be regarded as a monomania, how could this be reliably distinguished from a normal love that was also intensely passionate? Second, could we ever be sure that a single prominent symptom such as a delusion was in fact the only delusion present? Third, what were the implications of a particular delusion—about the secret police, for instance—turning up in quite different mental states and with varying levels of intensity?

And yet the concept of monomania facilitated the description of new disorders like obsessive-compulsive disorder that survive to this day. It was a necessary transitional concept. In its place, Falret suggested that clinicians needed to reach to the disease ground in which a variety of monomanias might take root and flourish. This disease ground might involve an expansion of behaviors as in classic mania or a contraction as in melancholia. This change in mood set the stage for the separate description by Falret and Jules Baillarger in the 1850s of a new disease—*folie circulaire* or *folie à double forme*—the first descriptions of bipolar disorder or manic-depressive illness.

A second part of Falret's critique spoke to the growing interface between psychiatry and the law. Esquirol's volitional monomanias, and in particular his concept of homicidal monomania, posed huge legal difficulties. If we diagnose an insanity just because someone has done something "mad," we set up a medicolegal crisis. If patients were raving mad, the legal system knew what to do, but if they were only partially mad, should they be executed or pardoned? Falret argued that the grounds for finding a patient not guilty or less responsible must lie in the clear demonstration that the patient had a disease rather than just an irresistible impulse.

INSANITY AND THE LAW

Although it is beyond the scope of this book to chart the evolution of medical jurisprudence as it relates to insanity,[45] it is useful to recognize a set of watershed developments that took place in the nineteenth century, during the same years in which the concept of manic-depressive illness took shape.

Unless human nature has changed, simply on the basis of population, murders must have been less frequent through the nineteenth century than they had been before, and insanity was less frequent, and murders by madmen less frequent again. If only for this reason, there was less pressure on any society from the Romans through the developing democracies of the nineteenth century to work out a set of rules to manage the trial and disposition of such cases. There was also no body of specialists to offer views on how individual cases and on how medicolegal issues in general should be viewed.

The prototypical case involved a senseless murder by someone in a frenzied or delirious state or by someone who was an idiot from an early age. Many delirious states led on to death, and so that the risk of further offending was not a salient issue. Where death appeared less likely, committal to prison would follow, often without a trial. These offenders were quite alienated from their wits and would have been unable to defend themselves in court. The judgment of many societies was that they were sufficiently punished by their insanity or their idiocy to make further punishment unnecessary. In all other cases, no matter how eccentric the defendant, if he was not grossly alienated from his wits, his conviction for murder was likely to lead to execution.

Courts at the time had to deal with a series of offenses not typically found today. In the sixteenth and seventeenth centuries, issues in which the question of sanity came to the fore included witchcraft, blasphemy, and heresy. These accusations were intensely political in the sense that blasphemers or heretics threatened the social order. Were these returning Messiahs deluded or political? In England, a Puritan revolution, based on what for Church of England believers was heresy, had brought down Charles I.

In attempting to deal with the problems facing them, judges formulated the issues in a manner that suggests there were considerable developments in thinking about insanity taking place outside of the asylums. For example, Matthew Hale, England's lord chief justice in 1676, anticipates many of the difficulties Esquirol and Falret struggled with and seems to be speaking a much more modern language than many later alienists :

> There is a partial insanity of mind . . .; some persons that have a confident use of reason in respect of some subjects, are yet under a particular dementia in respect of some particular discourses, subjects or applications; or else it is partial in respect of degrees; and this is the condition of very many, especially melancholy

persons, who for the most part discover their defect in excessive fears or grief, and yet are not wholly destitute of the use of reason; and this partial insanity seems not to excuse them in the committing of any [capital] offence; for doubtless most persons, that are [suicides], and others are under a degree of partial insanity when they commit these offences. . . . It is very difficult to define the indivisible line that divides perfect and partial insanity . . . the best measure that I can think of is this; such a person as laboring under melancholy tempers hath yet ordinarily as great an understanding, as ordinarily a child of fourteen hath, is such a person as may be guilty of treason or felony.[46]

Hale distinguished mental illness from witlessness that existed from birth and noted that mental illness could be caused by "distemper of the humors of the body, as deep melancholy or adust choler; sometimes from the violence of a disease, as a fever or palsy; sometimes from concussion or hurt of the brain, or its membranes or organs."[47] He also noted the possibility of witlessness induced by drink or drugs and distinguished levels of responsibility depending on whether the person himself or the doctor had administered the drug.

In Hale's time the maxim was that the mad could have no guilty intention. Clearly this principle applies to the delirious, but, as Hale's observations hint, the issue of homicides in which the apparently mad had an intention to kill were becoming an issue. As a result, the test applied was whether the madman had the capacity to know right from wrong to any greater extent than, for example, a child of fourteen might have. On the basis of an inability to tell right from wrong, it might be legally justifiable to excuse a madman who appeared to have intended his act.

The key drivers of change were a series of prominent homicidal acts in the eighteenth century in which the defendant did not seem furiously mad. In 1723 Ned Arnold attempted to murder Lord Onslow. Arnold had been eccentric from a young age, was a vagrant, and was widely noted by local villagers to have believed for some years that Onslow was a source of all his troubles. He was reported as having attempted at times to tear out his breast in order to release Onslow from inside of him where he was

wreaking mischief. On the day of the crime, however, he had prepared for the offense. He had bought shot and, after establishing
Onslow's likely route, made sure he was lying in wait.

In summing up, Mr. Justice Tracy stated: "A man that is an
idiot, that is born so, never recovers, but a lunatic may, and hath
his intervals; and they admit he was a lunatic. You are to consider
what he was at this day, when he committed this fact. Then you
have a great many circumstances about the buying of the powder
and the shot; his going backward and forward; and if you believe
he was sensible, and had the use of his reason, and understood
what he did, then he is not within the exemptions of the law, but
he is as subject to punishment as any other person."[48] The jury
found Arnold guilty, and he was sentenced to death. Onslow intervened, and Arnold was imprisoned for life.

The key trial was that of Mathew Hadfield, who shot at
George III as he entered the royal box at Drury Lane Theatre on
May 15, 1800. Hadfield was apprehended and questioned by the
king's brother, the Duke of York, who later stated in court that
"he said he was tired of life, that he thought he should certainly
be killed if he were to make an attempt upon his Majesty's life."
Hadfield had been injured in action against the French. A wound
to his head had penetrated his skull to such an extent that the
jury was able to inspect the membrane of the brain itself. Offi-
cers from his regiment testified that before he had been wounded
he had been an excellent soldier but that afterwards he had been
incoherent and had clear symptoms of derangement. Alexander
Crichton, called for the defense, said: "When any question concerning a common matter is made to him, he answers very cor-
rectly; but when any question is put to him which relates to the
subject of his lunacy, he answers irrationally. . . . It requires that
the thoughts which have relation to his madness should be awak-
ened in his mind, in order to make him act unreasonably."

The case posed problems for Hadfield's attorney, Erskine, in
that his client clearly knew right from wrong, and this act should
lead to his execution. Erskine argued that, in the cases that gave
rise to real difficulty, "reason is not driven from her seat, but dis-
traction sits down upon it along with her, holds her, trembling
upon it, and frightens her from her propriety." The madman rea-

soned from premises that were false: "not false from any defect of knowledge or judgment, but because a delusive image, the inseparable companion of real insanity, is thrust upon the subjugated understanding, incapable of resistance because unconscious of attack."[49] Hadfield, Erskine argued, had a delusion "that he must be destroyed, but must not destroy himself."

He went on to state: "The prisoner, for his own sake, and for the sake of society at large, must not be discharged; for this is a case which concerns every man of every station, from the King upon the throne to the beggar at the gates; people of both sexes and of all ages may, in an unfortunate frantic hour, fall a sacrifice to this man, who is not under the guidance of sound reason; and therefore it is absolutely necessary for the safety of society that he should be properly disposed of, all mercy and humanity being shown to this most unfortunate creature."

While Hadfield was committed to an asylum, the defense of insanity had been accepted in someone who was not delirious and, once accepted, carried the implication that an accused might walk free if he had a remitting disorder that mitigated the guilt at the time of the offense.

The dominating case of the nineteenth century involved Daniel McNaughton, the illegitimate son of a Glasgow wood turner.[50] McNaughton had expectations of becoming his father's partner, but after the two fell out, he set up shop on his own. He became increasingly eccentric and believed he was being persecuted by the police—a newly established institution set up by Prime Minister Robert Peel. In an effort to escape persecution, he went to France but found he was still persecuted there. His delusion became focused on Peel. Moving back to London, he bought a pair of pistols. Hanging around Whitehall near Peel's office, he appears to have mistaken William Drummond, Peel's private secretary, for Peel himself and on January 20, 1843, he followed Drummond and shot him in the back. Drummond died five days later.

The trial and not guilty verdict were controversial and led to a formulation of a set of rules, since called the McNaughton rules. These permit a not guilty verdict in the case of partial insanity but do so on very strict provisions. An individual who hears the voice of God telling him to kill someone is clearly insane, but

under the rules hearing the voice of God telling you to kill someone when killing is against the law of the land does not excuse a
crime. Hearing the voice of God say that an individual was just
about to try to kill you would provide a defense on the basis that,
whether insane or not, self-defense is a legitimate defense to a
charge of murder.

This rule skirted a key question, which is how many of us
would be able to gainsay the voice of God if we heard it. Five
years before the McNaughton trial, the American alienist Isaac
Ray argued that insanity has generally such a destabilizing effect
on the mind that it is simply not possible to say that the insane
individual formed the intent to commit a crime in the usual way.
Ray argued against the notion that patients should be acquitted
only if there was a very clear link between their delusions and the
event for which they were charged.[51] As he put it in his treatise in
1838,

> Insanity was a much less frequent disease than it is now and the
> popular notions concerning it were derived from the observation
> of those wretched inmates of the madhouses whom chains and
> stripes, cold and filth, had reduced to the stupidity of the idiot,
> or exasperated to the fury of a demon. Those nice shades of the
> disease in which the mind, without being wholly driven from its
> propriety, virtuously clings to some absurd delusion, were either
> regarded as something very different from real madness, or were
> too far removed from the common gaze, and too soon converted
> by bad management into the more active forms of the disease, to
> enter much into the general idea entertained of madness. Could
> Lord Hale have contemplated the scenes presented by the Lu-
> natic Asylum of our own times, we should undoubtedly have
> received from him a very different doctrine for the regulation of
> the decisions of after generations.[52]

The severity of the rules appears to have been a means of as-
suaging public anger at the apparent shift toward diminished
criminal responsibility in the cases of Hadfield and McNaughton.
The public disquiet at the trial and the growing difficulties in
the domain of deciding criminal responsibility in the case of the
mad were fueled by an increasing series of books dealing with just

these issues. All of the major alienists from John Haslam at the start of the century through Isaac Ray to Emil Kraepelin at the end of it gave lectures on and wrote on forensic issues.[53]

For all of these alienists and for society, the new brain and its nerves raised specters. The discussion was moving beyond irresistible impulses and command hallucinations to a faulty or degenerate neurobiology. The term *degeneration* had been introduced in 1857 by one of Falret's students, Bénédict Morel. It referred to the passing on of a biological taint from parents to children that would lead to alcoholism, criminality, and insanity. This notion became one of the dominant themes of the new social sciences and of psychiatry.[54] Degeneracy underpinned the mental illnesses that were taking shape in midcentury, but it was also a first attempt to account for social problems in terms of biology.

Degeneracy was the key theme in the definitive book of the period, published in 1876: Cesare Lombroso's deeply shocking *L'uomo deliquente* (*Criminal Man*).[55] This work, rather than Prichard's moral insanity, presented the first picture of the psychopath, the unfeeling and remorseless criminal, the Hannibal Lecter–like figure who continues to stalk our imaginations and policies. The shock came in Lombroso's bald statement that there was no hope of reform for these individuals. This claim at once undercut religious notions of redemption, which hold that all sinners can be saved, as well as secular hopes of salvation through educability and then medical hopes of a cure.

Shortly after the publication of the first edition of *Criminal Man*, in 1881, Charles Julius Guiteau assassinated President James Garfield in Washington, D.C. Guiteau was undoubtedly insane but how much did his insanity contribute to the crime? The court heard about the work of Lombroso and the latest links between criminality and heredity, along with indicators that Guiteau could not be regarded as responsible for his actions. But the issue of responsibility lies at a profound intersection between biology and social order. To accept Guiteau was incapable of doing otherwise suggested to the court a materialism that was not acceptable. Despite a distinguished slate of experts for the defense, and an American tradition as exemplified by Isaac Ray of regarding insanity as exculpatory, Guiteau was convicted and executed.[56]

In an effort to diagnose the psychopath, Lombroso, in keeping with the science of his day, assembled a visible set of physiognomic and behavioral signs that made the diagnosis more probable. Such soft signs are widely used in psychiatry today, but his efforts to quantify the Mark of Cain were disparaged as no more robust than Gall's phrenology had been, by a later generation trained by Freud to interrogate the subject in new ways rather than to look at him. Although the dominant figure at the end of the nineteenth century, someone to whom alienists like Kraepelin looked, Lombroso vanished from the stage in the first half of the twentieth century.

But if human beings are ever going to fit fully into their bodies, the question of the causality of evil is clearly a key matter. Can cohesive societies emerge from biology? The psychopath is a figure that stalks the secularism that the new biology brought in its train, a symbol for fundamentalists that secularism breeds amorality. These issues are not yet resolved. Pleas today that some murderers are genetically predisposed to commit a criminal act are likely now to lead to guilty verdicts—and execution on the basis that the propensity cannot be changed.[57]

The profound dilemmas facing jurists, medical experts, and the public when Guiteau was put on trial can be recaptured by considering the issue of treatment-induced homicide now. There is little question that many antidepressants can increase agitation in the period immediately after treatment has begun, and that this can lead to violence. But it is also clear that jurisdictions faced with homicide cases involving possible treatment-induced violence are bewildered. The law has not evolved to handle such cases.[58] If drugs can contribute to an increase in risk, do we know enough to distinguish the real situation in which they do contribute from inappropriate "treatment-induced" defenses? And how frequently would real treatment-induced problems have to happen before the requirements of the social order would trump the rights of an individual to a fair defense? As Hale noted, if a man's toxic state is due to the unskillfulness of his physician, what then?

Whatever the humane and medical impulses of the early asylum builders might have been, there is no extricating psychiatry from the law. At some fundamental point, psychiatry is involved in the government of the people by the people. The hope of nineteenth-century alienists was that a new science of insanity would make the process of distinguishing guilt and innocence more rational. As Jean-Pierre Falret had suggested, the hope lay in finding a set of diseases that might form a middle ground between biology and old-style insanity.

This hope almost certainly played a great part in the willingness of the profession and later the public to embrace manic-depressive insanity and dementia praecox (schizophrenia) when these were proposed by the German alienist Emil Kraepelin in 1899. Clear mental diseases involving a potentially remediable disordering of biology offered a possible way to reconcile biology and society. If one of those diseases was linked to substance misuse, personality problems, and irresponsible behavior and it could be treated, the specters raised by Lombroso might be laid to rest.

CHAPTER THREE

Circular Madness

❊ ❊ ❊

The creation of manic-depressive disease lay seventy years in the future when, in 1830, Rufus Wyman, then the superintendent of McLean Hospital, described the following case:

> In diseases of the pathetical states or functions, there may be exaltation or depression of one or more of the passions. . . . Exaltation, and depression of passion, are sometimes manifested alternately in the same individual. [One of my patients] has been for several years subject to alternations of these states, without disease of the intellectual powers. During the state of depression he talks little—scarcely answers questions—goes to bed early—sleeps well—rises late—takes food regularly—is indifferent about his dress—refuses to walk, or ride, or to attend church—writes no letters—reads no newspapers—discovers no interest in any person or kind of business. He is not anxious, or distressed on any subject—is perfectly quiet and inoffensive.
>
> After being depressed for two to five weeks he gradually becomes more active, gay and full of business. As a first change, he begins to smile, and answer questions; then to sit up later, sleep less and rise earlier—walks, and rides when requested. In a few days he begins to converse freely, read newspapers and play at chess. Next he calls for his best clothes—is anxious to attend church, visit every where, and see every body—plans voyages—is

full of business—writes letters to all parts of the United States, to England, France, Holland etc.—becomes gay—dances—sings— is irascible—offended when opposed—passionate and violent— tears his clothes—breaks windows, swears, strikes, kicks, bites, dashes drinks in the faces of attendants and sometimes says "I would send you to hell if I could"; but instantly, sensible of the inhumanity of his wishes, and becoming calm adds with good feeling, "but I would remove you to heaven in one minute." The paroxysms of passion, in various degrees are repeated many times in a day, from the most trifling causes, and without malice.

In this case, the changes from depression to exaltation of passion are usually sudden, and sometimes instantaneous. The paroxysms are, almost universally free from any apparent disease of the intellectual powers. His letters are well written, his plans of voyages are judicious, and the whole discovers an intimate knowledge of business. When the transitions are gradual he appears, during the intervals, quite well for several weeks, and is a kind hearted, intelligent, agreeable man.[1]

Wyman's case looks now like a wonderful description of manic-depressive disease, but this is not what it was. He was supporting Esquirol's notion of monomanias by describing an individual with severe impairments of functioning in the absence of any intellectual disturbance.

In 1837 James Prichard, when describing moral insanity, wrote:

The most frequent forms, however, of the disease are those which are characterized either by the kind of excitement already described, or by the opposite state of melancholy dejection. One of these is, in many instances, a permanent state; but there are cases in which they alternate or supersede each other; one morbid condition often lasting for a long time, and giving way, without any perceptible cause, to an opposite state of the temper and feelings. . . . When this habitude of mind is natural to the individual and comparatively slight, it does not constitute madness; and it is perhaps impossible to determine a line which marks a transition from pre-disposition to disease; but there is a degree of this affection which certainly constitutes disease of mind, and that disease exists without any illusion impressed upon the understanding. A state of gloom and melancholy depression occasionally gives way after an uncertain period to an opposite condition of preternatural excitement. In this form of moral derangement the disordered condition of the mind displays itself in a want of self-government, in continual excitement, an unusual expression of strong feelings, in thoughtless and extravagant conduct. . . . Not infrequently, persons affected with this form of the disease become drunkards.[2]

Descriptions like Wyman's and Prichard's indicate that alienists had cases of manic-depressive illness in their care before the disease was first described. In this sense, the issue of priority in the discovery of manic-depressive disease is almost irrelevant—this was a disorder clamoring to be described. But the question of who discovered manic-depressive illness, or bipolar disorder, gave rise to one of the most celebrated priority disputes in psychiatry. The fact that both Jean-Pierre Falret and Jules Baillarger could ignore earlier precedents and dispute the priority between them brings home the fact that, despite compelling clinical appearances, there were fundamental conceptual problems that had to be overcome before the new disorder could be recognized.

Celebrated though the contributions of Falret and Baillarger now are, there are a number of puzzles to the evolution of the new disorder they were the first to describe. One is the fact that neither Karl Kahlbaum or Emil Kraepelin whose later work laid the basis for the modern forms of both bipolar disorder and manic-depressive illness appear to have been significantly influenced by either Falret or Baillarger. A second, as we shall see, is that although cases of the new disease were undoubtedly present in the asylums, they were in fact quite rare.

WAR IN PARIS

Jules Baillarger was born in 1815, twenty-one years the junior of Jean-Pierre Falret. After training in medicine, he moved to Charenton to study with Esquirol. Like Esquirol, who had been the first to consider hallucinations in detail, Baillarger pursued research on hallucinations, winning the Prix de l'Académie in 1842. In 1840 he was appointed to the Salpêtrière, where Falret was also working. He moved to the asylum at Ivry a few years later. In 1843 he established the *Annales Médico-Psychologiques*, which became the leading French psychiatric journal. In 1852 he established the Société Médico-Psychologique, the first scientific association for French psychiatrists. He held the organs of power in French psychiatry and was offered the first chair in French psychiatry when it was created in 1875 but declined on the grounds of age.[3]

Falret was born in Marseille in 1794. Beginning the study of medicine at age seventeen, he came under the influence of Pinel and Esquirol and became an alienist. He was *chef de l'hospice* at the Salpêtrière from 1831. Falret's interests overlapped heavily with Baillarger. Following Bayle, during the 1830s both Falret and Baillarger studied brain anatomy in the hope of pinpointing other disorders, before concluding that postmortems were unlikely to yield further breakthroughs. Both focused on hallucinations in the 1840s. In 1841 Falret began teaching a clinical course in the Salpêtrière that was to provide the basis for his claims to priority when the two collided over their subsequent area of mutual interest.

Baillarger made the first public move. "All the writers on mania have considered the transformation of mania into melancholia or vice versa to be fairly common. They have also all perceived these facts to be two different disorders, two distinct attacks, which succeed each other more or less within a single patient. This is an opinion, which I have sought to combat. Indeed I would like to demonstrate that we have here not two diseases but a single one; the two supposed attacks are nothing but two stages of a single attack."[4]

Baillarger's first presentation of his ideas was at a meeting of the Académie de Médicine de Paris on January 30, 1854. The academy was an exclusive society, which at the time probably had about eighty elected members, including Baillarger and Falret.[5] Baillarger's lecture was published in the *Bulletin de l'Académie*, almost immediately afterward.[6] A few months later it was published in the *Annales Médico-Psychologiques*,[7] and the main ideas were outlined in the *Gazette hebdomadaire*, on February 3, 1854.[8]

There are no states which show more marked differences from one from the other and more striking contrasts than melancho-

lia and mania. The melancholic is weak and irresolute; his life is
spent in inertia and mutism; his conceptions are slow and confused. The maniac by contrast is full of confidence, of energy
and audacity; he deploys the greatest activity and his loquacity
has no limits. It would therefore seem, in theory, that two states
so opposed must be foreign one to another, and that a great
distance must separate them. This is not however that which
is demonstrated by observation. Indeed we see, in many cases,
melancholia succeed mania and vice-versa, as if a secret bond
united these two diseases. These singular transformations have
often been reported.[9]

After noting that Pinel, Esquirol, and Guislain cite comparable transformations, Baillarger says that the fact seems to him
not to have been sufficiently studied:

By bringing together and comparing a certain number of observations, it becomes clear that there exist quite numerous cases
in which it is impossible to consider in isolation and as two distinct disorders the excitation and the depression which succeed
each other in a single patient. This succession, indeed, is not a
matter of chance, and I have been able to confirm that there exist connections between the duration and the intensity of the
two states, which are clearly nothing other than two periods of a
single attack. The consequence of this view is that these attacks
properly belong neither to melancholia nor to mania but that
they constitute a special kind of mental alienation, characterized
by the regular existence of two periods, one of excitation and the
other of depression.

He then describes a series of cases to illustrate the key features
of *folie à double forme.* The first involves the twenty-eight-year-
old Miss X who had several attacks of mania from the age of sixteen and from the age of twenty-one had a fairly constant illness
during which in the first fifteen days she would have a profound
melancholia followed by a mania, which would then last for the
same time. She might then have an intermission of short duration
lasting a few days, or at the most two or three months, before a
new attack began.

The second case was a man he had heard about from Esquirol, whom Baillarger describes as having attacks of mania that would last ten to twelve days followed by a period of despondency, usually happening with no transition and often during his sleep. This differed from Miss X's case only in terms of the slightly shorter duration of attacks.

Third was another case seen by Esquirol, that of a woman who had an episode of melancholia at the age of twenty-eight and nothing else until the age of thirty-six. She then began to have attacks, which would begin with a melancholia that lasted six weeks and was then replaced by a general excitation, insomnia, and agitation, which would last for two months before the patient recovered, and she would then remain well for eight months. Every year the attacks recurred with similar symptoms at the same time of the year.

The fourth case was that of Mr. X, who had had a twenty-year period of alternating excitation and depression. He would fall into a state of melancholia lasting several months, and then would gradually recover his animation and pass through a very short interval of reason before his activity increased to a point of a furious excitation. "Although very old, he is at times affected by attacks of priapism and goes as far as to run around his garden prey to a lascivious fury." This period can last three months before he gradually relapses back into a "splenetic state."

These cases differed from a larger group in which patients alternated between six months of depression and six months of overactivity, exemplified by the twenty-four-year-old Miss M, who began with a melancholic episode when she was twenty. These came on in a regular pattern starting in May and lasting to October, when she would appear to recover before then passing into an excited and manic state. At the time of the lecture, Miss M had had four cycles of this kind.

Finally Baillarger described the case of a twenty-five-year-old man, who became excited and grandiose every autumn for three years running, who then in spring calmed down and sank into states of depression during the summer months.

Commenting on these cases, Baillarger mentioned that other cases showed much shorter durations. One patient had been re-

corded as showing signs of melancholia, followed by signs of mania, which alternated every two days. Other patients had attacks
lasting six or eight days. The briefer the episodes, he claimed, the
more precise the correspondence between the length of attacks of
mania and of depression. Some patients with brief episodes regularly went to bed melancholic and woke up manic. These correspondences, he suggested, cannot be seen as clearly when the melancholic or manic periods last for up to five to six months before
any transition between one state and another. In these cases, transitions often take place much more slowly and imperceptibly.

One of the critical problems for Baillarger, which brings out
the conceptual difficulties he faced in establishing the new disorder, lay in a group of patients who achieved equilibrium between
episodes of mania or melancholia. They no longer showed signs
of delusions. He describes coming to the wrong clinical judgment
on a number of occasions in letting patients go home, when it
was clear retrospectively that signs of their next illness episodes
were already there.

That Baillarger felt a need to account for patients who had
intervals of a month or more apparently well before relapse is il-
luminating. The theoretical problem that lengthy euthymic intervals posed was that they left him open to the claim that, if patients were well for such a long period, was it not more reasonable
to see in this two distinct diseases that succeed each other rather
than two phases of the same illness. "Is there not here in fact an
intermission? And is this intermission not sufficient for one to
admit two attacks and not one alone?"

For Baillarger, this issue raised in profound form the question of what is madness. At this point, he distinguishes between
lesions of the intelligence and a loss of awareness of these lesions
and argues that it is the loss of awareness that a belief is delusional
rather than the presence of a bizarre or intensely held belief that
constitutes madness. On this basis, he argues that patients who
are not apparently deluded or hallucinating for a period of some
weeks may nevertheless still be mad, or at least may not have returned to their premorbid mental state.

He gives the example of one of his patients whom he had let
go home, but who still retained a slight tendency to isolation and

to taciturnity that was not natural to her. This difference from normal, however, did not prevent her from having excellent manners and being very hardworking and seeming to be in every way reasonable. But the fact that she relapsed quickly after discharge provided the grounds for thinking that the equilibrium of her faculties had not been entirely restored, which was something, he suggested, that her relatives could have told any clinician who had cared to ask them.

A further problem lay in the agitated overactivity that might be present at the start, at the end, and in the course of the disorder, giving rise to apparent cycles of activity. In contrast to the regular periods of the disorder itself, he argued, agitation appeared irregularly.

After reviewing the clinical picture, Baillarger outlined a number of different patterns. Some patients might have only one attack of melancholia brought to an end by an attack of mania or vice versa. Others might have attacks that recurred up ten times at intervals of two, four, or six years. A third group had intermissions at regular intervals. And a final group had attacks without any intermissions. "The disease, which usually lasts for several years, can thus be compared to a long chain in which each attack is one of the links." He concludes:

> Outside monomania, melancholia and mania, there exists a special type of madness characterized by two regular periods, one of depression and the other of excitation. This type of madness occurs in the form of isolated attacks, or recurs in an intermittent fashion or the attacks can follow each other without interruptions. The duration of the attacks varies from two days to one year. When the attacks are short the transition from the first to the second period takes place in a certain manner and ordinarily during sleep. By contrast when the attacks are prolonged it takes place slowly and by degrees. In the latter case patients appeared to enter convalescence at the end of the first period but if the returned health is not complete after fifteen days, six weeks at the most, the second period breaks out.

On February 14, 1854, two weeks after Baillarger made his presentation, Falret began his presentation to the same academy:[10]

At our last meeting, our honorable colleague, Dr. Baillarger, read a paper on a new type of insanity—*la folie à double-forme*. I must tell you, Gentlemen, that to me this type of insanity is not new. I have been aware of it for a long time, and for more than 10 years I have described it in my lectures at the Salpêtrière. Many similar cases have been presented by the students there and discussed in our clinical seminars. We even gave it a name because, in our opinion, it is not a mere variant but a genuine form of mental illness. We call it *folie circulaire* because the unfortunate patients afflicted with this illness live out their lives in a perpetual circle of depression and manic excitement, which is typically brief but occasionally long-lasting.

He then quoted from his lecture series in the Salpêtrière that had been running for several years and that had been published a few days before Baillarger's presentation:[11]

The transformation from mania to melancholia, and vice versa, has always been considered merely adventitious. However, not enough attention has been paid to the fact that there is a certain category of patient who continually exhibits a nearly regular succession of mania and melancholia. This seemed sufficiently important to us to serve as a basis for a specific mental disorder, which we call *folie circulaire* because these patients repeatedly undergo the same circle of sickness, incessantly and unavoidably, interrupted only by rather brief respites of reason. Of note, however, is that these two states, which in their continual succession comprise *folie circulaire,* are neither melancholia nor mania in the usual sense of these terms. It is as if the basic features of these two conditions are present without their extremes. First of all, there is no incoherence of ideas, as in true mania, but simply manic exaltation, that is to say, mental hyperactivity with a constant need to move and markedly disorganized behavior.

Falret's presentation was very different from that of Baillarger. He described no cases but rather instead the features of mania and depression. Arguing that these manias and depressions were not as serious as full-blown mania or melancholia, he claimed nevertheless that their conjunction produces a disorder that is worse—a disorder in which "we have never observed a complete cure, nor even a lasting improvement." He distinguished *folie circulaire* from mania:

> In ordinary mania one occasionally sees melancholic states of varying degree and duration. Sometimes, manics exhibit a more or less prolonged state of depression before they explode; or, before their recovery is complete, a period of prostration may ensue, which is probably due to nervous exhaustion. . . . But, in order to be called *folie circulaire,* depression and excitement must succeed one another for a long time, usually for the whole of the patient's life, and in a fashion very nearly regular, always in the same order, and with intervals of rationality, which are usually short compared with the length of episodes. . . .
>
> We believe it constitutes a genuine form of mental illness, because it consists of a group of physical and mental symptoms which stay the same for any of the respective phases that succeed one another in a determinate order so that, once the symptoms are identified, the subsequent evolution of the illness can be predicted. Indeed, it is a more authentic category of disease than either mania or melancholia because it is not based on a single cardinal symptom—the degree of delirium, sadness, or agitation—but is instead founded on the conjunction of three specific states occurring in a determinate, predictable, unalterable order.

Just as Baillarger had, Falret tackled the lucid interval:

> At this point, the patients present such a contrast with the state which is just ending that they do seem reasonable by comparison. Some of them are sufficiently in control of themselves so as to no longer exhibit any thought disorder that may have been present only temporarily. They often hide certain wild ideas that are left over from the phase of exaltation, while other ideas begin to surface that herald the coming phase of depression. To appreciate their actual condition, one must look for what is missing rather than to what is manifest. Then one sees that the patients do not speak, or do much of anything, as one would expect if they were in a normal state. These negative findings are of con-

siderable value when it comes to the question of whether or not these patients are in a lucid interval. . . . one will find exceptional cases where their thinking seems to have been restored to its former state, but this state lasts only briefly, even in circular insanity with long phases.

Is it a frequent form of mental illness? Judging by what little attention such cases have received up until now, and by the small number of cases one finds on the wards, it does not appear especially common; but there are many causes that interfere with an accurate appreciation of the actual frequency.

One of these factors he notes is the existence of milder forms that never reached the asylum:

Moreover, since this form of mental illness . . . does not ordinarily present the degree of intensity found in true mania or in partial insanity, properly speaking, it follows naturally that such patients often remain in society. We are convinced of this by direct observation; in fact, we were asked to examine some patients who had long been afflicted with this disorder, but who had never aroused sufficient concern in their parents for the latter to make the decision to hospitalize them.

The parents find it a simple matter to conceal from others the condition of their child because their relatives are similarly unable to see in the patient a state of insanity. When the patients get excited, the way one gets during a particular phase of intoxication, then people exclaim that they are having their "happy hour"; the parents rejoice in their vitality, in their high spirits, and everyone goes along with this interpretation of the situation. When their mood changes and they are disorderly or mean, people say that they are in a bad temper, that they are acting strange, restless, are difficult to live with; but it is only on occasion, and without much insistence, that anyone calls them crazy.

Falret noted that the disorder appeared to have a large hereditary component and that it was up to three times more common in women. He also pointed out several advantages of knowing that this was a disease and that it had a natural history, even if the prognosis was poor. It meant that the clinician would be in a better position to decide if any therapeutic intervention made any difference to this course. It also meant that clinicians faced with a patient charged with a crime would be able to predict for the court what would happen next to the patient, thereby side-stepping the irresistible impulse problem and demonstrating that many of the behaviors of the affected person truly stemmed from a disease and were not under his or her control.

Baillarger responded to the lecture in acrimonious terms[12] and disputed the priority for the rest of his life, whereas Falret barely made reference to it again.[13] In 1894 busts of the two men were placed at the entrance to the Salpêtrière during the same ceremony. Opinions in French psychiatry have oscillated regarding the allocation of priority, with majority opinion favoring Baillarger for a long time and more latterly favoring Falret.

But does any of this matter? The bitterness of the priority dispute seems out of proportion to the issues. Given that manic-depressive disorder looks like it would have forced its way onto the clinical radar at some point, was the contribution of either man particularly gifted? Rufus Wyman's clinical description is more convincing to the modern eye. Indeed, perhaps out of a need to establish the novelty of the new entity, both men stressed the regularity of cycling between poles of the disorder, and how it was possible to predict when patients would change from one state to the other, in a manner that now seems simply wrong.

The condition was also, by both men's admission, rare. For a disorder that was fundamentally incurable, it was odd that between them they had no more than a handful of active cases—Falret notes four at the time of his lecture, and Baillarger seems to have had no more, even though these two men could call on the resources of two large asylums.

Neither Falret's nor Baillarger's presentation in fact secured the niche that was later occupied by manic-depressive disease. A profusion of terms swirled around French psychiatry for decades thereafter, with Billod in 1856 using *folie à double phase*,[14] and others using *folie alterne*. The concept did not become established even in Paris until the mid-1880s, when the Academy sought submissions on the issue and awarded a first prize to Ritti, whose presentation on the issue was titled *folie à double forme*.[15]

What happened in Paris had little effect in Germany. When Emil Kraepelin outlined the new concept of manic-depressive disease in 1899, he cited neither Baillarger nor Falret. There were good reasons for this in that manic-depressive disease was not something that he posited had regular and predictable periods. Indeed, Kraepelin's disorder might not involve any cycling at all. It was only in 1966, when oddly once again two academics described a new disorder at the same time, bipolar disorder, that what had happened in Paris a century earlier once again became relevant.

There is, however, another continuity. A key feature that united Falret, Baillarger, and Kraepelin was a new emphasis on the course of the disorder. This aspect, perhaps more than anything else, justifies focusing on the watershed years of the 1850s in Paris. In this sense, Falret in particular departed from what had been there before and heralded what was to come.

KARL KAHLBAUM AND CYCLOTHYMIA

In reaction to the Enlightenment, a romantic movement dominated German psychiatry from the early nineteenth century. The romantics were keenly interested in the place of the soul in illness and regarded all forms of madness as having a common root in disordered passions. By 1860 Wilhelm Griesinger emerged as the leading figure in an alternative or biological tradition. Griesinger was a figure very like Laycock in Britain, who in the 1840s posited that a great deal of brain functioning might be based on reflexes and that all mental disease was likely to be brain disease, with the additional specification by Griesinger that there was essentially one brain disease. Taking the example of general paralysis of the insane (GPI), which typically gave rise to melancholic, manic, and demented states in the course of the disorder, Griesinger argued that patients might progress through various stages yet still have the same disease. Neither Griesinger nor the romantics put much emphasis on the clinical observation of patients. This was the background facing Karl Kahlbaum, whose contributions to our story start in the 1860s.

For more than fifty years Western psychiatry has credited Emil Kraepelin as being its founding father. The creation of *DSM-III* was supposedly an expression of a neo-Kraepelinian movement, which sought to return psychiatry to its clinical roots in detailed observation of patients, after an interlude in which the discipline had dallied with psychoanalysis. But arguably psychiatry is now neo-Kahlbaumian, and perhaps the main reason neo-Kraepelinism came into fashion is that no one knew anything about Kahlbaum.

Kahlbaum is an intriguing figure for many reasons, one of which is the difficulty in learning anything about the man. Born on December 28, 1828, in Prussia to a family who could sponsor his education and subsequent work, he was a liberal Catholic in a conservative Protestant state, at a time when these things counted enough to block his entry into the university establishment.[16] He moved instead to a sanatorium in Görlitz near Dresden, which he bought and transformed from an institution for epileptics to one for psychiatric patients. There he was joined by Ewald Hecker, another whose career path was blocked by politics[17] and whose sister Kahlbaum later married at the age of fifty.

Between them, Kahlbaum and Hecker introduced fashionable reforms, such as greater patient freedom and the removal of restraints. But when discussing their patients, they eschewed fashion and described their cases in a new way. Central to this was a consideration of the longitudinal course of the patient's condition, an approach, Kahlbaum argued, that should give rise to clinical entities or syndromes.[18] This concept was a much fuller version of the idea that Falret had put forward in 1854.

When he first presented his ideas in an academic forum, it seems he was ridiculed so badly that he deferred publication of a new syndrome—hebephrenia—that was based on these ideas. This ridicule might prompt the suspicion that Kahlbaum was a singularly poor presenter of material, and perhaps this accounts for his later obscurity. However, his later work reveals another reason for the rejection. To appreciate his ideas, the reader or listener needs to "free oneself of the authority of a certain philosophical axiom . . . namely, the axiom of the unity of the soul. Even the most important truths may become substantial obstacles to scientific progress if interpreted narrowly or excessively generalized. . . . The concept was derived from only a single phenomenon of the mind, the unity of self-awareness . . . [it] has had a disastrous impact."[19]

This mission statement ran smack up against the central tenets of both Romantic psychiatry and popular sentiment and embraced all of the difficulties entailed in embodying the mind, described in the preceding chapter. This was not just a matter of whether certain lunatics could become partially insane. If asked to locate their selves, most of his audience would have referred to their souls. If Kahlbaum was now arguing that souls might not be continuous from one moment to the next, or that selves and souls were not the same thing, what did that mean for the self? Locke's and Hume's attempts to explore these issues in the eighteenth century had thrown up a series of paradoxes that remain unsolved today.

A great deal of what we know about Kahlbaum comes secondhand through Hecker. Whether because of an innate shyness or unfavorable reactions to his ideas or because his academic background would not have been seen as respectable, Kahlbaum rarely presented material and wrote only sixteen articles. It fell to Hecker to outline his ideas on hebephrenia and later cyclothymia.

The difficulties in getting to know Kahlbaum would perhaps be of interest solely to an academic historian were it not for the fact that his ideas on hebephrenia, catatonia, dysthymia, and cyclothymia as well as his methods for investigating clinical syndromes shaped the Kraepelinian template. To add piquancy to this issue, Kahlbaum is a central figure in Kraepelin's memoirs, and catatonia and hebephrenia were the two disorders Kraepelin thought about most. It is also clear that early in his career Kraepelin considered going to train with Kahlbaum but was advised that this would be a bad career move.

Hecker later in 1871 published the first account of hebephrenia and launched the term into the psychiatric literature, where it was to have a key place for a century.[20] This disorder affecting young men primarily was characterized by severely disorganized behavior. The patient was often silly and fatuous or apparently unable to plan and execute behavior. Instead, he might copy the actions of the examiner, repeating words and phrases or gestures.

He might or might not have delusions or hallucinations. This condition had a very poor prognosis. The syndrome was the first building block in Kraepelin's later dementia praecox.

In 1874 Kahlbaum described another syndrome—catatonia.[21] This syndrome became a key in the evolution of both dementia praecox and bipolar disorder. Catatonia is one of the most extraordinary conditions in psychiatry. It was first described by Galen 1,700 years beforehand and given the name cataplexy. In mild forms, the patient may simply be stuporous. In severe forms, patients often can lie or stand motionless in odd sometimes seemingly physically impossible postures for hours or days, defecating and urinating on the spot, inaccessible to human contact. Kahlbaum outlined overactive and underactive forms of the disorder, which he saw as a motility psychosis—a madness affecting the motor areas of the brain. These states were usually episodic, with the underactive forms lasting more than a year on average and the overactive forms more likely to resolve within six months. Some forms could be periodic.

While many catatonic patients spontaneously recovered, others became chronic. Most psychiatrists, up to the 1960s, had seen patients of this type, who had been mute and inaccessible residents of a hospital sometimes for decades. From 1900, however, under the influence of Kraepelin, this syndrome had become catatonic schizophrenia, and, as such, the failure of these patients to recover was not so surprising—unless one knew that this was not what Kahlbaum had described. Catatonia was an extraordinary as well as fearsome condition that appeared to have vanished by the 1960s, so that today's clinicians may never have seen a case. Its disappearance is commonly attributed to effective early treatment with antipsychotics, even though the development of antipsychotics involves screening tests in which agents that trigger catatonic states in animals are selected for further investigation.[22] There are no grounds to think that antipsychotics would lead to the disappearance of catatonia.

Where Kraepelin subsumed catatonia for the most part into schizophrenia, an alternative German tradition stemming from Karl Wernicke, and later championed by Karl Kleist and Karl Leonhard, saw catatonia as a prototypical bipolar disorder and as a condition that exemplified the need for a new concept—that of cycloid psychosis. It was this tradition that gave rise to the birth of bipolar disorder in 1966 (see chapter 5).

Within the psychotic domain, Kahlbaum also described a condition he termed paranoia. Far from the classic picture of insanity, an individual with paranoia could appear perfectly normal. He would be able to reason and argue logically on a wide range of issues until the questioner touched on a sensitive point. Then, the interviewer would become aware that on certain issues a passion had engulfed the individual and there was no reasoning with him. Formerly, the term paranoia had been a synonym for insanity or mania, but in Kahlbaum's hands it was transformed into a partial insanity that emerged at vulnerable life points.

In 1882 Kahlbaum outlined two affective disorders—cyclothymia and dysthymia—against a background of circular or cyclic insanity. Circular insanity was a severe disorder, which led to hospitalizations for both manic and depressive episodes, in which the patient was typically psychotic.[23] He suggested that this condition was by then widely accepted in psychiatry, with general agreement that it was marked by a stability of symptoms during recurrences. But, although arguing the condition was widely accepted, he makes no reference to Falret or Baillarger.

Cyclothymia, in contrast, was a pure mood disorder, which showed minimal intellectual derangement and typically did not require hospitalization. Patients cycled from an excess of vitality to a lack of vitality—that is, from hyperthymia to depression, a state that might today be called bipolar II. Dysthymia, a word used by Hippocrates to describe the woman at Thasos, similarly was a pure state of depression without compromised intellectual functions. Cyclothymia and dysthymia were "a partial disturbance of the mind, a primary mood disorder. The other group involves a complete disturbance of the mind . . . ending in a state of degeneration." Cyclothymic patients recovered, whereas circular insanity patients did not.

In describing Kahlbaum's work on cyclothymia,[24] Hecker notes that cyclothymia might be relatively common among people who remain in the community and never need to be admitted to an asylum. One of the key features about the disorder in these community cases was that other physicians, relatives, or even the patients themselves commonly did not recognize any abnormality. Everyone seemed much more likely to think of the excited phase as being one in which the person was back to normal. Kahlbaum suggested that most cases of periodic depressions were likely to be cases of cyclothymia.

The fifth edition of Kraepelin's textbook had been released in 1896 just as Hecker outlined Kahlbaum's thinking on cyclothymia, and Hecker read Kraepelin's emerging views as supporting this position. He also notes with excitement a German translation of a monograph by Carl Lange of Copenhagen,[25] in which Lange described periodic depressions in patients who had never been in an asylum and described them in a way that distinguished them from classic melancholia. Hecker claimed that he was seeing just the same kind of mood disorders in the community "very often," and he went further and argued that Lange was probably describing the depressive phases of cyclothymia. As we shall see in the next chapter, Lange also claimed that this disorder responded to treatment with lithium.

Hecker went on to note that even the depressive phase of cyclothymia may go unrecognized, because patients complain primarily of somatic symptoms that were diagnosed as neurasthenia. In his article, he gives classic descriptions of endogenous and bipolar depressions. These patients, he noted, have psychomotor retardation, stemming from an inhibition of activity, and an indifference to things that formerly brought interest and enjoyment. Even though they have had prior episodes from which they recovered, they are typically hopeless as to the possibilities of recovery, leaving them at risk of suicide. "When observing these states, one cannot help thinking of a machine whose oil has completely dried up, so much so that the gears can move only with great difficulty and rub each other painfully."[26]

Kahlbaum described the exalted phase of cyclothymia as hyperthymia to emphasize the novel concept of a disorder in which only mood was affected. Kraepelin later referred to these states as hypomania, a term popularized by Mendel in the 1880s.[27] In this phase, Kahlbaum and Hecker described patients as being expansive and often more talented than they might be when well. Patients who were not usually very musical might sing and play instruments with some proficiency. They often showed poetic talents or a more stylish taste in clothing than would be normal for them. Hecker described a patient who became engaged to be married in every euphoric phase, only to break off the engagement in the following period of depression. These features, though, could be very subtle, and only a proportion of cases resulted in symptoms that everybody could recognize as illness—such as when the patient began to show an "urge to purchase things" and to squander money, or a boisterous tendency to play tricks and to become engaged in atypical activities.

Having described the depressive and exalted phases, Hecker went on to note that many cyclothymic patients have a "moral deficiency" that leads to a tendency to lie, become intoxicated, keep bad company, and the like. This observation of an increased frequency of substance abuse and features that might now be described as personality disorder has been borne out by subsequent studies. A linkage between bipolar disorder and substance abuse is widely accepted, and many physicians would now implicate a bipolar process in the generation of some personality disorders, as we shall see.

It was important for Kahlbaum and Hecker to be able to distinguish between the depressive phase of cyclothymia and melancholia. They argued that patients with cyclothymia had a complete lack of delusional ideas and that depressed patients often slept in a way that was not typical of patients with melancholia, for whom insomnia was much more likely to be a symptom. Cyclothymia also had a younger age of onset than melancholia, which started in later years.

Hecker argued against vigorous treatment during the depressive phase of the illness because "the consequence of such an approach is only a worsening of the excited phases of the disorder." He believed that "the primary aim of treatment should be to limit the manic exultation as much as possible."[28] To do so, he suggested using a depressive episode to explain the nature of the disorder to patients and to encourage their efforts to control themselves. By recognizing the emergence of a phase of exultation, patients could try to suppress it as early as possible.

EMIL KRAEPELIN AND MANIC-DEPRESSIVE INSANITY

Emil Kraepelin was born in northern Germany in 1856,[29] the same year as Freud, two years after Falret and Baillarger's celebrated dispute. He studied medicine in Würzburg and then moved to Leipzig where he worked with Wilhelm Wundt, widely credited as being the first psychologist. Wundt's research was on the cerebral reflexes posited by Laycock and Griesinger. He studied the time it took one word to elicit another, in order literally to localize them on the basis of reflex associations. Kraepelin's contribution to this research was to investigate the influence of drugs on these processes, for which he coined the term *pharmacopsychology*.[30]

Kraepelin then moved as a physician to the Estonian asylum at Dorpat, and five years later to Heidelberg, where he spent twelve years before moving to Munich. He began writing a textbook of mental medicine in 1883 while still in Leipzig, because he wanted to marry and needed the money.[31] While in Dorpat and Heidelberg, his interest turned to the clinical trajectory followed by his patients. "I soon realized that the abnormalities at the beginning of the disease had no decisive importance compared to the course of the illness leading to the particular final state of the disease, just as happened with the various forms of paralysis (syphilis)."[32] This appreciation played a growing role in the successive editions of his textbook, becoming the key issue in the sixth edition published in 1899 in which he used it as the central criterion on which to differentiate manic-depressive insanity and dementia praecox.[33]

Kraepelin never completely abandoned his prior interest in psychological research. He continued to have an eye for fundamental brain mechanisms, such as inhibition and disinhibition, which might play a part in disease processes, but by the mid-1890s, he had become scornful of brain mythologies. His focus on the disease course put him on a path that was distinctively different from Vienna's more neurologically oriented Theodore Meynert, Breslau's Karl Wernicke (see chapter 5), and later the emerging dynamic psychologists linked to Freud. In 1895 Freud and Josef Breuer had published *Studies on Hysteria,* which inaugurated a new era. This work had minimal impact on Kraepelin, who was dealing with a patient group that was entirely different from Freud's.

The drama in Kraepelin's 1899 textbook lies more in the emergence of dementia praecox, later schizophrenia, than it does in the appearance of manic-depressive insanity. In the fifth edition published in 1896, he had maintained a separation between hebephrenia, catatonia, and the paranoid psychoses, but in light of the new criterion of disease course in 1899, he included hebephrenia, catatonia, and a range of paranoid psychosis within dementia praecox. This new disease was characterized by its progressive dementia. Disease course in Kraepelin's hands was being used as advocated by Kahlbaum and as is typically still used today. For instance, the initial clinical presentations of Alzheimer's dementia and Jacob-Creutzfeld disease may be the same, but in Jacob-Creutzfeld disease the decline is precipitate, and this distinction underpins the assumption that there are two different pathological processes at play.

Manic-depressive insanity had its place in the 1899 edition of the textbook as a foil to dementia praecox rather than as a condition developed in its own right. In order to bring out the importance of the disease course for his new system, Kraepelin had to have a contrasting disorder that did not lead to cognitive and clinical decline. Manic-depressive disorder provided that contrast, and, almost by definition, as a result affected patients had to get better.

In constructing the category, Kraepelin adopted Kahlbaum's circular insanity and cyclothymia, as well as dysthymia: "Over the years, I have convinced myself more and more that all of the described pictures are simply manifestations of a single pathological process. . . . it is utterly impossible to find any definite boundaries between the different clinical pictures which have so far been kept apart."[34]

Simple alternation between excitement and stupor could not be a classificatory principle because this pattern occurs in dementia praecox and general paralysis of the insane. But periodic, circular, and simple manias could all be regarded as manifestations of the one illness if they all showed a remitting course. Kraepelin argued that it was impossible to find sufficient regularity among the various different clinical presentations to distinguish them as different affective disorders. He argued that, far from being consistently up or down, even in the course of one day many patients cycled through depressive and manic states or had mixed pictures, such as agitated (overactive) depression or inhibited mania (manic stupor) or querulous mania. He also noted that patients can have a mixed condition in the sense of being manic one day and depressed the next. They can therefore alternate rapidly from pole to pole and also be disinhibited in relation to some activities but inhibited in others.

One of Kraepelin's collaborators, Wilhelm Weygandt, had first outlined this concept of a mixed state.[35] Weygandt argued that the brain had independent affective, associative, and activity faculties and that each of these faculties could vary independently—either up or down. This variation gave rise to the possibility of elevations of mood, for instance, but inhibition of activity. The states predicted from the model can be read into real clinical situations to some extent. It may have been Weygandt's work that finally led Kraepelin to include a number of disorders that had previously been viewed separately into the category of manic-depressive illness in the absence of any basis for distinguishing them.

Postpartum or puerperal psychoses, for instance, were included in the manic-depressive mix. Some forms of puerperal psychosis, Kraepelin argued, might become chronic cases of dementia praecox, but for the most part these were considered cases of manic-depressive illness. He came to this view despite providing some of the most compelling descriptions of the distinctive features of puerperal psychosis, under the heading of acute confusional insanity.[36] His descriptions argued strongly for the possibility that puerperal psychoses, which clinically often resemble a steroid psychosis much more than either classic manic-depressive psychosis or schizophrenia, might be independent disorders. But the fact that the conditions remitted made them manic-depressive.

The fate of Kahlbaum's catatonia was most curious. Kraepelin recognized that catatonic features occurred with some regularity in manic-depression. These he seems to have passed off as consequences of the mixed states that manic-depressive disease could give rise to. The occasional cases of enduring catatonia for him trumped the fleeting presentations found in mood disorders, and as a result catatonia was subsumed into dementia praecox.[37] Just as with postpartum psychoses, the possibility that it might be an independent disorder almost vanished as the concepts of dementia praecox and manic-depressive illness took hold.

Postpartum psychoses and catatonia hint at a limitation of Kraepelin's method. Kraepelin's clinics in both Heidelberg and later Munich were relatively selective in the patients they took, and while he did follow up patients in the local asylums, he was not able to follow up systematically the cases of patients who never returned. A large number of frank but transient and single-episode psychoses accordingly were never likely to be given the weight that they might have in a classification system based on a follow-up of all cases.

One key disorder—the involutional melancholias—suggests that Kraepelin's thinking became unduly rigid, with disease course being a criterion that trumped everything. These classic depressive psychoses have their onset after age fifty, and patients typically present a striking picture of disturbed sleep and appetite, diurnal variation of mood, and either paranoid, nihilistic, or guilt-laden delusions. In 1899 Kraepelin thought that these patients were much less likely to recover than other patients with mood disorders. As clear mood disorders, these should have been added to manic-depressive illness, but their failure to respond suggested lumping them in with dementia praecox. He was unable to decide and opted to let involutional melancholia stand as a separate disorder until the eighth edition of his textbook, when he finally included it in the manic-depressive group.[38] This makes it clear that the classification system was based on a very simple criterion—whether the patient recovered or not. According to contemporaries such as Karl Wernicke, the system was overly simple.

The idea of manic-depressive illness met with a muted response internationally. When Kraepelin's work was discussed in the English-speaking world, it was in terms of dementia praecox. Manic-depressive illness was all but ignored. By the end of the chapter, it may be somewhat clearer why this should have been the case.

In America, Adolf Meyer initially welcomed Kraepelin's new orientation to clinical course as the breakthrough for which psychiatry was waiting.[39] But Meyer, who later emerged as the leading figure in American psychiatry, shifted his ground between 1910 and 1920 and began to criticize Kraepelin as being too neurological and as failing to take into account that the patient's disorder took place in the context of her life story. Simply writing patients off as having an inevitably deteriorating condition was not good medicine. Meyer preferred to talk instead of paranoid, hebephrenic, catatonic, and simple parergastic reactions and in terms of manic and depressive thymergastic reactions.[40] Following the publication of an English translation of Eugen Bleuler's work on schizophrenia in 1950, parergastic reactions and dementia praecox diagnoses were subsumed into schizophrenia, a much more commodious concept capable of extension to include a wide range of odd behaviors. There was a vogue to see many artists as incipient schizophrenics, just as there now is a trend to see them as manic-depressive. Only after the emergence of schizophrenia was manic-depressive illness free to develop in its own right.

In Britain, the reception of Kraepelin's ideas was mixed. An early criticism came from the Dublin physician Connolly Norman, who rejected dementia praecox as overinclusive.[41] Indeed, Norman was one of the first to highlight the risk that institutionalization might confound the clinical picture, by creating a misleading impression of degeneration or dementia.

Thereafter, there were regular references to Kraepelin at psychiatric meetings in Britain, but all were in terms of the validity of dementia praecox; some disliked the term dementia and some disliked praecox. Manic-depressive illness was rarely raised.[42] An English translation of Kraepelin's work did not become widely available until after the First World War.

The reaction to Kraepelin was probably also colored by the war, when hostility to his concepts was fueled by hostility to all things German. Some traces of this can be seen in the writings of Michael Shepherd, who features prominently later in this story, and who as late as 1995 argued that Kraepelin was an unimaginative German nationalist, whose thinking contributed to later Nazi eugenics.[43] Shepherd found it unbelievable that having deposed one idol, Freud, American psychiatry would have replaced him with Kraepelin.

The French were also reluctant to embrace Kraepelin. The key issue here again was dementia praecox. They were unwilling to accept that all psychotic disorders had the common degenerative clinical course that Kraepelin proposed for dementia praecox.[44] Whereas dementia praecox was at least considered in France, manic-depressive disorder made no inroads on *folie circulaire*. But the greatest resistance came from Germany itself, as will be outlined in chapter 5.

Ultimately, however, when it came to manic-depressive insanity, the somewhat unimaginative Emil Kraepelin had picked a name that worked. Names as well as concepts have survival value. They contribute to what might now be called branding. From this point of view, dementia praecox was as poor a choice of name as possible, but manic-depressive disease worked in that everyone could bring to it what they wanted.

But why manic-depressive illness? Why not manic-melancholic disease, given that almost all the depressions he was faced with were melancholic in terms of their severity and clinical features? The answer lies in another quirk in the man—he had a partiality for novelty. Melancholia was an old-fashioned word. Depression was creeping into use; the first major paper on depressive illness was Carl Lange's in 1886. Despite being encrusted in Latin, dementia praecox was also a relatively new concept.

Most clinicians, if now asked to picture a classic case of manic-depressive illness or bipolar disorder, can do so just as readily as they might conjure up an image of Parkinson's disease. In the midst of the concepts that have swirled around this disorder, then, there seems to be a pure form that has stabilized a variety of quite different concepts. These concepts speak to competing views as to what constitutes a disease. Does it primarily hinge on some ideal form, or is the clinical course its primary characteristic, or does it hinge on treatment responsiveness? The various formulations outlined in this chapter from Falret onward have all at one point claimed that without a close approximation to the true disorder, it would not be possible to find out what treatments really work. One of the key issues for the remainder of the book is the converse of this—if one of the affective disorders responds to some treatment, can we then assume we have found a distinct disorder?

If a treatment works, might it help us decide whether Falret, Baillarger, Kahlbaum, or Kraepelin was closer to the mark? But before moving on in the next chapter to the role of lithium, we can look at whether any of these concepts put forward by the professoriate impinged on the real world of asylum medicine. The French and Germans refused to use each other's concepts. If asylum physicians elsewhere used neither French nor German concepts, and indeed were reluctant to take up any concepts put forward by academics, then none of these debates would have much impact on the lived experience of patients.

A WINDOW ON THE PAST

Emil Kraepelin traveled widely in Europe and Asia. He was not however an Anglophile and came to Britain only once, where he visited two places. Despite his travels, his memoirs are among the most tedious books ever written. One of his few passionate moments is when he describes London: "I thoroughly disliked [London] and the way of life with its endless uniform rows of houses, its lack of beautiful buildings and views, its confusing masses of people, its dull air, monotonous, tasteless cuisine and bleak Sundays." The only other place he visited was North Wales: "It was a pleasant feeling to leave the noisy, foggy city of London and to arrive at the ancient city of Chester. From here we made a 4 day journey through North Wales, mostly on foot, visited Llandudno, Betws-y-Coed . . . and climbed Mount Snowdon in the rain."[45] Unfortunately, while he visited Bedlam in London, he does not appear to have visited the asylum at Denbigh in North Wales.

The asylum that opened in North Wales in 1848 was representative of most nineteenth-century asylums in the Western world from California to Estonia. The reasons for its construction were repeated elsewhere, the cases it took were identical to those taken elsewhere, and the trajectory of its history maps onto popular and academic notions of the rise and fall of these institutions.

Before there was an asylum in North Wales, parishes raised money to assist relatives to look after idiots and the insane at home. To a twenty-first-century eye, this might seem like a model of community care, but what struck those concerned about the plight of the mentally ill in the nineteenth century was the scope in this community system for gross abuse in some cases and a more general deprivation of access to medical advances that it inflicted on all patients. The advocates of medicalization had no reason to suspect that institutionalization might be anything other than a good thing.

Around 1800 the British economy was changing. Industrialization and a new pattern of landowning was creating a laboring class, where before there had been peasants. For the purposes of looking after each other, the peasantry had been linked through parishes, and it was the parish that offered financial support if a family member was mentally ill, by giving funds either to relatives for care or to institutions for boarding out.

With a labor market came the need to consider the question of poor relief for laborers who were laid off and did not have a farm to return to for subsistence. A new system of poor relief built workhouses for the indigent poor and reorganized parishes into poor-law unions, which were administrative units large enough to support the building of a workhouse.

A Madhouses Act of 1828 made it obligatory for parishes to return an annual list of lunatics, especially dangerous lunatics. The Poor Law of 1834 recommended that such patients be removed to madhouses or asylums rather than catered for in the workhouse. In France in 1838 a comparable law drafted by Esquirol mandated the building of asylums across the country.

When the Metropolitan Lunacy commissioners surveyed lunatics countrywide in 1842, Samuel Hitch, then one of the leading medical campaigners for asylums, came to survey North Wales. He reported that there were 664 lunatics in North Wales of which 19 pauper lunatics were in English asylums, 32 in workhouses, 303 living with relatives, and 310 farmed out to strangers. He estimated only 6.5 percent of Welsh lunatics received care in an asylum compared with 42 percent in England.

The differences between Wales and Ireland were instructive in this regard. In Ireland the English felt free to deal with social issues in an interventionist way, using Ireland as a test case for social measures.[46] As a result, many of the earliest and biggest asylums in the new United Kingdom were established in Ireland, specifically in Dublin. Wales in contrast was part, albeit a peripheral part, of the emerging British market economy, and social measures such as asylums had to take root in the native soil. It needed a set of reformers to raise consciousness of a problem and to agitate for change.

The reformers' strategy was to discover and trumpet cases where the traditional system had failed. One such case involved Mary Jones, who was discovered by the lunacy commissioners in an attic near Denbigh. She had been confined on a foul pallet of straw for more than fifteen years in a room with a stagnant and suffocating atmosphere from the stored urine used in the family business for the treatment of wool. Her "chest bone protruded five or six inches beyond its natural place; and there was an excoriation of the parts below. The legs were bent backwards, and the knee-joints were fixed and immovable. . . . She was emaciated to the last degree, her pulse was feeble and quick, and her countenance, still pleasing, was piercingly anxious, and marked by an expression of despair."[47]

Lord Ashley presented Mary Jones's case in Parliament in July 1844 and again when he presented a bill making it a requirement for all counties to have an asylum. This was needed, he said, because in the case of Mary Jones her doctor testified that had she been caught in time there was a possibility for a cure. Cases such as hers provided impetus to the cause of those who wanted to provide asylums to rescue their fellow human beings from degraded treatment and who believed that a regime of humane custodial care could in many cases restore wits to the senseless.

Whereas Mary Jones was confined to an attic, wandering lunatics might be handcuffed and leg-locked. But the community often resisted sending people away to the asylums because of the costs involved. In North Wales, if local patients were to be hospitalized, it would be in English asylums where the attendants and doctors spoke a foreign language. This was politically unsustainable. The remedy was to build an asylum in North Wales at Denbigh.

The choice of Denbigh was dictated by the geography that dictates all Welsh political and institutional developments. Four-fifths of Wales is formed of rugged folds of hills and mountains, so that 90 percent of the population is forced onto northern, western, and southern coastal strips.[48] In the North, the mountains are highest rising to Mount Snowdon and the coastal strip is thinnest.[49] The asylum builders opted for Denbigh, a central Tuscan-like town sitting on a hill and dominated from the Middle Ages by an impressive castle. Denbigh offered reasonable access to everyone from North Wales.

Building began in 1844, ten years before Falret and Baillarger's dispute. The story that unfolded was typical of asylum building everywhere. Within ten years of opening in 1848, an apparently reasonable provision of 120 beds seemed like a serious underestimate. The hospital almost from the start ran at maximum occupancy. As early as 1860, further building was mooted. By 1862, when Kahlbaum was setting down his ideas on the importance of the clinical course for establishing disease entities, an extension of 200 beds was approved. This was completed by 1866, but by 1868 the asylum was full again.

Through the following decades, new wings were added to the hospital to accommodate these extra patients, and the hospital grew just as other asylums in America and Europe were growing. The end-of-year hospital census increased year on year from an initial 100 up to 1,000 by 1914, peaking in 1948 at 1,500 patients, the year before lithium and a cornucopia of newer physical treatments were discovered and a process of deinstitutionalization began.

The North Wales asylum offers an extraordinary opportunity to look at manic-depressive and other mental illnesses that cannot be reproduced elsewhere. When social scientists or historians look at the old asylums, they see institutions that had been built in the countryside but which by the twentieth century were almost all engulfed within cities. Asylums that began dealing with relatively small rural communities drawn from one ethnic group by the end of their life were dealing with multiethnic urban communities that, in terms of population growth, were many multiples of the communities that had been there before.

In contrast, around 1900, three-quarters of the admissions to Denbigh came from individuals with classic Welsh surnames such as Jones, Roberts, Pritchard, Williams, Evans, and Parry. In 2000 more than two-thirds of the admissions still came from individuals with Welsh surnames. The overall size of the population furthermore is almost precisely the same in 2000 as it was in 1900. There are variations so that there were more children in the 1890s, and fewer people over the age of sixty-five, where now the ratio is reversed, but this difference is of lesser consequence when it comes to manic-depressive illness and schizophrenia, which typically begin between the ages of fifteen and fifty-five; this section of the population was the same size in 1900, to within 1,000 people, as it was in 2000.

Anywhere else in the world, both because of geography and rising wealth, a growing number of people had a choice of hospitals, but in North West Wales, because of enduring poverty and by virtue of being hemmed in between the mountains and the Irish Sea, the insane had nowhere to go except to Denbigh. Because of the choices that opened up to people elsewhere, it is very difficult to know how representative patients ending up in the public or private asylums across the Western world between 1800 and 1950 were of the mental illness happening in their communities of origin, but this is not an issue for North Wales.

North West Wales did not urbanize. The area was desperately poor 150 years ago and remains one of the poorest regions of Britain today. There was effectively no private practice 150 years ago, and there remains very little today. While people are much more mobile now and can travel to get ill elsewhere in Britain, because of the regulations of the National Health Service patients with severe mental disorders are typically sent back to their point of origin for treatment.

The resulting asylum records shed light on three issues. One is the question of Kraepelin's involutional melancholia—was he right or wrong to include it in manic-depressive illness? The second is just how common was the new disease, manic-depression. And the third is when did the new disorder begin to be diagnosed in an asylum like Denbigh. On this score, it needs to be noted that the Denbigh asylum was progressive, being one of the first to open a pathology laboratory in Britain, and extraordinarily quick to adopt convulsive and other therapies when they became available in the late 1930s. If manic-depressive illness had any traction as a concept, there is every reason to believe that the asylum at Denbigh would have picked it up relatively early. Later in chapter 5, we will see what happened in North Wales to the postpartum psychoses that Kraepelin added into manic-depressive illness. Finally, in chapter 7, we will look at the age of onset of manic-depressive illness, as reflected in the asylum's records.

On the issue of involutional melancholia, there were 658 admissions from 568 individuals for severe depression, or melancholia—17 percent of all admissions. Of these, 57 percent were women. This gives an admission prevalence of 5.7 per 100,000 per annum, compared with an admission prevalence of 8 per 100,000 for severe depression today.

If we break these 568 patients down by age group and look at length of stay and rates of recovery, we find that patients admitted in their thirties had a 76 percent recovery rate and a median length of stay of 224 days. Patients admitted in their forties had a recovery rate of 72 percent and a median length of stay of 285 days. The patients with classic involutional melancholia had an onset of a similar disorder in their fifties or sixties and older. For these patients the recovery rates were 65 and 56 percent, with lengths of stay of 261 and 203 days, respectively. Overall, patients admitted in their thirties or forties were 1.2 times more likely to recover than patients admitted in their fifties or sixties. This outcome hardly fits the picture of two different disorders.

The main difference between younger and older age groups was an increased death-in-care rate. This rose from 10 percent for patients in their twenties to 44 percent in patients in their sixties. This result, however, was not based on death after an extended and refractory treatment course but often death rather early in the course of the disorder. The data strongly suggest Kraepelin got the recovery rates of older patients wrong, and as a result he inappropriately separated involutional melancholia from the rest of manic-depressive illness.

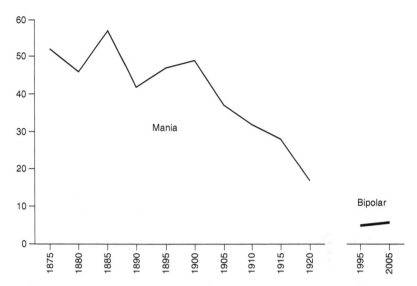

Figure 3.1
Mania as a Percentage of All Admissions to the North Wales
Asylum between 1875 and 2005

But, the key things for us to look at are the rates of diagnosis
of mania and the point of impact of Kraepelin's concept of manic-
depressive illness on British clinical practice. The first thing that
strikes any reader of the records is that most patients apparently
had mania. As late as 1900, patients who were suicidal, patients
with senility, and patients with what now would be called schizophrenia were all labeled as manic. More than 55 percent of the
diagnoses are for mania (see figure 3.1). Either this illness was dramatically more common 100 years ago than it is now or else the
word mania has been used in a completely different way from the
way it's being used now. Around 1900, the use of mania as a diagnosis begins to fall, and it falls progressively to the current rate of
less than 5 percent.

A further large group of patients, 35 percent of all those who
were admitted to the asylum, were diagnosed as having melancholia. Retrospectively, these patients appear to have had a severe
depressive disorder only in very few instances—10 percent. Most

patients, then diagnosed as having melancholia, would now be diagnosed as having schizophrenia, or even senile dementia.

As regards diagnosis, the picture in the Denbigh records begins to change in the early 1900s with cases such as that of WT, who was admitted in 1891 at the age of forty-five, having been looked after at home for a number of years. He had been a businessman, who had spent a great deal of time traveling back and forth between Wales and Argentina. His family wondered if his first breakdown seventeen years previously, from which he had recovered at home, had stemmed from an engagement to a Catholic woman, or whether it had been triggered by the general alarm that had accompanied an outbreak of yellow fever. He had recovered but was never quite the same. He continued working until his early forties, when his family committed him to the asylum where he remained until his death twenty-three years later.

On admission, in contrast to most patients, he seemed almost normal—far from manic in the sense of agitated or overactive. After some days, the grandiosity and probable delusional beliefs became apparent. These periods of elation alternated with mute and almost catatonic states, and he settled down to a cycle of episodes of depression, followed by overactivity and periods of lucidity. In 1904, thirteen years after admission, the notes indicate that his condition was then being viewed as circular insanity. Despite a wealth of detail, WT is in fact one of the most difficult patients to diagnose from the asylum, but the reference to circular insanity is the first of its kind from a North West Wales patient.

In 1906 a national conference on the classification of insanity in Britain introduced a new system of diagnosis to Britain.[50] This system proposed a new disorder, primary dementia, which was the equivalent of Kraepelin's dementia praecox.

Even before this conference, the North Wales records were recording diagnoses of dementia praecox. Thus, Bessie Hughes, a seventeen-year-old girl admitted on October 16, 1905, with hebephrenic and catatonic features, was noted to be a good case of dementia praecox, even though she was fit to leave hospital nine months later. The records indicate that, until then, a case like Bessie's would have been diagnosed as melancholia with stupor. The term dementia praecox came into use rapidly in North Wales, and primary dementia was never adopted to the same extent. Dementia praecox was not definitively replaced by schizophrenia in these records until 1949.

There could not be a greater contrast between the rapidity of the uptake of the dementia praecox concept and the use of manic-depressive illness as a diagnosis. The new national classification system subdivided mania and melancholia into recent, chronic, and recurrent mania or melancholia and introduced the term *alternating insanity*. But none of these terms were used with any regularity. The fall in the frequency of diagnoses of mania in the first instance stemmed from an increase in the use of the dementia praecox diagnosis.

The new classification had little effect on RO's diagnosis. Admitted in 1908 and discharged in 1909, RO was the first patient from North West Wales to be diagnosed with *maniacal depressive insanity*, a disorder not on the list. In fact, this odd use of words was a better description of his case as it was presented in the hospital records than a diagnosis of manic-depressive insanity would suggest, in that he presents on only one occasion and shows features of agitated depression without any alternation of mood.

RO was an exception. Patients with mania or melancholia when admitted continued to be diagnosed as having mania or melancholia, rather than alternating insanity or manic-depressive illness, until September 1920, when a thirty-year-old sailor, RP, was admitted with grandiose beliefs and violent behavior. He remained in the hospital for more than a year, during which time he had attacks of agitation at regular intervals. On discharge he was diagnosed as manic-depressive. RP was readmitted two years later and spent most of the following fifteen years as an inmate of the asylum, his case developing into one of *folie circulaire*. In 1931 he was noted to have a "manic-depressive phase well marked and alternate with complete cycle in about a month."

The diagnosis, however, did not come into regular use until 1924, when three women who were admitted were given this diagnosis. One was AA, whose records from 1924 describe a sixty-year-old woman who had two admissions for involutional melancholia or what would now be diagnosed as psychotic depression—no hint of mania. ER, also admitted and diagnosed in 1924 as manic-depressive, had a postpartum psychosis. Finally, WH had her tenth admission in 1924 and on that occasion was diagnosed as manic-depressive. She came much closer to the modern ideal type of a manic-depressive—there had been nine previous admissions starting from May 1900, mostly for mania, but none had led to this diagnosis.

Looking back through these records, it is relatively easy now to distinguish manic-depressive illness from schizophrenia or other disorders. One of the primary indicators lies in the use of the word *dementia*. Patients with schizophrenia came into hospital clearly mentally ill, having been in recent possession of their faculties, but in the course of the years after their admission, the hospital records show an increasing use of phrases such as "he has become quite stupid or quite demented," or he "is good for nothing." Manic-depressive patients in contrast got well and went home and on subsequent admissions to hospital were often described as being in exactly the same state that they had been in during the course of their previous admission. One of the great advantages of the North Wales Hospital records is that there were only two ward clerks who kept the records for close to a century, and the physicians in the hospital were also a stable group so that patients presenting successively over twenty or thirty years or more might regularly meet the same physician.

Sifting through 3,872 admissions from North West Wales between 1875 to 1924, it becomes clear that bipolar disorder patients are hard to find. Only 127 such patients were admitted for the first time during this period. This gives rise to 10 cases per million per year, a rate that remained constant across fifty years and continues to hold true to today.[51] If Kraepelin had not lumped them together with the other mood disorder patients, who composed more than 80 percent of the manic-depressive cohort, the bipolar patients would have been close to invisible.

From this perspective, the struggles for diagnostic priority in Paris appear an irrelevance. *Folie circulaire* and other labels were simply not used in a working asylum like Denbigh before 1900. Had they been used, so few patients were involved that the issue would still have been a minor one.

Of these bipolar patients, 60 percent in North Wales were female, compared to the 66 percent Kraepelin reported. The average age of first admission was thirty-two years old, with the youngest admission being for a seventeen-year-old. The average length of stay in hospital for any one episode was six months. Almost all patients went home well, with only a very small proportion having continuous fluctuations in clinical state that precluded discharge. This group of 127 patients had 345 admissions, and on average each person had four admissions every ten years.

Today the district general hospital unit serving the same area has a slightly higher proportion of female admissions for bipolar disorder. The average age at first admission is thirty-one years old. The average length of stay is a month. But people have 6.5 admissions every ten years. On any one day in the asylum, a visitor would have found on average of four patients with bipolar disorder, whereas now in the sixty-bed unit serving the same area they would find six patients with bipolar disorder. The rate of diagnosis of bipolar disorder in a comparable unit in America now is likely to be much higher for reasons that will become clearer in chapters 6 and 7.

One of the biggest differences is in the way people present. In the nineteenth century, more than 80 percent of the admissions were for mania. Today, more than 50 percent of the admissions are for depression. Either the presentation of the illness is changing, or treatment is having an impact on presentations, or we have a greater sensitivity to episodes of depression that would formerly not have led to admission. The remaining chapters look at the impact of treatment on this most dramatic of psychiatric disorders.

A number of reasons can now be offered for the muted academic reception and slow clinical uptake of the manic-depressive concept. The concept of manic-depressive insanity was a complicated one that, on the one hand, included disorders not usually lumped together and, on the other hand, at least initially excluded one of the commonest depressive disorders—involutional melancholia. The majority of patients with the disorder had a condition that was quite different from one implied by the disorder's name. Retrospectively, the disorder Kraepelin had in mind would arguably have been more appropriately termed severe affective disorder rather than manic-depressive disorder. Finally in opting for manic-depressive disorder rather than manic-melancholic disorder, Kraepelin wittingly or unwittingly endorsed the notion of a relatively discrete mood disorder, when most turn-of-the-century alienists saw insanity as involving a disorder of the rational faculty.

The bottom line must be that, while the "ideal type" of a manic-depressive patient now seems compelling, it does not appear to have seemed as compelling to clinicians at the start of the twentieth century and, paradoxically, was not what Kraepelin had in mind.

CHAPTER FOUR

The Stone of Madness

❀ ❀ ❀

The basic division of psychiatric disorders into mood disorders and schizophrenia continues to form the bedrock of classification systems, even though Kraepelin, who originated the distinction, later pointed to cases of patients with both strong manic-depressive and schizophrenic features.[1] This division shows up in the categorization of drugs. Whereas chlorpromazine and its derivatives were initially seen as neuroleptics or tranquilizers and iproniazid was identified as a psychic energizer, these drugs have all become either antipsychotics or antidepressants despite compelling evidence that the drugs called antipsychotics can be used to treat mood disorders, delirium, and anxiety disorders and that many antidepressants may be much more effective for anxiety states than for mood disorders.

The one drug that remained outside the conventional classification system was lithium, which is neither an antidepressant, antipsychotic, nor tranquilizer. As we shall see, lithium has acted as something of a rock disrupting the flow of the psychiatric and psychopharmacological waters around it. Although a psychotropic drug, it did not come from a pharmaceutical company and has been a major inconvenience to most companies wishing to break into the mood disorder marketplace. Its use provided a major stimulus to the development of clinical trials, but these trials have not succeeded in clarifying its niche. At a time when drug development has become a multinational collaborative enterprise, lithium's development stands out as being the result of the persistence of one man and his bitter dispute with another.

Lithium's use ultimately led to a transformation of manic-depressive illness into bipolar disorder. In contributing to the emergence of bipolar disorder, lithium helped to institute what has been termed a neo-Kraepelinian turn in American psychiatry, although arguably this turn was fundamentally anti-Kraepelinian. It was this movement that gave rise to *DSM-III*. Lithium has also been at the cutting edge of what many have bemoaned as a biological reductionism that has dehumanized psychiatry. Arguably, however, the stimulus lithium provided to the development of clinical trials has meant that it has had an even greater but less recognized role in the emergence of an informational reductionism, which has had a much greater impact on clinical care than any turn to biology.

THE EARLY HISTORY OF LITHIUM

Before 1850, physicians attempting to make diagnoses looked at the body—its tumors, and areas of discoloration. When it came to looking at what might be going on within the body, they were restricted to what came out—urine, feces, or blood. A common image portrays the physician holding a flask of urine up to the light scanning for the tiny crystals or other deposits, which were generically termed urates.

The production of urates appeared to be increased in gout and rheumatic conditions, giving rise to the notion of a uric acid diathesis. Some people, it was postulated, were predisposed to produce more uric acid than others, and this excess could lead to illness. For patients with gout, the hypothesis is essentially correct.

Around the 1830s, urea and uric acid had a mystique difficult to appreciate now. When Frederick Wöhler synthesized urea in 1830, this was the first creation of an organic molecule in a chemical laboratory. It seemed to bridge the gap between organic and inorganic matter, between biology and machinery. This laboratory step has been portrayed ever since as a death knell for vitalism— the idea that there is something specific and unique about human life that will never yield to the probing of materialist science.[2]

Work on the uric acid diathesis was therefore cutting-edge science in the mid-nineteenth century. Furthermore, the uric acid theories seemed to point the way to a therapy after it was discovered that a newly discovered compound called lithium dissolved urates.

Lithium was isolated from petallite, found in rocks off the Swedish coast. Working in the laboratories of the most famous Swedish chemist of the day, Jon Jacobs Berzelius, Johann August Arfwedson isolated the new substance from petallite in 1817 and discovered that it was an alkali metal. Berzelius suggested the name lithium in recognition of its origins in stone.[3]

This discovery gave rise to a lithium water industry. For more than fifty years, the usefulness of alkaline substances to treat gout or rheumatic conditions had underpinned the popularity of spa waters, which are generally alkaline. The great European spas quickly discovered that their waters also contained lithium, as Berzelius had suggested, or if not, they added the newly discovered alkali. As late as 1929 lithium was being added to new soft drinks or beers for similar reasons; in 1929 the soft drink 7UP started life as a lithium-containing beverage.[4] Lithium salts continued to be used to treat rheumatism and gout to the end of the twentieth century.

Lithium could be combined with other salts such as chloride to make lithium chloride, a salt substitute. A combination with bromine proved a popular means to deliver the bromide sedatives that entered medical and psychiatric care toward the end of the nineteenth century. These combinations brought lithium into mainstream medicine in more concentrated forms than was found in spa waters.

In 1843 the surgeon Alexander Ure reported that lithium carbonate could dissolve stones in urine.[5] Finding a means to handle renal stones was then one of the most salient tasks in medicine,[6] the equivalent perhaps of perfecting an artificial knee joint now. A wide variety of heroic measures had been tried. When Ure tried to inject lithium carbonate into a patient's bladder to dissolve kidney stones, however, weeks of repeated injections failed to dissolve it (perhaps because the stone he picked was too big), and the patient died.[7]

In 1859 Alfred Garrod suggested that lithium might be useful not only for gout but also for a range of linked conditions.[8] According to Garrod, lithium should combine with uric acid to form lithium urate, which, being soluble, would wash away in the bloodstream and be flushed out of the body in urine. Following this lead, Garrod became the first to give lithium orally as a therapeutic agent.

Garrod noticed that lithium produced diuresis, which made it of interest to both humoral and modern schools of medicine. Humoral practice aimed at mimicking the mechanisms the body employed to treat itself, so that anything that caused diuresis would be used widely. But lithium was equally a Paracelsian medicine par excellence. It was a pure and simple element.

While using lithium to treat gout, Garrod reported that patients often showed a general sense of well-being. Physicians noted something similar in the 1960s when treating patients who had epilepsy with a variety of anticonvulsants (see chapter 6). In just the same way, therefore, as the psychotropic effects of many of these later drugs were discovered, a recognition emerged that lithium might have a more general effect aside from alleviating gout, although at this point its benefits were seen as providing general tonic rather than specific psychotropic effects.

Although medicine was changing and becoming more mechanical, the dominant conception of gout remained humoral. It was viewed as resulting from a humoral imbalance within the body. Therefore, while this disturbance led to precipitations in certain joints, it was expected that the same disturbances might interfere with functions elsewhere in the body, giving rise to "gouty" migraine, diarrhea, sciatica, morosity, and epilepsy. On this basis, lithium could be expected to improve not only gout but also the general humoral economy of the body and potentially to be prophylactic.

According to Garrod, "It would naturally be supposed that lithium salts might prove of advantage in the treatment of both acute and chronic forms of gouty inflammation, and likewise, when administered in the intervals of the attacks, might keep an auspicious state of the bloods so as to prevent the recurrence of such inflammatory action."[9] He believed that lithium's chief use "is in chronic gouty cases, to ward off attacks . . . It is likewise valuable when administered as part of the prophylactic treatment."[10] These humoral ideas mapped onto the morose and irascible clinical presentation of gout, which often got significantly worse prior to an attack of gout. Armand Trousseau, a professor of medicine in Paris in the 1850s, compared the picture to the equivalent of a premenstrual syndrome.[11] One of Trousseau's pupils, Antoine Gilbrin, argued that the uric acid diathesis affected the nervous system, where it led to nervous attacks, vertigo, hypochondriasis, mania, and delirium.[12]

These prodromal nervous syndromes were also linked to the irritable prodromal syndromes found before an epileptic attack. In the 1860s Jean-Pierre Falret, along with his pupil Morel, put forward the case that "larval epilepsy," or the disposition to epilepsy, might lead to "periods of excitation and depression, motiveless and explosive anger, irritability, amnesia for the aggressive episodes and gradual weakening of the mental faculties"[13]—an idea that reemerged in the manic-depressive story in the 1980s.

Bromides were also used to manage epilepsy, and this led in the 1870s to the use of lithium bromide to manage epileptic disorders, both within and outside asylums. In the United States, the use of lithium bromide was popularized by Silas Weir Mitchell.[14] When used for epilepsy, lithium also appeared to improve other features of the personality of the patient, making him feel generally better. This mode of entry of lithium-containing compounds into the asylums and their "psychic" effects foreshadow the later discoveries of the "mood-stabilizing" properties of valproate and carbamazepine. And, just as with these other drugs, lithium came to be used in patients with ever more frank nervous problems.

In New York no less than in Paris, alienists and other physicians treating nervous disorders began to use these compounds. Thus William Hammond, the surgeon general in the U.S. Army during the Civil War and, from 1868, the professor of nervous and mental diseases at Bellevue Hospital in New York, reported in 1871 that lithium was a useful sedative agent for nervous problems.[15] Hammond was a therapeutic activist who later went on to advocate the early treatment of incipient cases of insanity in the community, against the opposition of many of his colleagues who

believed that the earliest possible institutionalization was the better course of action.[16]

By 1886 John Aulde in Philadelphia was advocating lithium
bromide for a range of nervous complaints and, indeed, prophylactic lithium to prevent nervous troubles recurring.[17] To support
his views, he quoted the comments that William Pepper made at
the first annual meeting of the Association of American Physicians in 1886: "The nervous system may be at the root of and may
be the real cause of all these disorders."[18] He also quoted John
Draper at the same meeting, who stated, "We have too much limited the gout by insisting on the deposit of uric acid in the joints.
. . . This is, after all, only an epiphenomenon of the disease."[19]

In Britain, Alexander Haig took the uric acid diathesis even
further. In a series of articles from 1884, although primarily focused on gout and other rheumatic conditions, Haig explicitly
correlated increased uric acid levels with the kinds of depression
that went with physical disabilities like gout and suggested that
lowering blood uric acid levels would raise spirits—the word
mood would have been rarely if ever used at this point.[20] Gout and
rheumatism are classically periodic illnesses. They flare up and
then abate to some extent. Because lithium then had an established place in the prophylaxis of gouty problems, the notion of
giving it for periodic nervous problems is not so surprising.

The key individual in the emergence of a prophylactic use of
lithium for mood disorders is Carl Georg Lange. Born in 1834,
Lange studied medicine at Copenhagen University and graduated
in 1859. He became Denmark's first neurologist and was appointed
professor of anatomy and pathology in Copenhagen. He had an impressive string of discoveries, but because he was Danish, his work
has been largely written out of history. He described aphasia at the
same time as Hughlings Jackson but is not recognized for it. He
pinpointed syphilitic destruction in the spinal cord as the cause of
tabes dorsalis but is overlooked for this also. He worked on conditioned reflexes twenty years before Pavlov but receives no credit.[21]
He was the first to describe depression, but no one knows this.

The main thing he is remembered for is "About Emotions:
A Psycho-physiological Study." Written in 1885, this work was
translated widely and made him famous, along with the Bos-

ton psychologist, William James, as one of the proponents of the James-Lange theory of emotions. The key element of this view, in contrast to orthodox views at the time, was that physical changes, such as increased heart rate in fearful situations, come first and our subsequent interpretations of these effects are what we normally call our emotions. This theory was counterintuitive to most people and repugnant to many, but it had the merit of focusing attention on physiological changes that could be measured in contrast to psychic changes that could not.

Lange came to study depression and lithium in the course of treating a large number of neurological patients, many of whom, he noted, seemed to have a general depression of function or of spirits. In an 1886 article, he outlined a new disorder—periodical depression.[22] This was the first use of the term depression for a medical disease. Lange may have had to use the word periodical to lift the lay term depression out of its quotidian use and make it suitable for use as the name of a disease. In this article, he outlines the classic picture of endogenous or vital depression. This condition, he said, was not melancholia, because melancholia involved psychotic features. A number of Danish alienists argued against him, saying that melancholia did not always involve delusions or hallucinations and that all he had described was melancholia without delusions.[23]

Both Lange and his critics were right. Looking at admissions for melancholia to the North Wales Asylum during this period, two-thirds had clear psychotic features. Of the remaining third, many were so stuporous that physicians could not determine whether they were deluded. The prototypical case of melancholia, therefore, did involve delusions, but there were sufficient exceptions to argue that what Lange was seeing was continuous with these other nondeluded cases. Psychiatry was slowly recognizing that there might be mental disorders in which patients were not deluded or hallucinating. But Lange suggested this possibility first for patients with depression, and his use of this word may have played a significant part in Kraepelin's favoring the term manic-depressive illness rather than manic-melancholic disorder.

Lange may have been biased toward seeing this new disorder because he had a number of relatives with what might now be termed mood disorders. But he also believed he was looking at a concomitant of neurological disorders rather than an illness that might exist in its own right. These depressed patients appeared to have a urinary sediment that led Lange to think that they might be producing excess urates, and this finding pointed the way to the use of lithium. He first reported on the benefit of lithium for "depression" in 1881.

In his 1886 monograph on the phases and treatment of periodic depression, he reported giving patients lithium carbonate, which he hoped would act prophylactically against the recurrence of clinical symptoms. A similar use of lithium for recurrent unipolar depressions later became the key issue in the lithium wars of the 1960s.

Carl's younger brother Frederick (Fritz) Lange was in charge of a provincial asylum at Middelfart. Taking his lead from Carl, Fritz gave lithium to several hundred patients with depressive features, in doses of the order of those used today. Reporting the results in 1894, he outlined benefits that appeared within a few weeks of starting treatment.[24]

Lange's discoveries, however, and the entire field of lithium therapeutics were soon to be eclipsed. The downfall came not because others demonstrated that lithium did not do what the Lange brothers claimed for it, but rather because the uric acid diathesis fell out of favor.

Medicine at the end of the nineteenth century resembles the end of the era of the dinosaurs. Hitherto dominant life forms, in this case the humoral models and fellow travelers like the uric acid diathesis, were abruptly extinguished and new groups rushed into the vacuum. The main driver for competitive success in the new medical economy was specificity. The emerging bacteriology of Koch and Ehrlich from the 1880s put a premium on distinguishing between infections and eliminating them specifically with magic bullets. At the same time, the development of anesthesia greatly extended the reach of surgery, and a host of specific corrections to the disabled human machine became available. An old era was buried and, with it, treatments that almost certainly did something but whose theoretical underpinnings were passé. Lithium was one of these.

Lithium was lost to psychiatry and drifted out of favor in the rest of medicine. In the late 1940s, it came into vogue as a salt substitute as a result of research indicating that salt might contribute to hypertension. This use of lithium was linked to cardiac difficulties, and it was banned by the Food and Drug Administration (FDA) in 1949.

Carl Lange died in 1900, and Fritz in 1907. Some forty years later, another Danish psychiatrist, Hans Jacob Schou, criticized the management of depression that the Lange brothers had advocated, which in addition to giving lithium had also involved mobilization of their patients. Schou argued that this treatment stemmed from their belief that mobilization would help remove uric acid from the system. But because the uric acid diathesis was discredited, clinicians should now know that depression was better treated by isolation and confinement to bed.[25] In addition to being a medical superintendent at a provincial asylum, Schou also had a *nervesanatorium,* where rest treatments were the order of the day.[26] After lithium's reappearance in the 1950s, Schou's son Mogens ran trials of lithium for patients with depression that failed to show it offered any benefits.

THE NEW MEDICINE

While treatments like diphtheria antitoxin at the end of the nineteenth century ensured the success of Koch and Ehrlich's revolution, the ultimate flowering of the new medicine came with the discovery of the sulphonamides in the 1930s and the mass production of penicillin and other antibiotics in the 1940s. These breakthroughs led on to diuretics, antihypertensives, and the first hypoglycemic agents, as well as the production of a variety of steroids in commercial quantities. Although there had been drugs in medicine before, few had eliminated diseases, saved lives, or provided the potential to alter life-styles. The new treatments were welcomed unreservedly as freeing the world from scourges that had plagued humanity for millennia. Few talked about new capacities to engineer human souls.

A new medicine was born. The culture of health changed radically. In psychiatry, a set of processes was instituted that would lead to the third edition of the *Diagnostic and Statistical Manual*

(*DSM-III*) in 1980. And the chemical companies that produced these breakthroughs formed pharmaceutical divisions, which, as they became profitable, branched off from their parents to become the most profitable corporations on the planet.

Many of the new drugs came from the synthetic dyes discovered in the second half of the nineteenth century, a number of which had effects on histamine, a hormone that mid-twentieth century research had targeted for its role in stress responses. This research led to the investigation of the phenothiazine methylene blue, and the iminodibenzyl summer blue. Methylene blue gave rise to the antipsychotics, and summer blue to the antidepressants.

The French company Rhône Poulenc discovered the antihistaminic properties of the phenothiazine nucleus, and in December 1950, in an effort to maximize the stabilizing effects of the phenothiazines on a variety neuroendocrine systems, Paul Charpentier synthesized chlorpromazine.[27] First conceived as a potentially useful adjunct to surgery, chlorpromazine produced a striking behavioral indifference that made its use in mental disorders all but inevitable.

The obvious states in which to try a new sedative agent were the manic and delirious states that cause so much disruption in hospital settings. It was just such a patient who was first given chlorpromazine in the Val-de-Grâce Military Hospital in Paris, at the suggestion of Henri Laborit in 1952. A series of thirty-eight such patients under the care of Jean Delay were independently given the new drug in the neighboring Sainte-Anne hospital a few weeks later.[28] Chlorpromazine's effects were stunning. Laborit and Delay later disputed the priority for the clinical discovery of the psychotropic effects of chlorpromazine in a battle at least as bitter as that between Falret and Baillarger had been ninety-eight years earlier—a battle that probably cost both men a share of the Nobel Prize.

Chlorpromazine produced its dramatic effects in manic and delirious states and in the acute psychotic states the French termed *bouffée délirante*, which would now be termed brief reactive psychoses.[29] It was much less obviously effective in schizophrenia or depression.[30] As it became clear chlorpromazine and its successors were more than simple sedatives, Delay and colleagues encapsulated these novel and distinctive features in the notion of a neuroleptic—an agent that acted on the extrapyramidal systems of the midbrain. There was no reason to call them antipsychotics, and they were decidedly not antischizophrenic agents.

In contrast, in America delirious states were regarded as psychotic, and many manic-depressive states as well as all acute and transient psychoses were diagnosed as schizophrenic. The response accordingly of "schizophrenic" states to chlorpromazine led to its designation as an antipsychotic or antischizophrenic agent. The fact that the new wonder cures were used widely for anxiety states and in office practice, far from the psychoses of the back wards, did nothing to inhibit this designation.

The new drugs completely surpassed the older sedatives. Patients treated soon after arrival in hospital could be turned around in weeks, and a proportion of even the most recalcitrant patients "awoke" and moved toward discharge. And, to crown a decade that transformed mental illness, a minor modification to the phenothiazine nucleus gave rise to the first antidepressants.

Seeking a new chlorpromazine, Geigy, based in Basel, made the closest replica of chlorpromazine possible from summer blue —imipramine.[31] This proved singularly ineffective in agitated or psychotic disorders, but its side effects hinted at a benefit in depression. In 1955 Roland Kuhn began giving imipramine to forty hospitalized melancholic patients, who might otherwise have been expected to respond only to electroconvulsive therapy (ECT). The response of the first patient convinced him that imipramine was a breakthrough.

Imipramine quickly led to amitriptyline and to the discovery that serotonin, norepinephrine, and dopamine were neurotransmitters. By the second half of the 1960s, Arvid Carlsson had proposed that selective serotonin reuptake inhibitors might be useful both clinically and as probes with which to analyze behavior.[32]

Right through to the end of the 1960s, the talk was of transformations and cures of the type brought about by the antibiotics and other new drugs. If not effected by the original molecules, these cures would certainly come from one of the host of psychotropic successors with which pharmaceutical companies flooded the market from 1955 through to 1970. No one seemed to notice the first articles appearing in the mid-1960s, whose references to the new chronic patients suggested the rock of psychosis might be reemerging from under the antipsychotic floodtide. And although from the very start a small number of European skeptics wondered if antidepressant cures might herald an increased rate of mood disorder recurrence, the notion that we might need prophylactic treatments, or mood stabilizers, was simply not part of the tenor of the times.

AGAINST THE PSYCHOPHARMACOLOGICAL GRAIN

The origin of the modern use of lithium in psychiatry in contrast to the almost rational engineering of chlorpromazine has the qualities of a fable. It is a story involving isolated investigators, in out-of-the-way locations, with a sprinkling of extraordinary ironies, taking on and subverting one of the most stunning breakthroughs of modern medicine.

It begins with John Cade, who was born on January 18, 1912, in Horsham, a small town north of Melbourne in Australia. After training in medicine, in 1936 he took up psychiatry. Enlisting during the Second World War, he was captured by the Japanese and held prisoner for three and a half years. During this time, apparently, on the basis of observing the emergence of mental disorders among fellow prisoners, he was persuaded that there must be a physiological link between these disorders and the physical conditions in which they were being held.[33]

After the war, Cade was interested to see whether he could pin down these physical inputs. Resuming clinical practice in Bundoora Hospital near Melbourne in 1946, he began an investigation using guinea pigs. The key experiment involved injecting urine from manic, depressed, and schizophrenic patients and from normal controls into guinea pig abdomens. The injections were often fatal, especially injections of urine from patients with mania. Cade pinpointed urea as the likely cause of the toxicity. Urea when injected led to a very similar death. The urea levels in the urine from patients, however, were much less than the urea levels needed to produce death. Cade thought that there must be another substance in the urine that enhanced the toxic effects of urea. One of the candidate substances for such an enhancer was uric acid. But to investigate uric acid, Cade had to find a way to produce soluble urates, and the best way to do this was to combine uric acid with lithium to produce lithium urates.

Expecting lithium urate to make urine even more toxic, Cade was surprised to find that urine containing lithium urate appeared less toxic than untreated urine. In order to determine whether this stemmed from the lithium urate or lithium, he switched from lithium urate to lithium carbonate, which when administered in urine also appeared to have protective effects. This chain of events set up the next step, which was to administer lithium carbonate without urine to see what lithium did in its own right.

> After a latent period of about two hours the animals, although fully conscious became extremely lethargic and unresponsive to stimuli for one to two hours before once again becoming normally timid and active. Those who have experimented with guinea pigs know to what extent a ready startle reaction is part of their makeup. It was thus even more startling to the experimenter to find that after the injection of a solution of lithium carbonate they could be turned on their backs and that, instead of the usual frantic righting behavior, they merely lay there and gazed placidly back at him.[34]

Retrospectively, given the doses of lithium he used in this experiment, far from discovering a psychotropic effect of lithium, Cade may have produced these effects by poisoning the guinea pigs. Thinking he had discovered a psychotropic effect, however, he tried lithium on himself, and finding that it was without problematic effects, and aware that it had been used for nearly 100 years in other areas of medicine, he embarked on a clinical trial with patients.

In a *Medical Journal of Australia* article, he gave details of ten patients, of whom three had chronic mania, six had episodic mania, and one was described as schizoaffective. A great deal of how the lithium and bipolar disorder story has developed in the close to sixty years since this article was published arguably hinged on Cade's witting or unwitting rhetorical skill in framing his cases.

In all the cases of mania, he reported lithium as producing a dramatic effect on the mental state of the patients within days, even in patients who had been ill for up to five years. These benefits were lost when the treatment was discontinued but were retrieved on reinstatement of lithium. Five of the vignettes end with the patient leaving hospital, taking up work, and seemingly unlikely to ever return to hospital. In the case of the schizoaffective patient, the affective symptoms improved but his delusions and hallucinations remained. Six schizophrenic patients had also been given lithium, and they became quieter but there was no real change in the core features of their illness. In the case of three depressed patients, there was no apparent response to lithium. Cade proposed that lithium had a specific antimanic action and even that mania stemmed from a "deficiency in the body of lithium ions."

The first manic patient treated was WB.

> A little wizened man of 51 who had been in the state of chronic manic excitement for five years. He was amiably restless, dirty, destructive, mischievous and interfering. He had enjoyed preeminent nuisance value in a back ward for all those years and bid fair to remain for the rest of his life . . . By the fifth day it was clear that he was in fact more settled, tidier, less disinhibited and less distractible. From then on there was steady improvement so that in three weeks he was enjoying the unaccustomed and quite unexpected amenities of a convalescent ward. As he had been ill so long and confined to a closed chronic ward he found normal surroundings and liberty of movement strange at first.[35]
>
> It was with a sense of the most abject disappointment that I readmitted him to hospital six months later as manic as ever but took some consolation from his brother who informed me that Bill had become overconfident about having been well for so many months, had become lackadaisical about taking his medication and had finally ceased taking it about six weeks before. Since then he had become steadily more irritable and erratic. His lithium carbonate was at once recommenced and in two weeks he had again returned to normal. A month later he was recorded as completely well and ready to return to home and work.[36]

WB had subsequent episodes of mania when lithium was discontinued following the development of toxic effects and subsequent responses to treatment when it was reinstituted. What could not have been reported in 1949 was that WB died of lithium toxicity some years later. A number of other patients described toxic effects of lithium, including anorexia, ataxia, malaise, and depression. At one point, the toxic effects so troubled Cade that he gave up using lithium. Far from becoming a committed lithium advocate in later years, Cade subsequently experimented with a number of other minerals and claimed in the case of strontium that it had an anxiolytic effect that was demonstrable in both healthy controls and patients with a variety of psychiatric disorders.[37]

In the 1949 article, these complications of treatment lay in the future. The benefits, in contrast, had something of a Lazarus-like quality of awakening from the dead, being persuasive by virtue of both the response of chronic patients and also the loss of benefit when treatment was stopped only to have the benefit reappear with renewed treatment. Cade also managed to position lithium as having an almost specific curative effect, while the title of the article—"Lithium Salts in the Treatment of Psychotic Excitement"—belied any impression of specificity.

Despite this glowing testimonial, the reception of lithium was mixed, even within Australia. Cade's original article noted that cardiotoxicity had been recognized as a possible problem from fifty years before—in 1909. It was widely known that the FDA had just banned lithium because of possible cardiotoxicity. In 1950 a Dr. Roberts in the *Medical Journal of Australia* reported a fatality using lithium.[38] On the eighth day of treatment, the patient began to convulse, went into status epilepticus, and died from cardiovascular collapse. This was the first fatality linked to lithium's use in psychiatry.

Roberts's report drew a response from Val Ashburner, who already had treated more than fifty patients with lithium in Sunbury Mental Hospital in Victoria, some of whom had shown minor toxic manifestations, none of which were problematic.[39] Ashburner had been present at a meeting with a dozen clinical colleagues in 1949 where Cade had first presented his findings. Going back to his hospital pharmacy, Ashburner learned that there were copious amounts of lithium carbonate in stock, owing to its continued use for rheumatoid and other conditions.

The question of toxicity highlighted the need to establish a safe dose and to be able to monitor treatment. Coincidentally, the first moves to solve this problem also took place in Melbourne. The Beckman company had just produced a new flame spectrophotometer that made it possible to analyze levels of sodium and potassium in soil samples. Victor Wynn in the department of physiology in Melbourne conceived of the possibility of applying the same technique to monitor blood and tissue potassium and sodium levels—something that is now a mainstay of general medical practice. Using a machine he purchased himself, Wynn and colleagues published their first results in 1950.[40]

Another member of the department was Bert Trautner, a German émigré who fled the Nazis. Aware of Wynn's work and the problems with lithium, Trautner persuaded a psychiatric trainee, Charlie Noack, to recruit patients, whom they would treat and whose blood lithium levels they would monitor. They treated 100 patients, reported that lithium was indeed beneficial specifically in manic states, and proposed a first set of indicators for safe lithium blood levels, although in fact blood monitoring made no difference in any of the cases they reported.[41] The importance of this article probably lay in the fact that it provided a much larger sample of patients, that it was linked into a university department, and, only secondarily if at all, that it offered a means of monitoring treatment. When later users of lithium referred to reports of its use in Australia, it was often this article they were citing.

In contrast in Western Australia, Glesinger reported on 104 cases, of whom 7 had chronic mania; 14, recurrent mania; 39, classic schizophrenia; 12, hebephrenia; 6, epileptic disorders; and 26, diverse states. Unlike others, he found 45 percent showed a good response, regardless of diagnosis, a further 28 percent showed some response, and 27 percent had no response, of whom 11 percent had toxicity troubles.[42] Glesinger's article also bucked the trend by suggesting that sophisticated methods of monitoring lithium levels were not needed, despite reporting on two deaths that seemed linked to lithium toxicity.

But by this time chlorpromazine and its progeny had just arrived in Australia and were about to sweep all before them. Trautner and colleagues produced one more article on lithium, focused more on the issue of measuring its disposition than on its therapeutic benefits.[43] This was essentially the last Australian publication on lithium, other than a chapter by Cade in 1970 outlining the discovery of lithium.[44] There can be two discoverers of a drug—the person who uses it first for some new purpose and the person who persuades the world there is something new to which it should pay heed. While Cade may have been the discoverer in the first sense, he was not the person who put lithium on the map.

LITHIUM ON THE MARGINS

Publication in the *Medical Journal of Australia* was unlikely to excite the psychiatric world in 1949, and it is hard to detect any impact of Cade's work in the English-speaking world. Russell Murdoch Young, working in Parkside Hospital in Macclesfield, England, began using lithium in 1950 apparently on the basis of Cade's article, later saying—but not reporting—that in his experience lithium could turn off the symptoms of mania after a few days treatment, as though a switch were flipped, where chlorpromazine might quiet the patient without any real change in the underling condition.[45] It is difficult to know how many other clinicians read the Australian articles and tried lithium.

In early 1954, Eliot Slater, the editor of the *British Journal of Psychiatry*, faced with a paper claiming to demonstrate a beneficial effect of lithium in mania by means of a double-blind trial, turned it down as not being of sufficient interest. The first British publication came in 1956.[46]

In the United States, the problems were even greater. Cade's article was published seven months after the FDA had banned lithium. Although later work suggested that efforts to reduce salt rather than lithium intake may have caused the cardiac problems,[47] the regulatory die had been cast. As a result, and combined with the fact that the early 1950s were a period when the newly ascendant psychoanalytic establishment put little premium on any biological treatment for nervous disorders, lithium was unlikely to be picked up in the United States. The first American article appeared in 1960,[48] authored by an Australian, Sam Gershon, who had previously worked with both Cade and Trautner. Nothing else was to appear for a further eight years.

The greatest interest in lithium was in France. In 1951 Despinoy and Romeuf reported lithium was useful in three cases of chronic mania, but not so useful in one case of agitated schizophrenia, two of confusional states, and four cases of stupor.[49] Reyss-Brion and Grambert reported little effect in mania.[50] In 1952 Mlle Deschamps, one of the first users of chlorpromazine in 1952, reported a benefit from lithium in mania and not in schizophrenia.[51] These observations all refer to Cade's article.

In 1953 Duc and Maurel reported on thirty cases.[52] They were drawn to lithium, they stated, because of its convenience compared to electroshock, insulin coma therapy, or deep sleep therapy, which needed specialist staff and facilities. Two grams of lithium carbonate produced a noticeable calming within twenty-four hours in most cases and in three to five days in the most severe cases of agitation. Their first case was dramatic. Antonio M, a seventy-year-old manic-depressive who had been hospitalized regularly over a twenty-year period, who had not responded to electroshock or deep sleep, and whose bouts of mania were coming with increasing frequency, responded almost overnight to lithium. Their second case was that of Josephine R, a twenty-two-year-old woman with a puerperal psychosis, who also responded only to lithium. In contrast to the others, Duc and Maurel found benefits in states other than mania, and not always in mania.

Intriguingly, these investigators also reported that lithium slowed the brain waves on an electroencephalogram (EEG) in the same way as convulsions did, tempting them to compare the effect of lithium to that of a classic convulsive therapy. As we shall see in chapter 6, these early observations fit in with the very latest theories about how mood stabilizers work. But, as Duc and Maurel noted, in all likelihood these EEG changes reflect toxic effects of lithium rather than offer hints as to its therapeutic mode of action. Modern investigators seem less discriminating.

In 1954 Carbère and Pochard reported dramatic responses in an agitated opiate addict, a thirty-year-old cycloid psychotic, two patients with mania, two patients with schizophrenia, and in a patient with brief reactive psychoses, in whom other treatments including electroshock, sedatives, and the newly launched chlorpromazine had been tried unsuccessfully.[53] Again as with Duc and Maurel, the response to lithium seemed relatively nonspecific.

In light of these results and comparably confusing results from other investigations, by 1954 the question of whether lithium was specific to mania or not had come center stage. Teulié, Follin, and Bégoin reported on twenty-five cases of mania, ten cases of schizophrenia as well as twenty-one cases of epilepsy, seven cases of chronic delusional states, and five cases of stupor.[54] They used lithium citrate or lithium carbonate for patients with mania or schizophrenia, and lithium bromide for those with epilepsy, on the basis of a note by Cade that lithium bromide had once been used for epilepsy and might have been discarded prematurely. They found lithium was effective for classic mania, poor for atypical mania, and without effect for psychoses.

While this result seemed specific, the findings in epilepsy were anything but. Here lithium was not aimed at controlling fits, but rather at treating the personality difficulties that were commonly seen as a concomitant of epilepsy. They reported two good results, seven cases with partial benefits, and eight cases with no benefit. On this basis, they switched to lithium carbonate in treating six more epileptics and had one stunning improvement, two good results, and three with no apparent benefit. The key point here is that they were reporting on a benefit in what would now be thought of as personality problems.

In contrast, others continued to report strikingly good results in cases of mania, with minimal benefits in other states.[55] In a doctoral thesis presented in 1955, Massin suggested that "lithium citrate seemed in fact to be the best treatment for mania."[56] Where many other papers had reported brief courses of treatment, Massin stressed "the importance of prolonging the treatment because stopping treatment often led to a rapid relapse."[57]

Despite all this activity, and the fact that by the mid-1950s publications on lithium in French outnumbered all other national contributions combined, Plichet in a review of the use of lithium in *La Presse Médicale* said that Cade's article had little impact in France.[58] Lithium was a troublesome treatment that was contraindicated in depression and would not replace electroconvulsive therapy for mania. It might have some benefit in prolonging recoveries induced by ECT, but at a cost of possible deaths if not monitored closely.

But the real problem was that lithium was up against chlorpromazine. This was more than a competition between two drugs. No company could patent lithium, whereas the phenothiazines gave rise to a succession of patentable molecules. Hence, company promotion would never underpin lithium's use. Interest in lithium died out in France.

At a ward round at Allan Memorial Institute in Montreal in 1959, Ewen Cameron suggested lithium treatment for a patient with mania, referring to the one British article on the topic. Edward Kingstone, the senior resident, investigated the safety of lithium, finding that if patients did not become sodium deficient, it was probably safe. But he was anxious, nevertheless, because of lithium's dangerous reputation. Kingstone and colleagues treated seventeen patients over four months with the majority of patients who had mania responding to treatment. He sent their case reports to the *American Journal of Psychiatry*, which responded that his article would not interest readers of the journal. This would have been a first publication of the use of lithium for patients with mania in North America. Instead the article went to *Comprehensive Psychiatry*, a journal that had just been set up by the American Psychopathological Association (Cameron was on its editorial board).[59] Later that year Kingstone went on a fellowship to the Maudsley Hospital in London, where he found that lithium carbonate was not even considered for possible use.

Some indication of the perilous position of lithium can be gleaned from looking at its place in the programs of the psychopharmacological meetings of the time. Following the discovery of chlorpromazine, the major companies essentially created the first psychopharmacological organizations.[60] The meetings of these new organizations in the late 1950s and early 1960s celebrated the dawn of a new era in psychiatry following the advent of antipsychotics and antidepressants.

The first such organization was the Collegium Internationale Neuropsycho-pharmacologium (CINP), whose inaugural meeting was held in 1958. All of the big names in world psychiatry and emerging neuroscience converged on Rome for this meeting. The program covered the biochemical and neurophysiological aspects of psychiatric disorders and the significance of the efficacy of the new antipsychotics, antidepressants, and tranquilizers. In a set of proceedings that ran to 720 small-print pages, there was only one four-page piece on lithium—from Mogens Schou of Denmark.[61]

In this paper, Schou notes that at this stage he and colleagues had given lithium to 157 patients with a favorable response in 80 percent. The response seemed to be specific to mania. He noted that there could be problems with toxicity but stressed that these probably stemmed from reduced sodium intake rather than from lithium intake. At this stage he said that they had patients maintained safely on the treatment for four years.

The second CINP conference was held in Basel in July 1960. Again all the leading lights from world biological psychiatry and psychopharmacology were present. The meeting gave rise to a 520-page publication of the proceedings, in which there is not a single mention of lithium.

The third CINP meeting in Munich in September 1962 resulted in a 600-page-long set of the proceedings. Lithium was given one page—the final page. Here Schou states:

> Through its title and the communications so far given, this morning's discussion seems about to create the false historical myth that 1962 is the tenth anniversary of the psychopharmacological era. This, however, is neither true nor fair because in 1949 the Australian, Cade, discovered the therapeutic efficacy of lithium salts against manic phases of the manic depressive psychosis.
>
> There may be a number of reasons for the unjustified neglect of this drug during the years. One is its rather narrow spectrum of indication, namely the typical manias and especially the chronic ones; but a high specificity of a drug ought not to detract from the appreciation of it. Furthermore, it is known that lithium may under certain extreme conditions produce kidney damage . . . but the main reason for the neglect of lithium may be quite simply that lithium salts are so inexpensive that no commercial interests are involved. This drug has therefore completely lacked the publicity that is invariably given to drugs of higher money earning capacity.

It is indeed conspicuous that lithium does not appear in any of the many general surveys, in spite of its therapeutic value being proved in a group of patients, which was resistant to most other therapies. This may conceivably be due to mere ignorance but such a suggestion is perhaps impolite. I would rather think that lithium is omitted from these schemes, because it is chemically completely unrelated to any of the other drugs used in psychiatry. I am therefore in complete agreement with what Dr Akimoto has just said. We must not let schemes and terminology, however beautiful and logically satisfying they may be, rule our thinking and obscure our observational powers. If, because it is easy or out of a desire for systematization, we adhere to a too categorical classification of drugs, we run the grave risk of distorting truth and hampering scientific progress.[62]

All this was about to change. Taking into account all possible articles on lithium from the chemical, physiological, and therapeutics literature in all languages, there had been 28 articles up to 1899. Thereafter, the pace of production stepped up to reach 4 per year by 1949. There were 20 articles per year through the 1950s, stimulated in part by concerns about toxicity and efforts to monitor physiological levels. In the 1960s the rate increased to 30 per year, hitting 100 per year in 1966, and finally peaking at 200 per year around 1968–69—when lithium became embroiled in controversies about its mood-stabilizing properties.[63]

MOGENS SCHOU AND THE DISCOVERY OF LITHIUM

Mogens Schou was born in Copenhagen on November 24, 1918, the son of Hans Jacob Schou. Schou studied medicine in Copenhagen from 1937, his interest having been stimulated by his father and the experience of seeing distressed patients in the family sanatorium while growing up. In 1939 the first beneficial effects of ECT were reported and he remembers his father telling him about how it looked like it might be a treatment for both mania and depression and furthermore might lead to an understanding of the basis of mental disorders.[64]

After graduating from Copenhagen in 1944, Schou began research in the new field of clinical chemistry at the St. Hans Hospital in Roskilde and then at the Dikemark Hospital in Norway, made famous by Rolv Gjessing. Gjessing had described various forms of catatonia including periodic catatonia. His work suggested there must be a physiological or biochemical explanation why patients cycled between poles of stupor and intense overactivity.[65]

Gjessing's work on the periodic catatonias contributed hugely to two later research programs in psychiatry. One was an interest in circadian rhythms, which blossomed in the 1970s and 1980s and reached popular attention in the concept of seasonal affective disorders. The other was a research program during the 1960s, which saw neuropsychiatric disorders as something close to inborn errors of metabolism, whose treatment involved looking for either a missing chemical to be replaced or one present in an excessive amount that needed to be eliminated.[66]

This approach had its greatest triumph within the broader domain of the brain disorders in the case of phenylketonuria, now readily detected and treated at birth, and in the demonstration that dopamine was lowered in the brains of patients who had Parkinson's disease and that a replacement strategy with L-dopa could produce dramatic benefits. A very similar mind-set underpinned the emergence of the famous catecholamine hypothesis of depression in 1965 (chapter 5).[67] With a host of new instruments that became available after the war, such as spectrophotometers and chromatographs, researchers in America and Europe set about analyzing the bodily fluids of patients with nervous disorders.

After working with Gjessing, Schou had a stint in New York working with Heinrich Waelsch, at Columbia University's Psychiatric Institute. Waelsch and Derek Richter from Britain were the leading pioneers of the emerging discipline of neurochemistry.[68] Waelsch's links to Schou underpinned later American studies of lithium conducted at Columbia.

But the key influence on Schou was Eric Strömgren. Strömgren had become the head of the psychiatric hospital in Risskov near Aarhus by the time Schou completed his training. It was Strömgren who arranged for him to undertake research in Norway, Copenhagen, and finally in New York. Strömgren was internationally known. He had been offered the chair of psychiatry at

Copenhagen when it fell vacant, but declined in favor of staying at Risskov and building up an institute that would have strong departments in all areas of psychiatry from child to old-age psychiatry, including neuropathology, social psychiatry, genetics, and psychotherapy. It was this breadth of vision that attracted Schou to Aarhus, where he was to remain for the rest of his career.

When later asked about how events unfolded, Strömgren said: "Of course . . . knowledge of the old Danish lithium treatment may have prepared me unconsciously and made me sensitive to any new information concerning lithium. To the conscious parts of my mind, however, it looks as if I was convinced by the first report from Australia that here was really a thing to be taken seriously. . . . I found it extremely fascinating if lithium salts which are chemically so simple could have a therapeutic effect in psychiatry, especially so if they are active against just one disease, which could tell us much more about that disease than lots of information concerning the therapeutic effects of complicated compounds [chlorpromazine] which had no clear preference with regard to the different disorders they were used."[69]

Strömgren brought Cade's article to the attention of Schou, who planned a controlled trial to evaluate its effects. Pinning down Schou's interest in using controlled methods is difficult. This was something he said was in the air at the time.[70] But, in fact, few double-blind trials had then been reported. One of the other influences Schou points to lies in Gjessing's attempts in treating patients in catatonic states. In these states, the condition appeared to be relatively unvarying, and therefore any change following the institution of treatment could be regarded as evidence of a treatment benefit. Chronic manias did not show quite the invariant picture found in catatonia, but Schou proposed to explore the effect of treatment by alternating lithium and placebo in this chronic group. In contrast to the treatment of patients with a more episodic and classic manic-depressive course, he simply gave continuous lithium. In the case of the chronic patients, neither the clinicians involved in assessing the effects of treatment, Eric Strömgren, Niels Juel-Nielsen, and Holger Voldby, nor the patients, nor the nursing staff knew whether a patient was taking lithium or placebo.

The novelty of Schou's assessment procedure alarmed the nursing staff. Because some of the nurses apparently were unhappy at the idea that violent manic patients might be given a placebo, they broke the tablets and tasted them in an effort to identify the placebo, but Schou had made the lithium and placebo both look and taste the same.

The study began in 1952, a few months after his father had died. The results came through in 1953. From the records kept of the patients' disease course, it seems that those patients with chronic mania improved on lithium and got worse when switched to placebo, whereas the patients who had recurrent disorders who had been put on continuous lithium showed a sustained improvement.

Among the patients treated with lithium, one who had rapidly recurring manias and depressions appeared to have neither highs nor lows. This response led to a trial of lithium to treat people who were depressed, but it produced no obvious benefits and was terminated early by Schou and colleagues on the basis that lithium did not work for depression. The results were never published.

The alternative interpretation that, rather than being an antidepressant in this patient, lithium might in fact have been prophylactic did not occur to Schou. Others using lithium later had similar experiences and concluded that the absence of depressive episodes might point to a possible prophylactic effect. One of these was G. P. (Toby) Hartigan from Britain and the other was Poul Baastrup from Denmark. Both wrote to Schou, who then visited them.

In 1957 Baastrup began a trial of lithium at Vordingborg Hospital. He treated fifty-six patients and concluded that lithium was beneficial for mania.[71] As part of the trial, he followed up patients who had been discharged from hospital. They had been asked to stop taking lithium. But eight of the bipolar patients had continued to take lithium despite his advice, and two of them had even given it to manic-depressive relatives. The reason for continuing with the treatment they claimed was that continuous lithium treatment prevented relapse.

Baastrup had mixed feelings about patients disobeying his

instructions. At this stage, lithium was an unknown quantity, of which one of the few things known for certain was that it could lead to physical complications. Intrigued by the observation, though, Baastrup looked back over the three years during which these patients had been on lithium and compared the rate at which they had been having episodes during these three years with their previous rate. It appeared that the rate of new episodes was reduced compared with previously.[72]

At the same time, Toby Hartigan had given lithium to a group of twenty patients of whom nine had chronic or intermittent manic episodes and four had alternating manias and depressions, while the remaining seven had recurrent depressive episodes. The intriguing finding came in this last group. As Hartigan put it, "I have been experimenting with lithium on a group of seven patients with frequent recurrent depressions. There is little in the literature to suggest that depressive syndromes are improved by the drug and it is certainly not to be advocated during the acute depression episode but I have been using it as a prophylactic against further depressions in these patients and have had very promising results in five of them, although admittedly follow up has not so far been long enough to be very convincing."[73]

In 1960 Hartigan sent a draft paper to Schou, who encouraged him to publish his results. Schou again wrote to Hartigan in November 1961 and February 1962. In September 1962 he suggested to Hartigan that Eliot Slater, the editor of the *British Journal of Psychiatry*, would be interested in a paper on these observations because Slater, although uninterested in even reviewing Schou's first paper on lithium in 1954, was now convinced of the advantages.[74] Neither Baastrup nor Hartigan, however, were academics, and both were slow to publish, doing so only in 1963 and 1964.

By then Schou's thinking had changed quite dramatically. At the CINP meeting in 1962, Schou heard a talk given by Haruo Akimoto, the professor of Psychiatry in Tokyo, in which Akimoto claimed that imipramine could produce benefits in both mania and depression. Consequently, Schou began to think that both lithium and imipramine might be mood normalizers. This led to a publication in the *British Journal of Psychiatry* in 1963, in which Schou proposed that lithium might be a normothymotic or "mood normalizer."[75] In later life, he all but disowned this article as overenthusiastic.

In addition to these emerging clinical hints, there was another influence at play for Schou. He had a brother who from the age of twenty had suffered from repeated attacks of depression, which periodically made him unable to work. "The attacks usually lasted some months, and then disappeared, but they reappeared again and again, year after year, inevitably. Then, about 14 years ago [in the mid-1960s], he was started on maintenance treatment with lithium, and since then he has not had a single depressive relapse. He still needs to take the medicine to keep the disease under control, but functionally he is a cured man. You will understand what such a change meant to himself and to his wife and children, and how much of a miracle it appeared to us in the family."[76]

Baastrup and Schou went on to study high-risk manic-depressive patients put on lithium six and half years earlier. This study, published in the *Archives of General Psychiatry* in 1967,[77] reported that the frequency of episodes in patients after lithium was much less than it had been before and that the total length of time spent in hospital was also much less. This article and the articles by Hartigan and Baastrup, pointing to a prophylactic benefit of lithium not only in classic bipolar manic-depressive illness but also in recurrent unipolar illness, provoked an explosion. The fuse was set at a meeting at Göttingen in 1966 at which Schou and Michael Shepherd participated.

THE LITHIUM WARS

Michael Shepherd was born in Swansea in 1922.[78] Having trained in medicine, he moved to the Institute of Psychiatry, which under Aubrey Lewis was on its way to become a global player in psychiatric research. In the early 1950s, when reserpine and chlorpromazine were becoming available and the first pharmaceutical company representatives were visiting psychiatric hospitals, Shepherd engaged Lewis on the issue of how they would ever know that the drugs were actually working.[79]

In 1947, faced with repeated claims, which later turned out to be unfounded, that a variety of agents could cure tuberculosis, Austin Bradford Hill and colleagues on behalf of Britain's Medical Research Council had conducted a trial of streptomycin for treating patients with tuberculosis. This is generally cited as the first randomized controlled trial (RCT) in medicine—although it was not placebo controlled. After this, the notion of controlled trials began to take shape. One of the first to adopt such trials in psychiatry was Linford Rees. From the late 1940s, as the resident medical superintendent of Whitchurch Hospital in Cardiff, where he had access to hundreds of patients, Rees undertook some of the first clinical trials to test whether new treatments for which extravagant claims were being made at the time, such as deoxycortisone for schizophrenia and electronarcosis, were as effective as their proponents claimed. Rees's trials showed they were not. This was a powerful demonstration of just what clinical trials were designed to do. They were not designed to show that treatments worked. Clinical trials were aimed at identifying unsuccessful therapeutic interventions and bringing bandwagons to a stop.

In the course of 1952–53, Shepherd began to recruit patients to two clinical trials. One compared reserpine and placebo in a group of patients who were depressed,[80] and the other compared reserpine and placebo in a group of patients who had schizophrenia. These trials are the closest to the type of RCT now undertaken. They were parallel group trials rather than crossover trials. Rather than have patients alternate between active treatment and placebo, there were two groups of patients: one got active treatment throughout, and the other got placebo throughout. Because of this design, randomization was a critical feature of Shepherd's protocol in a way that it had not been for Schou, or Rees.[81]

Schou had alternated patients between placebo and lithium on a random basis. The investigators were blind to which treatment the patient was on, and the subsequent design of the trial aimed at seeing whether the clinical ratings showed better mental states clustering during lithium treatment periods with deteriorations during the placebo period. It is now clear that, if there is a withdrawal syndrome linked to treatment, this trial design is not optimal.

On the basis of his early clinical trials and the patronage of Lewis, Shepherd became secretary of the Medical Research Council's new clinical trials committee. This convened first in 1959 under the auspices of Bradford Hill. The group liaised closely with Jonathan Cole's Psychopharmacology Service Center based at the National Institutes of Health (NIH) in Bethesda, Maryland, and one of Cole's assistants at the time, Gerry Klerman, spent time with Shepherd in London hammering out the first protocols for multicentered trials.[82]

The group led by Shepherd ran a trial comparing ECT, imipramine, phenelzine, and placebo in depression. In this trial ECT was clearly the best treatment, and imipramine was also better than placebo, but phenelzine, a monoamine-oxidase inhibitor (MAOI), was not. The trial reported in 1965 at just the same time as a potentially lethal hazard of the MAOI group of drugs was outlined—the cheese effect. When patients on MAOIs ate cheese or drank wine, they risked a dramatic increase in blood pressure and possible stroke. The combination of Shepherd's trial and the cheese effect finished off the MAOIs. In fact, Shepherd's trial almost certainly used too low a dose of phenelzine, which brings out one of the hazards of trials.

On the basis of his trials, Shepherd was deeply involved in psychopharmacology. He was a founder of the CINP and, in 1962, the vice president of the organization. He was present at all the early meetings, but as an active participant in the plenary sessions, he had little if any contact with the small group of clinicians interested in lithium centered around Schou. The early lithium symposia at these meetings rarely attracted more than a dozen participants. The notion that lithium might be a useful treatment for mania was not widely disputed. But mania, while interesting, formed a small proportion of the mental hospital workloads, and even for mania the neuroleptics in any event were the first line of treatment. Schizophrenia and depression were much more important problems, as indeed were alcoholism, substance misuse, and other conditions.

Following early meetings on lithium, which aired claims that lithium was of benefit in mania, later meetings had moved on to discussing even less interesting issues, such as monitoring lithium levels to enable its safer use. This topic was not designed to arouse curiosity or entice in the otherwise unoccupied. In almost complete contrast to other drugs, and especially recent drugs, the complications of lithium were the main focus of attention.

At the meeting in Göttingen in 1966, Schou and Shepherd were slated to present on the same program for the first time. Schou presented the results from Baastrup and Hartigan's work, indicating that lithium might have a prophylactic effect for recurrent mood disorders. But this presentation ran smack up against the points made by Shepherd at the same meeting, who argued that the judgment of the clinical investigator needed to be subject to the rigors of an impersonal trial that would establish whether a specific effect of treatment could be shown. Many patients got well simply by being seen. Did more patients get well by taking this treatment than got well simply by being supported by their clinician? Shepherd was asked to comment on Schou's idea that lithium might be prophylactic. His response, that these observations were interesting but remained to be confirmed, was taken to indicate that he relegated mood stabilization to the realm of fantasy.

After the exchanges, Schou's wife, Netta, took issue with Shepherd for being too hard on her husband. Schou joined them and in the course of the conversation made the problem worse by revealing he had a brother who, on the basis of Baastrup's results, had begun taking lithium for a recurrent depressive disorder and, since taking lithium, had experienced no recurrences. This revelation confirmed for Shepherd his suspicion that Schou was a "believer" in lithium prophylaxis and that Schou thought further studies were not needed.

At this point, Baastrup and Schou had drafted their 1967 manuscript.[83] Shepherd claims that Schou sent him an early draft of this paper and that he made suggestions that Schou incorporated into the manuscript in a twisted form. Schou disputes this.

When Schou's paper was published, Shepherd and Barry Blackwell responded in a paper in the *Lancet* under the heading of "Prophylactic Lithium: Another Therapeutic Myth?"[84] After this opening salvo, they noted that Cade's open study suggested that 80 percent of manic patients might respond to lithium, whereas Schou's own controlled trial showed that only a third of manic patients responded. Generally they reported that almost all authors, including early Australian proponents of lithium, had indicated that depression responded poorly to lithium and that in the only controlled trial of lithium for depression, which Schou himself had undertaken, the trial had been discontinued when only one out of twelve patients responded.

They noted that Baastrup, after treating eleven patients with recurrent manic-depressive illnesses, declared "they cannot do without lithium." But "these patients formed the residual 18 per cent of 60 patients," of whom "some did not respond to therapy, others did not reappear."[85] In their second paper, Baastrup and Schou had selected 88 patients from among 156 who had received lithium during a six and a half year period and had selected the patients based on those who had been on lithium for a year or more who had a documented history of prior episodes of mood disorder, contrasting the frequency of episodes before and after lithium. But, as Blackwell and Shepherd pointed out, most of these patients had got well with ECT or antidepressant drugs in the first instance. The problem here was that, "in view of the natural history of affective illnesses and their fragmentation by physical methods of treatment, several patients could have had single rather than recurrent illnesses."[86]

They pointed out that if you took any group of patients with recurrent mood disorders and followed them for a period of time, you were likely to find similar results almost regardless of what they were treated with. Blackwell and Shepherd presented results from a group of Institute of Psychiatry patients that suggested that almost anything, including phenelzine, was prophylactic for recurrent mood disorders, when in fact Shepherd's 1965 trial had seemed to show that phenelzine simply was not an antidepressant. This suggested that Schou and Baastrup's patients had self-selected themselves as lithium responders and that, had they been randomly assigned to a controlled trial, the benefits would have not been apparent.

This heavy-handed response criticizing Schou for his research methods engaged the psychopharmacological establishment on the side of Schou and lithium, against Shepherd. What the proponents of psychopharmacology heard in the attack was the voice of therapeutic skepticism—something that threatened all of them.

In response to an editorial by Nathan Kline in the *American Journal of Psychiatry*, which was run as part of a campaign to get lithium licensed, Barry Blackwell wrote that the editorial "will be highly prized by collectors of original enthusiasms tempered by subsequent experience. Only time will tell whether your author's eulogy will earn him the fate his analogy deserves—to join Cinderella's godmother in the pages of mythology. To transform 'just plain old lithium' into the elixir of life, on the evidence available is an achievement second only to converting a pumpkin into a stagecoach." Kline replied that "Dr. Blackwell's delightful letter reads as though it were written by one of Cinderella's spiteful sisters. . . . There is even a feeling of faint personal familiarity with Dr. Blackwell's warning which reminds me of some of the caveats concerning the introduction of both antipsychotic and antidepressant agents. Of course it may also be that Dr. Blackwell is also not convinced that any of these drugs have been demonstrated to be of any use."[87]

Schou and Shepherd met only one more time, at a meeting in Yugoslavia in 1973. Here Shepherd indicated that, had Baastrup and Schou's paper been submitted to his journal *Psychological Medicine*, "it might well have been accepted as a preliminary communication in a suitably modified form." He went on to say, "the problem created by Professor Schou was of his own making: he appears to have believed so firmly in his own judgment as to have concluded that independent assessment was unnecessary. The evidence which he presented was certainly incomplete, as we pointed out at the time, and the history of physical treatment in psychiatry has unfortunately demonstrated too often the folly of relying on uncontrolled studies alone, however eminent and enthusiastic the clinical observers. Mention need only be made of deep insulin coma therapy and pre-frontal leucotomy in this connection. For this reason I am personally very glad that Professor Schou eventually felt able to overcome his scruples and to accept the widely accepted ethos of the scientific community."[88]

The scruples Shepherd refers to here lay in the concern Schou and others had that patients with manic-depressive disorder, if randomly assigned to placebo, would be at a real risk of suicide. For Schou, the idea of randomly assigning his own brother to placebo would have been unethical. It was one thing to use a placebo in an acute study, but was it ethical to continue giving it for several years, when there was strong suspicions that the alternative treatment was effective? Heinz Lehmann, for instance, broke the blind during a World Health Organization (WHO) lithium study, following a number of serious suicide attempts, and found that all the suicide attempts had been in patients on placebo.

Schou at this stage had come to the attention of Nathan Kline, then one of the key figures in American psychopharmacology. This led to invitations to a series of annual meetings held in the Caribbean, sponsored by a wealthy patient of Kline's, at which Kline organized informal workshops drawing in investigators from both Europe and the United States. At the meeting in April 1966 in Haiti, Schou met Jules Angst. Angst was a psychiatric epidemiologist who had just spent time on a research fellowship with Shepherd and Lewis at the Institute of Psychiatry. He also had an article in press advocating a renewed emphasis on distinguishing between what would come to be called unipolar and bipolar affective disorders. He was initially skeptical that lithium could have prophylactic effects.

But after meeting Schou, Angst contacted Paul Grof, who had been working in a mood disorder clinic in Prague since the early 1960s. Grof had shown that imipramine was ineffective in the prevention of recurrences in bipolar patients. How would lithium compare with imipramine? As Grof's early data ran counter to Schou's idea that both lithium and imipramine might be mood stabilizers, he was skeptical. But Angst persuaded Grof to travel to Aarhus and meet Schou.

Back in Prague, Grof set out to see whether the recurrent mood disorders that had not responded to imipramine might respond to lithium. The first problem he faced was that the director of the unit, Professor Hanzlicek, had flirted briefly with lithium in the 1950s and there had been some fatalities among those treated. Grof understood that if anything went wrong he would be dismissed from his post. But in contrast to the effects of imipramine, lithium did seem to reduce the frequency of relapses.[89]

The study, however, had a built-in assumption that came from Angst: "On average endogenous affective psychoses show a regu-

lar decrease in the length of the cycles with increasing number of
episodes. If one cuts the course of an affective psychosis at any
time one has to compare identical spaces of time on both sides of
this cut. One can expect that there will be more episodes after the
cut than before."[90] The natural course of the disorder supposedly
was such that intervals between episodes decreased with age and
the number of previous episodes. This mirror image approach
offered one way around the randomization problem. Baastrup
and Schou had assumed this, as did Angst and Grof in succeeding studies, and by taking this approach it appeared that lithium
had a prophylactic effect but that imipramine did not.[91] Baastrup
and Schou also ran a discontinuation study, randomly assigning patients who responded better to either lithium or placebo,
and found that those remaining on lithium did much better than
those switched to placebo.[92]

Still, Shepherd remained unimpressed. Until patients were
entered randomly into a placebo-controlled, double-blind study,
there could be no proof that lithium did what was being claimed
for it, despite Angst's assumptions about the natural history of
bipolar disorders. And indeed Angst's assumption now appears
incorrect; the natural history is not for episodes to get more frequent. The findings from the discontinuation study, Shepherd
argued, might simply be caused by lithium withdrawal.[93] With
the benefit of three more decades of experience, it appears that
lithium has a withdrawal syndrome that may trigger deterioration
after discontinuation.

The upshot was a series of further controlled trials. In two of
these, it appeared that the administration of lithium did indeed
lead to a reduced frequency of further affective episodes.[94] But
Shepherd and colleagues in two further trials showed that amitriptyline was also prophylactic in recurrent depressive disorders[95]
and that lithium and amitriptyline produced apparently comparable prophylactic effects when given to patients with recurrent
depressive disorders.[96]

This controversy dragged lithium out of obscurity and made
it one of the stars in the psychotropic firmament. It established
the idea that a drug might—in terms that came later—stabilize
mood. But, in the process, almost everything got turned inside

out. The original boost to lithium's trajectory was its apparent specificity to mania; now it was moving into orbit on the basis of a quite different action. It stabilized rather than cured, but did it do so in any way other than the way many other psychotropic drugs did?

As all this was happening, a further study eroded the notion of lithium's specificity. Michael Sheard, assessing a prison population, reported that lithium reduced levels of aggression in prisoners generally,[97] a finding that was quickly replicated.[98] This result could be seen as an all-but-complete contradiction to Cade's original 1949 report. Alternatively, if lithium responsiveness defines bipolarity, the Sheard result could be reinterpreted as evidence that many patients with personality disorders had in fact unrecognized bipolar disorders. This latter interpretation is the one that current advocates of mood stabilization now opt for.

The Aftermath of the Lithium Wars

In the short term, the argument between Schou and Shepherd did more for Schou and lithium than for Shepherd. Lithium defied the laws of psychopharmacological gravity. It had no company to push it. As of 1977 there were forty-four different versions of lithium on sale between the Americas and Europe. If there had been forty-four companies producing fluoxetine, Lilly would have had no incentive to market Prozac or later Zyprexa, drugs that would reach iconic status. But the issues raised were something that every meeting wanted to feature on its program. This was partly because Schou's allies were among the most influential figures in psychopharmacology.

Following the use of lithium by Gershon and Gerard at Ypsilanti State Hospital in Michigan in 1959, Rowell Laboratories, a small Minnesota company, began to provide lithium to investigators, and soon the FDA found that it was giving investigator licenses to an ever-increasing number of clinicians keen to use it.[99] Pressure began to build for its registration in America. In 1969 the American Psychiatric Association set up a lithium task force aimed at getting FDA approval for the use of lithium for mania. The members of the task force included Biff Bunney, Robert Prien, Joseph Tupin, and Samuel Gershon.

Despite all these "investigators," however, the American data remained sparse and unsophisticated. A second American study was undertaken by Ronald Fieve, who after graduating in medicine from Harvard in 1955 came to Columbia's Psychiatric Institute to train in psychiatry at the height of the psychoanalytic ascendancy. Fieve found himself in analytic training but was disillusioned by it. The head of his department, Laurence Kolb, suggested that he should investigate reports from Australia and Denmark on lithium. He began an open trial with lithium along with Ralph Wharton, a fellow resident, liaising with Heinrich Waelsch to monitor lithium and blood electrolyte levels. There was resistance to the use of lithium, but its beneficial effects in controlling symptoms of mania gradually brought about a change in atmosphere. This enabled him in 1966 to set up the first lithium clinic in North America.

Fieve's study came out in the *American Journal of Psychiatry* in 1968. It involved twenty-nine depressed patients. After starting with placebo, seventeen of the patients received lithium and twelve imipramine. Both treatments were linked to benefits, although imipramine appeared somewhat better than lithium. Despite these limitations, the study had an impact.[100] Biff Bunney and Fred Goodwin at the National Institute of Mental Health (NIMH) published another "study" that had only two patients. Lithium restored both patients to normal, and in nine of the ten times that placebo was substituted for it, their mania increased within twenty-four hours.

Kline and others meanwhile had begun to work on public opinion through television and radio to generate interest in the compound. Kline pushed the American College of Neuropsychopharmacology to apply for a license for lithium, in default of a company application—an unheard-of move. Finally, both Smith-Kline & French, in part, it is said, because of its acknowledged lead role in American psychopharmacology following the introduction of chlorpromazine, and Pfizer submitted applications for registration to the FDA in 1970 and lithium was approved for use in mania in the United States—but not for prophylaxis.

Lithium by this time was having an impact beyond therapeutics. While chlorpromazine was thought to be useful for everything from schizophrenia to mania and depression, there was little incentive for American physicians to distinguish among the psychoses. Almost all psychoses were diagnosed as schizophrenia. But the demonstrations of lithium's efficacy threw into relief emerging observations of discrepancies in the rate of diagnosis of schizophrenia in the United Kingdom and the United States. This led to the international pilot study of schizophrenia.[101] The United States was diagnosing more schizophrenia than any other country in the world except Russia. While everybody used chlorpromazine as the frontline treatment, this variation in practice was interesting but of little consequence. But if lithium was a more specific treatment for manic-depressive illness, if some patients responded to it where they had not responded to chlorpromazine, and, in particular, if it were prophylactic for mood disorders, then getting the diagnosis right made a difference. Across the United States, regional differences in the use of lithium went hand in hand with differences in the rates of diagnosis of manic-depressive illness.[102] And this was a big trigger to *DSM-III*, which went even further and carved bipolar disorder out of the corpus of other mood disorders, as we shall see in the next chapter.

In addition to lithium's role in distinguishing between unipolar and bipolar depressions, it also led to a recognition that not only were there bipolar I disorders, which involved hospitalization for mania, but there were depressions that might be accompanied by mood elevations that did not require hospitalization—bipolar II disorders. Where bipolar I disorder, or *folie circulaire*, was a rare disorder with an incidence of 1 per 100,000 per year, bipolar II, it was discovered, might affect up to 5 percent of the population depending on how one interpreted the affective instability in personality and other disorders. If ever a new generation of "mood stabilizers" were to emerge, they need not "lack the publicity that is invariably given to drugs of higher money earning capacity."

The Lithium Wars: The Ironies

In an anonymous review of an edited volume by Strömgren and Schou in 1980, Shepherd wrote: "The essence of the story is contained in the first two chapters, both by Schou, one an historical account of local 'lithium research' and the other a list of some 250

Risskov publications on lithium over a 25 year period, to many of which his name is attached. Now that the lithium bubble is bursting, such information may prove to be of some value to the future student of the natural history of over-valued treatments in psychiatry."[103]

This almost desperate hope that the lithium bubble would burst points to the tragedy of the story. Two men, with similar retiring personalities, and very similar concerns for careful clinical observation and data, who shared not only initials but also doubts about the pharmaceutical industry, and who both found their conflict intensely painful, ended up on opposite sides of a bitter conflict and both were ultimately undone by the very things they put their trust in.

While Schou came center-stage in psychopharmacology in the short term as a result of the conflict, Shepherd left the field. He retreated to focus on the epidemiological studies he had started at the Institute of Psychiatry in the early 1960s. The impetus to these studies was his realization that no one really knew what nervous problems the average person in the street might have. In the asylum era, people kept their inner lives to themselves, and it was only when inner lives toppled over into dangerous public spectacles that those affected came to the attentions of the alienists and their psychiatric successors. What we knew about mental illness was based almost exclusively on those of us who came to the attention of the doctors in this way.

Shepherd created psychiatric epidemiology, but this led to studies that, having adopted ever looser screening criteria, and side-stepping any notion of disability, have led in recent years to claims that half of all Americans will have a mental illness at some point in their lives. If they are ill, and if treatments work, as randomized controlled trials appear to show they do, the logic is that people who might not suspect they are ill should be detected and treated. This intervention in people's lives has won unqualified support, even at the highest levels of Republican administrations, and led to mandatory screening programs for children, as the proponents of treatment argue that intervention will reduce the national burden of alcoholism, drug abuse, suicide, divorce, and absenteeism. At a time when the global economy has become increasingly competitive, who can spurn these advantages?

Jules Angst came to the Institute of Psychiatry to train with Shepherd in the mid-1960s. The example of Shepherd's work and this training stimulated Angst to work on mood disorders in Zurich, and this work in 1966 led to a resurrection of the concept of bipolar disorder, as we shall see. By the late 1980s, Angst's work suggested that 5 percent of the population could be seen as bipolar.

But while Shepherd was marginalized by developments and found his work being used to fuel the bandwagon of therapeutic enthusiasts, Schou and lithium's star remained for only a short while longer in the firmament. Once the notion of mood stabilization was established, a further tide of mood stabilizers have come in and swept lithium off the psychiatric beach. The Columbia lithium clinic, the first in North America, survived until 1995, when it closed after being swamped by the increased use of valproate and other anticonvulsants, as we shall see in chapter 6. Lithium was skewered by the psychopharmacological forces and therapeutic enthusiasts, whose influence Shepherd was so keen to resist.

The incoming tides can transform the look of a beach. As Paul Grof put it in 2002, reflecting on the history he had lived through: "Long term treatments given to virtually no-one thirty years ago are now prescribed for nearly everyone with recurrent affective disorders to the point that the natural course of the illness is not known any more. With the use of lithium the concept of affective disorder has dramatically broadened and mood symptoms rather than comprehensively assessed psychopathology have become the center of psychiatric assessment. Having observed these changes, I have a deep appreciation of how many similar cycles psychiatry must have undergone in the past, and how much more in psychiatry we still have to clarify and to learn."[104] These issues will occupy us for the next three chapters.

INFORMATIONAL REDUCTIONISM

This chapter opened with a specter, namely that lithium brought an informational reductionism in its wake that has had more profound effects on the practice of psychiatry than any biological reductionism. If so, such a claim is ironically at odds with the unique and human story of the lithium protagonists outlined here.

In the struggles over lithium, Shepherd made clear his belief that the trials he did so much to pioneer would have stopped prefrontal leucotomy and insulin coma therapy in their tracks, and might have done the same for lithium had Schou agreed to proper trials. While the controversy helped sell lithium, it also sold randomized controlled trials.

But these earlier treatments did not come to a stop because trials showed they did not work. Quite the contrary, it was individual clinical judgments made by clinicians who were much more impressed by the advantages of chlorpromazine and imipramine that led to the demise of insulin coma and prefrontal leucotomy. And chlorpromazine and imipramine were not discovered through RCTs. So it is not immediately clear what RCTs actually do show. Do they show that drugs work?

This is a supremely important issue in that most commentators endorse the notion that modern evaluative methods have put medicine and psychiatry on a solid footing and in a position to build incrementally on advances made. This is sometimes called the epidemiological paradigm, sometimes evidence-based medicine. The leading journals in the field will now publish only clinical trial papers and have given up taking case reports. For proponents of this approach, the only remaining role for history is to document the sequence in which "facts" are established. Indeed, history is deeply suspect, as historians make no attempt to assemble all the information but rather obviously select the data to suit their argument. Many would regard argument as too good a word for the anecdotes or stories historians relate.

But the epidemiological paradigm makes a mistake of extraordinary proportions as regards the nature of clinical trial evidence. Philosophically, RCTs are constructed on the basis of a null hypothesis. When the null hypothesis is refuted, it means that it is not right to say a treatment has no effect. This is not the same as saying the treatment "works" and therefore should be given.

RCTs were initially designed to stop therapeutic bandwagons

in their tracks. This function is still best demonstrated when trials cast doubt on clinical enthusiasms about new treatments rather than when they demonstrate treatment effects of dubious significance. But, in a complete inversion of their original role, as we shall see in later chapters, RCTs have become the primary marketing tool of pharmaceutical companies. They are the fuel that powers bandwagons, helped by the fact that company trials in which the drug fails to beat the placebo commonly do not see the light of day.

We can make these abstract issues more concrete. On average, antidepressants or mood stabilizers have effects in 50 percent of patients in trials, whereas the placebo has comparable effects in 40 percent (see figure 4.1).[105] This is taken to mean that the drug works. And the money and culture in medicine follow this message.

But consider what makes for a placebo response. The natural history of mood disorders means that many will improve within a few weeks whether treated or not. It is also widely thought that sensible clinical advice on matters of diet, life-style, alcohol intake, and work and relationship problem solving may make a difference. It is suspected that patients' perceptions that they are being cared for by a medical expert may make a difference, and this effect may be enhanced by being given a substance they think will restore some chemical balance to normal—even if that imbalance is mythical and the substance is a placebo. The fact that the patients present themselves for treatment may also make a difference. All of these factors are reflected in the placebo response. But it is not possible to quantify the distinct contribution of these components—how much, for example, the natural history of the disorder contributes compared to advice about life-style.

The very same factors also contribute to the response for those on an active drug. But in contrast to the difficulties in quantifying the components of the placebo response, RCTs allow us to quantify the contribution made by the drug. In figure 4.1, four out of five, or 80 percent, of the treated patients would have improved had they received the placebo. One out of ten respond specifically to the drug, whereas two in every five respond to placebo—and at much less risk of side effects. If the money and culture in psychia-

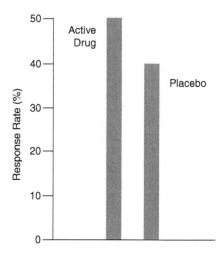

Figure 4.1
Antidepressant Rating-Scale-Based Response Rates: Drug versus Placebo

Source: The data for this figure come from an FDA review of all antidepressant placebo-controlled trials. Stone M, Jones L (2006). Clinical Review: Relationship between antidepressant drugs and adult suicidality, p. 31. www.fda.gov/ohrms/dockets/ac/06/briefing/2006-4272b1-index.htm

try followed the evidence, we should try to enhance the placebo response rather than try to ensure everyone is put on treatment.

Doctors and patients think they see one in two responding to the drug, and this seems impressive. They treat the results from antidepressant trials as though these drugs worked in a manner equivalent to penicillin in fulminant pneumonia. If a doctor failed to give penicillin in a case of pneumonia, or activated charcoal for strychnine poisoning or insulin for a diabetic, relying on their bedside manner to do the trick, most of us would be quick to sue if things went wrong. But, of course, RCTs are not needed for treatments like penicillin in a case of pneumonia, where patients who should die get up off their bed and walk, as do catatonic patients treated with barbiturates or ECT. We need RCTs primarily when it is uncertain if a treatment has an effect.

In fact, the situation is even worse in that in trials of mood stabilizers and antidepressants there are also five people who do not respond to either the drug or the placebo. Thus, in any sample of ten patients, with drugs like the mood stabilizers, the clinical trial data suggest one responds to the drug while nine do not. In preferentially accepting RCTs over case reports, journals seem to be making two mistakes. First, all of the major discoveries in medicine have involved case vignettes from Hippocrates through to Cade's ten patients on lithium, and on through the thirty-eight responses to chlorpromazine described by Delay and Deniker and the forty patients responding to imipramine described by Roland Kuhn to the patients being treated for cardiovascular conditions who noticed an interesting side effect caused by Viagra. The breakthroughs as regards new syndromes, new treatments, and new hazards still involve case reports, and if they fail to take these reports, journals are likely to miss out.

But of equal importance, while rejecting case reports as anecdotal, by preferentially taking RCTs of drugs like the psychotropic drugs given to mongrel syndromes like those recruited to clinical trials, journals are privileging the experiences of the one specific drug responder over the ninefold larger pool of other responders or nonresponders. They are engaged in a more problematic anecdotalism, in that RCTs garland these atypical responses with a claim that they will generalize to others given the treatment in a way that was never claimed for traditional medical case reports.

Michael Shepherd's first trial published in 1955 in which he demonstrated reserpine was an antidepressant provides a wonderful symbol for the changing character of medical journals and the new pitfalls of evidence-based medicine.[106] Shepherd undertook this trial, stimulated by reports of patients with hypertension feeling better than well on reserpine. The trial would have transformed psychopharmacology—had its results registered.[107] There might not have been any Prozac and certainly would not have been ideas about serotonin deficiency or chemical imbalances, as reserpine lowers serotonin levels and was an antidepressant. Shepherd put the failure of the study to register down to the fact that clinicians had never seen anything like it. The focus on statistics and the effects of a drug on a group rather than its effects on individual patients was unprecedented in a scientific article.[108]

But reserpine was also used as an antihypertensive, and, in fact, the two articles in the *Lancet* preceding Shepherd's article re-

ported on patients with hypertension becoming suicidal on reserpine.[109] Reserpine can induce an agitated state called akathisia, a
then unknown complication of treatment, in which patients can
become suicidal or homicidal. The case reports of this new hazard
were compelling. It was these and other case reports that gave rise
to the notion of a chemical imbalance in depression.

The point here is that this combination of trials and case series
points to the fact that reserpine suits some people but not others.
The science from this point on should have been about attempting to tease out who responds to reserpine and what implications
this might have for our understanding of psychiatric syndromes.
But this is not what happened. Where once clinicians paid no
heed to RCTs because they could not understand them, now they
pay no heed to case reports because they cannot understand them.
Case reports of hazards and patients getting worse on treatment
are dismissed because RCTs have proved the treatment works.

With the triumph of RCTs, everything to do with them has
taken on a reflected validity, including rating scales. In the case
of the lithium trials, Schou at least looked at actual recurrences,
rehospitalizations, and dead bodies in the lithium and placebo
groups. Current trials of antidepressants, antipsychotics, and
mood stabilizers are short term and rely on rating scales to assess
outcomes. Scales can assess function in four broad domains—the
disease specific domain as rated by the clinician and as rated by
the patient and then the nonspecific domain of global functioning, again from both clinical and patient points of view. Treatments that work should demonstrate benefits across all these domains, but no psychotropic drug does. The benefits that lead to
drugs being licensed show up almost solely on clinician-rated,
disease-specific scales. Therefore, strictly speaking it should be acknowledged that treatments have been shown to have effects that
are apparent only from someone's point of view.[110]

The problem this suggests is compounded by the fact that
when it comes to dead bodies in current psychotropic trials, there
are a greater number of them in the active treatment groups than
in the placebo groups. This is quite different from what happens
in penicillin trials or trials of drugs that really work.

Rating scales are abstractions from clinical practice. They are now being imported into health care on the basis that they will reduce variability in the clinical encounter and make that encounter more scientific. Health care practitioners are encouraged to administer mania, depression, or other behavioral rating scales when seeing patients, and as we shall see in chapters 6 and 7, patients are now also being encouraged to mood-watch using rating scales because companies know that such data will lead to treatment.

The hazards of taking measurement technologies like these out of clinical trial context are multiple but rarely acknowledged. A majority of rating scales within the behavioral domain are simply checklists. Far from being information rich, they are information poor. The main advantage likely to accrue from their use is to ensure that a number of possibly irrelevant questions are checked off as asked. In time-limited clinical exchanges, if these questions are asked, other more important questions are likely to be sacrificed. The clinical gaze is captured by those whose interests are served by the measurement technology. Pharmaceutical companies understand this very well and now run symposia devoted entirely to introducing clinicians to rating scales that the company expects will lead to increased sales of their drugs.

Second, while rating scales generate data, when reliance is put on such data there is an informational reductionism that is probably doing more to dehumanize clinical exchanges than the biological reductionism more commonly complained about. If specific measurements lead to an oversight for context or for other dimensions of an individual's functioning or situation that are not open to measurement, or that are simply not being measured, we are not being modestly scientific by measuring what we can; we are being pseudoscientific.

Third, the abstraction, or informational reductionism, that rating scales bring with them has a double-edged potential. Having figures for weight can allow us to plot norms for healthy weight, and the feedback from such figures can offer potent feedback in a weight-reducing program. But while this is the case, the figures can also seduce both patient and clinician. In the absence of figures from other areas of a person's life, against which the figures for weight can be put in context, the risk for the patient is that the figures for weight will come to dominate their concerns, establishing a neurosis. The risk for the clinician is that she will treat the figures rather than the person, but we do not pathologize a clinician's figure-centeredness.

The proponents of evidence-based medicine follow Shepherd in their skepticism of industry. They see trials as a means of reining in the pharmaceutical industry, but in fact, as the next four chapters will show, industry has commandeered RCTs for marketing purposes. Failure to appreciate what is at issue leads psychiatrists to think that RCTs establish specific facts as solidly as cultures in a petri dish allowed Koch to link specific germs to particular infections and that established facts are now being piled on established facts, when no such progress is actually being made. The insistence on specificity and belief in progress in the face of uncertainty has all the hallmarks of the rigidity that led millennia of physicians to advocate bloodletting in the face of a looming epidemic.

In the years just before he died, Shepherd's view of RCTs turned inside out. From once championing their role in showing whether treatments worked, he moved to arguing that they showed how little psychotropic drugs in fact did and how much was placebo effect.[111] Just months before he died, he described the current investment in evidence-based medicine as close to a fetish: yet another simplistic solution to the complex problems thrown up by psychiatry rather than a genuine solution that gets at the heart of the problems.[112] And he increasingly came to blame Emil Kraepelin for modern psychiatry's focus on specific disease entities that in his opinion had put a destructive premium on specific treatments.[113]

CHAPTER FIVE

The Eclipse
of Manic-Depressive Disorder

❀ ❀ ❀

In much the way that politicians give their name to periods—for example, the Reagan era or Thatcherism—so Kraepelin put his stamp on twentieth-century psychiatry. When a "paradigm" such as Thatcherism or Kraepelinism is established, the person who was once perhaps first among equals, but no more than that, removes the spotlight of history from other gifted contemporaries. The "ism" can take on a life of its own, sometimes incorporating things that its progenitor might have radically disagreed with.

Whereas combinations of symptoms and course can produce cases that defy classification, nevertheless, when an entire set of hospital records is reviewed, the majority of cases fall relatively cleanly, as Kraepelin argued, into those which run a remitting course and those which show an enduring disability. But within the remitting disorders, there are cases that appear to have many of the symptoms of schizophrenia. This group has been the recipient of a profusion of diagnoses, including schizoaffective disorder, reactive psychoses, and cycloid psychoses. Within manic-depressive disease, there is also bipolar disorder, a syndrome Kraepelin explicitly rejected as a distinct illness. But a century after it was first described, bipolar disorder came back on the radar linked to the fortunes of lithium. It is to bipolar and the other cycloid disorders we now turn.

THE LONG WAR: WERNICKE AND KRAEPELIN

Although Kraepelin is a towering figure now, in Germany at the turn of the century he operated in the shadow of Karl Wernicke. Born in 1848, Wernicke studied medicine in Breslau before succeeding one of the greatest names in early German psychiatry, Heinrich Neumann, to the chair of psychiatry and neurology in Breslau. His accession to the chair at a very young age was based on his extraordinary discovery in 1874 of a receptive speech area in the brain, now called Wernicke's area. This discovery came from investigations into patients with strokes and other cerebral injuries, during which he noted that people with injuries of the left parietal lobe of the brain were able to speak normally but unable to understand speech. Wernicke's discovery came hard on the heels of Paul Broca's discovery in Paris of a motor speech center, now called Broca's area, damage to which left patients able to understand speech and think of what they wanted to say but unable to utter words coherently. Broca's and Wernicke's twin discoveries supported a newly emerging vision of how the brain worked, which claimed that cerebral functions were localized, a notion that was deeply controversial at the time.

This discovery led Wernicke to suspect that the psychoses would also turn out to be localized to brain areas. The new "localizers" had rapidly made huge inroads in linking vision to the optical cortex, hearing to the auditory cortex, and motor functions to a motor strip. But in between these primary sensory and motor areas, there are huge areas, which began to be called the association cortices. Wernicke and others suggested that in these areas sensory inputs were assembled into higher cognitive constructs. And it was to these areas that Wernicke turned for a site for the psychoses.

He had a model of brain functioning similar to that of Laycock and Jackson in Britain, based on the notion that mental functioning comprised nested sets of psychic reflex arcs. Clinicians from Wernicke and Freud to the present have ever been prone to press the latest biological research into the service of a clinical vision in what can perhaps best be called a biological heuristic. In Wernicke's case, this heuristic led to the notion that mental disorder might involve a literal loosening of the association fibers forming these reflex arcs. One of the key symptoms such a lesion might be expected to give rise to was perplexity, a symptom present in the cycloid psychoses, a symptom heavily stressed by localizers ever since.

This effort to localize the psychoses was not a forlorn exercise. Wernicke had triumphs to add to his discovery of the receptive speech area. In 1881 he described a disorder called Wernicke-Korsakoff psychosis. First described by Sergei Korsakoff in 1877, and linked to alcoholism, this mental disorder shows memory disturbances, confusion, and perplexity as well as motor disturbances, all consistent with a disturbance of associations. And it is now clear that this disorder does stem from a very specific local defect caused by thiamine deficiency, trauma, hemorrhages, tumors, or other brain disorders.

Like Kraepelin, Wernicke was influenced by Kahlbaum, but in quite a different way from Kraepelin. Noting catatonia came in underactive and overactive forms, Wernicke began referring to the motility psychoses. When it came to mood disorders, he also followed Kahlbaum in distinguishing between mood disorders rather than grouping them, and he especially stressed cyclothymia. Finally, in 1895, he described a further disorder—an anxiety psychosis.

Wernicke argued that while Kraepelin's emphasis on the course of the illness was important, psychiatry had to distinguish among mental disorders on the basis of more than course. Too great an insistence on the course of the illness to the neglect of all other clinical features was unnecessarily rigid. For Wernicke, symptoms that pointed to a possible brain localization came first and tracking the course of any resulting disorders came second. Kraepelin dismissed this as brain mythology.

The only time Wernicke and Kraepelin appear to have met was at a meeting of East German psychiatrists in Leubus in 1890. Kraepelin had just started on the trip that took him to North Wales. Kahlbaum was also there—with Wernicke. Kraepelin seems to have had no more than an introduction to him.[1]

Contrary to perceptions now, Kraepelin at the time was in the position of the outsider in Germany. In Britain up to 1950, there were only two chairs in psychiatry, one in London and one in Edinburgh, neither of which was filled by a man with any expertise in brain sciences. In Germany, twenty-one chairs of psychiatry had been filled by 1880, almost all of them by neuropsychiatrists, most of whom sided with Wernicke rather than Kraepelin. Commenting on this imbalance in 1918, Kraepelin wrote: "Discoveries relating to the anatomy of the brain contributed less than might have been expected to the science of psychiatry. Nevertheless, it was considered so important that chairs of psychiatry were occupied by men who had previously devoted all their attention to the physiology or anatomy of the brain." He went on to say: "This proves that psychiatry needed to be put on a firmer scientific basis; it also indicates that the importance of clinical practice was underrated."[2]

He could make this comment later. Around 1903, he was Wernicke's junior, with no original discoveries to his name and only a textbook to his credit. While the textbook now seems important, textbooks in the absence of any other discovery have never been seen as the hallmarks of creativity. Then in 1903 he moved to Munich. Meanwhile, Eduard Hitzig, who had been one of the foremost brain researchers in Germany and chair of psychiatry in Halle, slipped into a diabetic coma. Wernicke was approached to fill Hitzig's chair and arrived in Halle in 1904. A year later while out riding he was hit by a falling tree. Kraepelin's path lay open.

His competitor was eclipsed but not by any achievement of Kraepelin's. By 1920 it was clear that Kraepelin's focus on clinical practice had not led to the discovery of disease causes either—despite the presence of Alzheimer and Nissl in Munich. His clinical method simply did not work as well as he expected: "We have to live with the fact that the criteria applied by us are not sufficient to differentiate reliably in all cases between schizophrenia and manic depressive insanity and there are also many overlaps in this area."[3] Had it not been for the impression that he was seeking to localize diseases that his laboratories gave him, Kraepelin would have been in a very marginal position indeed in early twentieth-century Germany.

Nevertheless, around this time, Kraepelin still wrote that "the etiology of insanity profited but little from the progress of science, mainly because no serious attempt was made to relate a particular type of insanity to a specific cause. This was due in part to the absence of any clear-cut definition of the different types of mental illness. Classification was generally accomplished on the basis of symptoms alone, not the underlying processes responsible for the disease. Thus, even in the systems of men like Meynert and Wernicke, etiological considerations were brushed aside."[4]

Although only briefly at Halle, Wernicke had passed his torch to a junior assistant, a twenty-four-year-old from Alsace called Karl Kleist.[5] After Wernicke's death, Kleist moved to study in Munich with Kraepelin. But his formative experience came as a medical officer in the First World War, where he dealt with head injuries. What he saw convinced him that the conventional view that brain trauma gave rise to nonspecific psychosyndromes was wrong and that the injuries were often better explained in terms of localized disturbances.

In 1920 he was appointed the professor of psychiatry in Frankfurt. Once established there, he disinterred Kahlbaum's catatonia and hebephrenia from the schizophrenia in which Kraepelin had buried them. He resurrected Wernicke's notions of motility and anxiety psychoses and added in a new state—confusion psychosis. These three states led in 1926 to the concept of the cycloid psychoses—a set of states intermediate between but distinguishable from both schizophrenia and manic-depressive illness that came in the form of motility, anxiety, or confusion psychoses.[6]

Kleist also distinguished between monoform and multiform disorders. Some disorders present essentially the same way every time—these were the monoform or unipolar disorders. Others presented quite differently every time, and these were multipolar disorders. But Kleist's contribution on the genesis of multipolarity was distinctive. Within his framework, both mania and depression could be unipolar disorders—and, while rare, there are unquestionably some unipolar manias. Patients ended up with multipolar disorders when they had more than one disease—both mania and depression, for instance. If they have two disorders, the implication was that the genetic loading should be greater.

This line of thought is very much like arguing that there are two disorders, bronchitis and asthma, and that, while clinicians occasionally see pure forms of either of these, many clinical presentations, especially in hospital settings, involve variable mixtures of the two conditions. In this sense, Kleist was arguing for a series of manic-depressive syndromes rather than manic-depressive illness.

Such thinking led to ideas that the risk for psychosis might have a separate genetic coding, so that some people might get depressed or manic without becoming psychotic, whereas others with an extra genetic loading when depressed, manic, or schizophrenic would also become psychotic. All of this is quite consistent with modern genetic findings for these disorders.[7]

Kleist was joined in Frankfurt in 1935 by Karl Leonhard, who more than anyone else disseminated these ideas.[8] In 1957, after he had moved to Berlin, Leonhard developed Kleist's three cycloid psychoses—anxiety, motility, and confusion. The motility psychoses were multipolar in that they came in underactive and overactive forms, and the confusion psychoses came in forms in which incoherence alternated with lucidity, while the anxiety psychoses often showed a swing from anxiety to an excessive happiness or elation that could be distinguished from the euphoria of manic-depressive illness. Delusions when present in these states were often fleeting. The clinical picture tended to be very unstable and to show shifts from day to day. Right from the start, he picked out one group of patients as having a much higher proportion of cycloid disorders than others—women with postpartum psychoses. This group was—and is—truly multiform, often varying kaleidoscopically from day to day.

Whereas Kleist saw multipolar clinical syndromes, Leonhard saw a series of discrete disease entities. Whereas Kleist had been interested in the neurological underpinning of these disorders, Leonhard focused more on the genetics. Patients who had a history of mania, he argued, also had family histories of relatives affected by manic episodes. Patients with a history of recurrent unipolar depression had family histories that included depression but not mania.[9]

Leonhard's monopolar or recurrent unipolar depression is a concept very different from major depressive disorder as it is diagnosed now, and it would be a mistake to think that Leonhard was contrasting bipolar disorders with major depressive disorders. The modern concept of major depressive disorder includes what was once termed endogenous depression but also neurotic depressions, which up to 1980 were largely seen as a form of mixed depressive anxiety disorders. These anxiety states are far more likely to be chronic states than recurrent mood disorders are likely to be, and they will necessarily have a quite different heredity from either bipolar or recurrent unipolar mood disorders.

Monoform or unipolar forms of depression for Leonhard presented similarly on all occasions. Thus certain forms of paranoid schizophrenia that maintained the same presentation throughout or the systematized schizophrenias fell under the unipolar heading. So also did involutional melancholia and some forms of endogenous depression.

In this system, involutional melancholia, the disorder that had caused Kraepelin such trouble, played a key role. This disorder of the middle to later years presented in an entirely typical way with very little variation between people. Individuals displayed the classic features of anorexia, insomnia, retardation, and agitation, with these features often linked to a development of nihilistic or guilt-laden delusions. This form of depression did appear to be quite different from that with which younger people presented to the asylum system, which often appeared anxious in one episode, neurasthenic in another, before presenting later with a manic episode. In addition to having a different presentation, involutional melancholia seemed completely unlikely to transmute into mania, and many of these subjects had no prior history of mood disorder before their middle years.

In contrast to a disorder like this, unsystematized schizophrenias or mood disorders in which the presentations might be entirely different from one admission to the next, were better seen as multiform or bipolar disorders.

Compared with Kraepelin, therefore, there were a number of classificatory principles built into Leonhard's system. One was the criterion of remission. A second was the possibility of recurrences. The recurrent disorders could be broken down into conditions with periodic recurrences versus other conditions. A third criterion was whether there was consistency in the clinical presentations across recurrences. The upshot of all this was a system that baffles all but the converted.

The complexity of Leonhard's work was one reason why it remained unknown outside Germany. Another was the isolation of German psychiatry following the war. A third reason was the emphasis on genetics inherent in Leonhard's thinking. The postwar years were ones when nurture had triumphed over nature, and the inclination was to trace the root of mental disorders to disturbances of social conditions rather than to faulty genes.[10]

Finally, Leonhard's and Kleist's work remained untranslated. Some of Leonhard's work was translated but inaccurately. Not until 1999 was a proper version available. Such setbacks were not much different from the fates of Bleuler, Kraepelin, Jaspers, and others whose work took decades to appear in English, but by the time Leonhard's work appeared, the international classificatory mold had been set. A new way of thinking if it had been easy to understand might still have made inroads—but Leonhard's work was not easy to understand.

THE BIRTH OF BIPOLAR DISORDER

In 1966 Jules Angst[11] and Carlo Perris,[12] stimulated by Kleist's and Leonhard's notion that mania ran in families, published studies that appeared to support the independent existence of a bipolar mood disorder. Reading the bipolar disorder literature now suggests these studies were immediately seized upon as seminal. They were not.

Perris was more influenced by Leonhard than Angst, and his study was an explicit test of Leonhard's hypothesis. His monograph was more accessible, as it appeared in an English-language journal. Angst came to the issue as a consequence of the data he had collected, with no preconceptions in mind. He published in German. But both bodies of work coincided with the reintroduction of lithium and interacted with the possibility that there might be something distinctive about lithium treatment for manic-depressive illness.

Carlo Perris was born in Cosenza, Italy, in 1928. His father was an oculist. He went into medicine and qualified in 1951. Aware that his chances of a university career in Italy were minimal, as he had no people supporting him, an absolute necessity at that time, Perris decided to go to America. But while waiting for a visa, he got a letter from a friend who had gone to Sweden, and in 1960 he went to Sweden instead.

Based at the Sidsjöns Sjukhus in Sundsvall, he began his field-work on bipolar disorders. Having worked in Sundsvall for some years, he contacted Jan-Otto Ottosson at the University of Umeå in the north of Sweden, who was then emerging as a leading figure in Swedish psychiatry. Ottosson supervised the research, and Perris later moved to Umeå and was offered the chair there in 1971 when Ottosson moved to Göteborg.

In his monograph, Perris compared what is now called bipolar depression with the recurrent unipolar depressions that were once called involutional melancholia or endogenous depression. Leonhard claimed these conditions should be genetically different. Perris appeared to confirm this claim but not in any dramatic fashion. Bipolar patients were more likely to have relatives who also had a bipolar disorder, whereas unipolar patients were more likely to have a relative who had unipolar disorder. But the proposal did not hold up for unipolar mania.

There were more traumatic episodes in the childhoods of bipolar than unipolar patients and unipolar depressives were more likely to have a somatic trigger to their initial episode. Unipolar cases that came from broken or traumatic childhood backgrounds had an earlier onset of their illness. Both celibacy and divorce were more common in the bipolar groups.

Perris gave all his subjects a personality inventory, and bipolar patients scored higher on a factor called substability or cyclothymia. Unipolar patients scored higher on a factor called subvalidity, or neuroticism. None of this was remarkable. And across a range of physical body measures and neuropsychological tests, then thought to link to personality, there were no differences between bipolars and unipolars.[13] When bipolar and unipolar depressions were compared with neurotic (or reactive) depressions, on some measures the bipolars and unipolars were similar to each other and different from the neurotic depressions. These results led Perris to certain conclusions:

To explain the difference in test situations between bipolar and unipolar patients, the difference between them in personality qualities may be relevant. . . . Without additional information, bipolar and unipolar depressive psychoses could be expressions of the same illness with different colouring due to the patho-plastic influence of the personality. The higher mortality rate in bipolar patients than in unipolar patients can also be explained hypothetically by differences in personality structure. . . .

[But] the genetic part of the investigation shows however that the heredity is different between the two groups and, besides, specific within each group. This argues against the hypothesis that bipolar and unipolar psychoses are different expressions of the same illness, and supports the view that they are two dif-ferent nosographic entities. It would thus seem reasonable to assume that one inherits partly a specific tendency to disease, which determines the form and course of the illness, and partly a particular biological substratum which determines personality qualities to a large extent, and the type of reaction to various test situations.[14]

This summary reflects quite well current understandings of the genetics of disorders like postpartum psychoses and bipolar disorders. Increasingly, it appears that genes may code for the form in which a condition will present, and these may be quite separate from the genes that code for vulnerability to trigger fac-tors.[15] But this possibility does not establish that these disorders are distinct, any more than tuberculosis of the gut is a different disease than respiratory tuberculosis.

The bottom line is that there were minimal differences be-tween bipolar and classic unipolar depressive psychoses. As re-gards treatment, bipolar patients showed a greater tendency to relapse when treated with a combination of electroconvulsive therapy (ECT) and psychotropic drugs than when treated with other methods.

Slightly older than Perris, Jules Angst was born in Zurich on December 11, 1926. Angst's bipolar study involved 326 patients treated in Zurich, culled from a larger sample of consecutive ad-missions between 1959 and 1963. He reported that genetic and environmental factors have a synergistic impact on the etiology of endogenous depression.[16] Whereas men and women were equally represented among those experiencing bipolar depressions, female gender was more likely to lead to endogenous depression. He concluded that unipolar depression, including involutional melancholia, differed significantly from bipolar disorders in terms of genetics, gender, course, and premorbid personality.

Angst's study was in German and, although published a few months before Perris's study, was accordingly later in coming to the attention of the non-German-speaking world. But even within the German-speaking world, when he took the findings to Manfred Bleuler, Eric Strömgren, and Aubrey Lewis, the leading figures in European psychiatry, he was told that it was inconceivable that Kraepelin's manic-depressive illness could be wrong.

And in fact neither of these studies was compelling. Neither offered any pointers as to how a clinician might differentiate between a unipolar and a bipolar depression that had not yet thrown up a manic episode. When patients were depressed, both conditions looked identical. There was no suggestion here that they should not be treated with identical medications, except perhaps for the addition of lithium.

In terms of classification, Kraepelin's system remained the easiest. Take a woman with a psychotic depression in her twenties who gets treatment with ECT, and remains well on antidepressants and antipsychotics, only to have another treatment responsive episode in her thirties and again in her forties and fifties, until finally in her sixties she has a manic episode. In Kraepelin's system, there is no problem classifying this woman from the start— she has manic-depressive illness. If she is now to be considered a case of bipolar disorder, when does her bipolar disorder start? If bipolar disorders are to be treated with mood stabilizers rather than antidepressants, have we any reason to think forty years of treatment as though she were unipolar had done any harm to this woman? Could treatment have caused a "new" illness?

BECOMING BIPOLAR

The studies of Angst and Perris came on stream just as the first serious efforts to investigate the catecholamine hypothesis of depression got under way. This hypothesis, put forward by Joseph Schildkraut in 1965, proposed that there was a chemical imbalance in depression.[17] Between its initial and later incarnation as a serotonin hypothesis of depression, this notion has dominated contemporary consciousness for the past forty years in the way Freud's notions of libido did for the forty years prior to that.

The hypothesis saw mood disorders as something not dissimilar from inborn errors of metabolism like phenylketonuria (see chapter 4). The research response seemed clear. Investigate everything conceivably related to catecholamine or serotonin metabolism going into the body and everything coming out, and the answer to what was wrong in mood disorders should lie in the difference. The enterprise caught the imagination of the nascent biological psychiatry research community and led to the setting up of a Collaborative Research Study on Depressive Disorders in 1969 at the National Institute of Mental Health (NIMH).[18]

But it quickly became clear that investigating a hypothesis like the catecholamine hypothesis called for greater specificity in the delineation of nervous disorders than was then customary in American psychiatry. One of the first outcomes of this research program therefore was agreement on the need for the creation of operational criteria, the first set of which was published in 1975.[19] The biology of this twenty-year research program produced nothing, but as agreement on the need for operational criteria gave rise to *DSM-III*, this research program must be seen as one of the more culturally significant ever.

The kinds of distinctions that seemed needed were exactly like the distinction between bipolar and unipolar depression that Angst and Perris had identified. However, this particular distinction did not initially look very promising—for instance, to Eli Robins and Sam Guze of Washington University in St. Louis, who were more impressed with a need to distinguish between primary and secondary or endogenous and reactive or neurotic and psychotic depressions.[20] But there was agreement that the principle of collecting homogeneous groups of patients with a very similar disorder, which also appeared to run in their families, seemed to increase the chance of being able to find a biochemical needle in the clinical haystack.

As this research program rolled out through the 1970s and 1980s, the persisting failure to find a biochemical source was increasingly attributed to the failure of clinicians to make fine enough distinctions between the various subtypes of mood disorders. Successive failures put a premium on differentiating ever further subtypes of mood disorders.

The early driving force behind the classificatory side of the project came from the Washington University Department of Psychiatry, where Robins and Guze had created in the early 1960s perhaps the only bastion of biological psychiatry in the United States.[21] Though believers in biological psychiatry, the department's researchers had little belief in drug treatments for psychiatric disorders. The main research plank was follow-up studies of patients and family history studies—a politically acceptable way to bring the issue of genetics into the frame in the 1960s. One of the St. Louis group, George Winokur,[22] took a particular interest in manic-depressive illness and, using the family study method in 1967, reported findings that overlapped with those of Perris and Angst.[23] In a 1969 book, he and colleagues introduced the new bipolar-unipolar distinction to a wider American frame of reference,[24] at just the time when lithium was becoming a cause célèbre in U.S. psychopharmacology.

But where the unipolar-bipolar distinction might have initially seemed a necessary clarification for research purposes, problems began to emerge. It was one thing to allocate patients who had been hospitalized with mania to a bipolar group and those hospitalized only with depression to a unipolar group, but what about those hospitalized only for depression who had evidence of milder manic episodes that had not led to hospitalization? In 1976 David Dunner, formerly of St. Louis[25] and later of NIMH, but at this point working with Ron Fieve in Columbia,[26] suggested distinguishing between bipolar I and bipolar II disorders.[27] Bipolar I disorders referred to patients who had been hospitalized for both depressive and manic episodes. Bipolar II disorders involved patients who had been hospitalized for depression and who had also had hypomanic episodes that had not led to hospitalization. Dunner and colleagues claimed that these were separate groups of patients and that both groups bred true.

This distinction was later supported by Hagop Akiskal,[28] Jean Endicott,[29] William Coryell,[30] and others. Akiskal took the next logical step and began talking about patients who had both depressive and hypomanic episodes, neither of which might have required hospitalization. Bipolar II was evolving into a concept that overlapped significantly with borderline personality disorder, substance abuse disorders, and many others. Within the major depressive disorder group, patients of the kind that might formerly have been thought of as depressive neurotics could also be interpreted as meeting these new criteria for bipolar II disorders.

Bipolar II had only just been mooted when in 1978 the ninth edition of the *International Classification of Diseases* (*ICD 9*) came out. This edition continued to classify all mood disorders as affective psychoses, offering the further possibility to distinguish between circular and depressive types of affective psychosis. In contrast, in 1980 *DSM-III* became the first classification system to distinguish formally between bipolar and unipolar mood disorders.

It may seem ironic that *DSM-III*, now widely portrayed as a neo-Kraepelinian manifesto, should have contained a feature at clear odds with Kraepelin's position. In fact, the St. Louis group behind *DSM-III* felt uncomfortable with the branding exercise that led to them being seen as neo-Kraepelinian. The notion of neo-Kraepelinism had begun in fact as something of a joke—a joke that stuck.[31]

The *DSM* was in fact almost anti-Kraepelinian when it came to manic-depressive illness. It set in place the conditions that have led to a wholesale relabeling of American patients as bipolar. Where earlier classifications had viewed cyclothymia in terms of a personality type, *DSM-III* made it a disorder.[32] And in between bipolar II and cyclothymia, *DSM* inserted bipolar disorder NOS (not otherwise specified), so that anyone with a touch of what their clinician felt might be bipolarity could be included.

Outside formal classification systems, Akiskal and others outlined states they termed bipolar II½, bipolar III, bipolar III½, bipolar IV, bipolar V, and bipolar VI disorders.[33] There was also widespread reference to bipolar spectrum disorders and even to soft bipolar spectrums. Many considered that all personality problems might have a bipolar affective instability at their heart and should be treated vigorously as though they were bipolar.[34] Jules Angst and others described conditions variously called recurrent brief depressive disorder[35] and later recurrent brief hypomania,[36] which for most American clinicians still seemed better diagnosed as borderline personality disorder—and which many European psychiatrists following Sydenham might have diagnosed as hysteria (chapter 1).

As this was happening, estimates for the prevalence of manic-depressive illness and then bipolar disorder were changing dramatically. From the 1870s to the 1960s, new cases of the bipolar form of manic-depressive illness that involved a hospitalization for mania had occurred in Europe at a rate of ten new cases per million of the population, giving a prevalence of the condition at less than 0.1 percent of the population. In the United States the prevalence was even less, if only by virtue of the fact that most of those who could have been diagnosed manic-depressive in fact were diagnosed as schizophrenic.

The introduction of lithium led to a first change in U.S. prevalence estimates.[37] In 1985 the first big American epidemiological study, following on the path blazed by Shepherd in the mid-1960s, the Epidemiologic Catchment Area study, reported that 1 percent of the population had bipolar I or II disorder.[38] By this time even bipolar I criteria had loosened, so that patients could be diagnosed as bipolar I if they had a significant episode of mania—one that need not have led to hospitalization but did, in the opinion of the investigator, entail disability. On this basis, the National Comorbidity Study reporting in 1994 estimated that 1.3 percent of the American population had bipolar I disorder alone.[39] By 1998 Angst was reporting that 5 percent of the population had bipolar disorder of one or another sort.[40]

The Epidemiologic Catchment Area study of bipolar disorder threw up an issue that has never since been resolved. There was criticism that the estimates of bipolar disorders were wildly overinflated and, in particular, that leaving a decision as to whether there had been a manic episode to the judgment of a lay questioner with no prior training in mental illness could not be scientifically justified.[41] The argument is that symptoms without some evidence of disability cannot be the basis for claiming illness.[42] The response from Robert Spitzer, the architect of *DSM-III*, has been that we should not be so surprised to find so many people have psychiatric disorders—population surveys would find that more than half the population had a physical illness in any one year, albeit perhaps only influenza.[43]

In general, figures like this play to the division between the business and science aspects of medicine. Figures pointing to 15 percent lifetime suicide rates in depression or 5 percent of the population being bipolar are good commercially for both physicians and pharmaceutical companies, but they may be bad science.[44] Critiques of such approaches, however, have little influence. As of 2005, epidemiological studies continued to indicate that most Americans would be mentally ill at some point. In response, Dr. Paul McHugh, emeritus professor of psychiatry and former chairman of psychiatry at Johns Hopkins said: "Pretty soon, we'll have a syndrome for short, fat Irish guys with a Boston accent, and I'll be mentally ill."[45] In the face of such scorn, there must be powerful vested interests for findings like this to continue to command center stage in the public debate.

Bipolar disorder became fashionable in another way also. Kay Redfield Jamison, a professor of psychology at Johns Hopkins University, in a book *Touched by Fire,* presented a case that many poets of the nineteenth and twentieth centuries had manic-depressive illness, as had a large number of writers, composers, and artists.[46] She followed this work with a compelling autobiography, *An Unquiet Mind,* detailing her own manic-depressive illness.[47]

These books followed in a tradition linking mental illness with creativity that stemmed from Plato and Alexander Pope, who noted: "Great wits are to madness near allied." Another early exponent of the linkage was Havelock Ellis: "The prevailing temperament of men of genius is one of great nervous sensitivity and irritability," with a tendency to melancholia.[48] Freudians,[49] as well as those interested in the social origins of mental illness[50] and now biological psychiatrists, have all seemed keen to play this game.

Through the early 1990s, the dominant link between illness and madness was to schizophrenia.[51] Jamison's work usurped this order of things, and manic-depressive illness took the place of schizophrenia. However, there are good grounds to remain skeptical of all proposed links, whether to manic-depressive illness or to schizophrenia. Van Gogh and Schumann, who are typically offered up in this context, probably had neurosyphilis,[52] which is also a relapsing and remitting illness that will give pictures of individuals who at times appear to be depressed and at other times appear to be euphoric and indeed grandiose. But where Jamison's book was tentative, characterizations linking genius to manic-depressive illness based on her book have been marketed vigorously by companies selling mood stabilizers in the late 1990s, whose patient information leaflets, for instance, typically contained lists several pages long of all the artists who had supposedly "confirmed" manic-depressive illness.

As of 2000, the word manic-depressive had all but vanished from the American clinical map. This vanishing began in the mid-1990s. When Fred Goodwin and Kay Jamison published the largest monograph on the disorder in 1990, it was entitled *Manic-Depressive Illness.*[53] Jamison's 1993 and 1995 books also referred to manic-depressive illness rather than bipolar disorder. It took the development and marketing of mood stabilizers for everyone to become bipolar. This process began in 1995, when Abbott Laboratories received a license for valproate for the treatment of mania (chapter 6).

There is now an extraordinary amnesia about this change. Clinicians and the public seem unaware that the picture was so different just a few years earlier and that the term bipolar disorder would have been meaningless to most people until very recently. In part, this amnesia must stem from the assiduous promulgation of a message that bipolar disorder was nothing new—that everything had been well recognized as far back as the Greeks.

THE CYCLOID PSYCHOSES

Whereas Jules Angst embraced and pushed forward the unipolar-bipolar dichotomy, his 1966 twin Carlo Perris traveled in a different direction. Perris became increasingly interested in the cycloid psychoses, which provide an interesting foil to bipolar disorder.

There are as many people admitted to hospital for what could be diagnosed as a cycloid psychosis as there once were for bipolar I disorder when the latter required hospitalization for a diagnosis.

In a series of articles from 1974 to 1990, Perris repeated for the cycloid psychoses what he had done for bipolar disorder.[54] When *DSM-III* introduced the vogue for operational criteria, Perris provided operational criteria for the new disorder.[55] It should be of acute onset and in subjects between ages fifteen and fifty, should not be linked to drug use or trauma, and should show at least four of the following in a multiform picture: confusion-perplexity, mood incongruent delusions, hallucinatory experiences, overwhelming pananxiety, happiness/ecstasy with religious overtones, motility disturbances, mood swings but to a lesser extent than found in affective disorder, and a concern about death.

One of his primary coauthors in this work was Ian Brockington, a professor of psychiatry in Birmingham, England. Brockington was the foremost authority on postpartum psychoses.[56] This interest made it natural that he and Perris should link up, as the distinctive picture presented by the postpartum psychoses has traditionally been one of the strongest arguments in favor of separating out the cycloid psychoses from other disorders.

From Hippocrates to Kraepelin, the postpartum psychoses had been regarded as a distinct disorder. But in 1899, despite giving compelling clinical descriptions of the distinctive features of the nonfebrile postpartum psychoses, "its acute dreamlike confusion, illusionary and hallucinatory state with motor agitation,"[57] Kraepelin decided that "the overwhelming majority of cases that tend to have the name of hallucinatory confusion ascribed to them, in my opinion, really belong to maniacal depressive or catatonic insanity."[58] This interpretation became a tradition that most clinicians followed—postpartum psychoses were therefore seen as either schizophrenic or manic-depressive disorders,[59] and later bipolar disorders.[60]

If we look back through the records of the North Wales Asylum, of 1,100 women of child-bearing age admitted between 1875 and 1924, 101 women were admitted for 103 episodes of postpartum psychoses. This disorder accounted for 10 percent of all female admissions in women of childbearing age. And as these vignettes show, the clinical picture is distinctive in terms of symptoms and course.

On the admission of Sophie J, for instance, a twenty-four-year-old married woman, it was noted that she "screams out in fear saying she is being frightened. She has hallucinations of sight and hearing, she has a fixed anxiety to her former medical attendant saying that he had shot her brains out with physics and sent her mad and has also killed her husband with physics." The hospital record notes that Sophie had tried to strangle her baby and was refusing food. She also complained that her husband was putting her on fire and nailing her to a cross. During her stay in hospital she was noted to be "rambling and mixed in conversation and did not know where she was, very confused, restless and uneasy." After two months she developed partial stupor and then gradually improved, so that ten months after admission she was discharged recovered and never returned.

Or Lillian K, a twenty-eight-year-old married woman, who had no mental health problems until immediately after the birth of her second child when she had to be taken to the asylum because she "talked nonsense all day and had been excited all day and the night before had torn her clothes and was lying naked and tried to feed the 4-month-old baby with jelly." On the ward, she appeared to be very talkative and "recognised everyone as old friends of hers" (even though she had never been there before). Her conversation became "rambling and confused," and she had auditory hallucinations, hearing her husband's voice constantly talking to her. She was "impulsive at times and threw her food about. She mistakes the identity of those about her." After a couple of days, Lillian made a quick recovery and could be moved to the workroom where she took up sewing daily. Three months after admission, she was discharged and never returned.

Finally Mary W, a twenty-two-year-old unmarried woman who worked as a servant, was admitted to hospital a week after confinement, as she "has since been very violent and unmanageable. Her face is flushed, eyes sparkling, she is very restless and sleepless, becomes violent, uses most obscene and disgusting language; tears her clothes to pieces. She has various delusions and rambles in her talk, she disturbs the inmates and . . . she attempted twice to go through the window, tears her clothes and breaks everything in her room, fancies that there are rats about her, wanders about and acts most violent. She has tried to injure herself and has intentions to commit suicide. She is in a confused condition and she cannot reply to questions in an intelligent and rational manner or give any account of herself." She recovered and was discharged after ten months, but was readmitted on four further occasions until 1924 when she was diagnosed as having manic-depressive insanity for the first time.

These three cases map on to Leonhard's anxiety, confusion, and motility psychosis. More than 80 percent of these North Wales postpartum cases showed motility disorders—either stupor or frenzy or both. A further 80 percent showed confusion, being typically described as dazed. This confusion is not the well-recognized one that goes with delirium but is something closer to the incoherence and perplexity described by Wernicke, Kleist, and Leonhard. Forty percent of the sample meets Perris's criteria for a cycloid psychosis.

But despite a distinctive etiology, a distinctive clinical picture, and a distinctive course, it was impossible to get the notion of a cycloid psychosis to take hold even for postpartum psychoses. Roughly 20 percent of the admissions for serious mental illness to both the asylum and to the district general hospital that has now replaced it are for acute and transient psychoses that do not go on to schizophrenia or for single manic episodes that do not go on to bipolar disorder. A large proportion of these have symptoms and a course that map onto the cycloid psychosis template, raising the question why this concept failed where bipolar disorder flourished.

Could response to treatment define the validity of these syndromes? Perris suggested the cycloid states were lithium responsive, which implied they were bipolar—which, of course, they are according to Leonhard's thinking, but this does not mean manic-depressive. It was also widely recognized that postpartum psychoses respond to ECT, which might also suggest that they are affective disorders. But given the prominent motor disturbances in the postpartum psychoses, this argument can be turned on its head.

ECT works not so much for patients with depression as for those with conditions involving prominent motor disturbances, such as involutional melancholia or psychotic depression, and with catatonia, as well as with Parkinson's disease and neuroleptic malignant syndrome.[61]

The bigger treatment-related problem in the modern era, however, is that by the time the concept of the cycloid psychoses hit the English-speaking world, drug companies rather than authoritative psychiatric figures, or compelling data, have had the greatest power to decide whether a condition will become widely recognized. Syndromes such as compulsive shopping disorder can be picked up by interested companies, and when this happens, the *New York Times* will run up to a 4,000-word feature in its Sunday magazine.[62] Diseases get mongered.[63] But there was no one interested in mongering the cycloid psychoses. As in selling anything, it is always better to keep the message simple, and telling anyone, even psychiatrists, that there is more than one bipolar disorder would not have been a good marketing strategy (chapter 8).

Two other factors militated against selling the cycloid psychoses. The first is that the flagship disorder in the group, the postpartum psychoses, had all but vanished by 2000. This disappearance was first noted in Sweden in the mid-1990s, when studies of the incidence of postpartum psychosis demonstrated a steady fall from the mid-1980s.[64] This decline was initially put down to a lack of psychiatric beds, consequent on deinstitutionalization. But this explanation seems unlikely, as the reduction in psychiatric beds that took place in the 1980s and 1990s has in fact more generally been accompanied by a fifteenfold increase in admissions,[65] and given this, a dramatic and severe condition like postpartum psychosis was not likely to be refused admission—if it was happening.

In North Wales, we have collected data on all admissions for postpartum psychoses between 1994 and 2006. Psychoses still happen in the postpartum period in women who have prior manic-depressive or schizophrenic illnesses. But they have all but vanished in women with no prior history of mental illness. In the historical sample from North Wales, 80 percent of the admissions had been for women with no prior history of nervous troubles. A minority of women had a prior manic-depressive illness or schizophrenia.[66]

The possible disappearance of this disorder, albeit in response to some unknown factor, argues for its distinctive nature, just as the disappearance of general paralysis of the insane after the advent of penicillin confirms its distinction from other disorders. Alternately if one opts to categorize postpartum psychosis as Kraepelin might have done, as instances of manic-depressive disease with stupor,[67] the problem is that if one variant of the disease vanishes there would seem to be compelling implications for further research into what factors may have made a difference.

The second brake on the development of the cycloid psychoses was the eclipse of Carlo Perris. As one of the creators of bipolar disorder, Perris was widely cited, which gave him grounds to believe that when the chair of psychiatry at the Karolinska Institute in Stockholm fell vacant in the mid-1980s that he might be a successful candidate for the post. However, he was up against a neuropsychiatrist, Göran Sedvall, who had a background in neuroimaging. Perris's interests in Kraepelinian-style clinical research were perhaps less suited to the emerging genetic and neuroimaging research of late twentieth-century localizers. In making its choice, the Karolinska appointed a Wernicke rather than a Kraepelin.

Perris was unhappy at the outcome. As is common in the aftermath of such competition, the protagonists and others can read a lot into the dynamics of what happened, and bitterness can develop. Perris withdrew from biological psychiatry, influenced possibly by his wife's background in clinical psychology, but also by an awareness of his own background and how family dynamics in his own home, where his mother had died when he was twelve, had shaped him.

He became one of the first to treat schizophrenic patients with cognitive therapy.[68] Perhaps critically, he had begun to develop this latter work before applying for the chair in Stockholm. His first book on cognitive therapy for psychosis had been published in 1986.[69] He subsequently contributed a large number of articles in this area.

His interest stemmed from his first experiences as a trainee at a mental hospital. There he saw young psychotic patients transformed in a very short period of time from being fresh-faced and fit into obese robots after treatment with high doses of antipsychotics given by biologically oriented doctors. These results led him to advocate minimal dose regimens of neuroleptics. It made him someone who brought home small gifts, sometimes as trivial as ale labels, stamps, or foreign coins, from trips abroad to patients who happened to be collecting those things. He was someone who sent postcards with personal greetings to hostels to which former patients had moved.

The week before he died, he had returned to Italy, where he was marooned in a hotel without water or ventilation because of local floods. He had suffered from ill health for years, and his weakened condition probably made him vulnerable to Legionnaire's disease, which ended his life in 2000.[70]

YOUR NAME VANISHES, ONLY YOUR WORK LIVES ON

The struggles between Kraepelin and Wernicke and later Perris and others have centered on questions about what makes a disease. Does etiology count more than symptoms? Does treatment course count more than response to a therapeutic agent—are these two sides of the same coin? It is not the role of history to answer this question. The role is to note what answers the field opts for at any one point in time. Or history can note that diseases, or disorders, or variants can vanish, as perhaps with postpartum psychosis, or that, as in the case of catatonia, a disorder may present at a constant rate but the field can oscillate between estimating that up to 20 percent of patients have it to figuring that it has vanished completely.[71]

Catatonia and the cycloid psychoses bring out a point worth noting. No one has argued about catatonia's status as a psychiatric syndrome. The argument has hinged on whether this syndrome was a manifestation of an underlying disease like schizophrenia and specific to that disease, so that all that is important is the etiology or treatment of schizophrenia, or whether it makes sense to seek out the etiology of the catatonic syndrome and perhaps a treatment for it.

Ventricular fibrillation, for instance, is an undoubted syndrome—a lethal one. It probably arises in most cases on the back of other disease processes. However, the etiology of those diseases, or even the nature of those diseases, is relatively unimportant once ventricular fibrillation sets in. At this point, treatment is aimed not at the underlying disorder but rather at the syndrome. In the case of ventricular fibrillation, treatment is with cardioversion, something that bears a passing resemblance to ECT, which is the most effective treatment for catatonia.

A great deal of medicine involves the treatment of syndromal events that arise on top of predispositions. Is the syndrome or the predisposition the disease? Was Kraepelin seeking the etiology of these underlying dispositions rather than the etiology of specific syndromes, thinking that this would lead to treatments? If so, there is no guarantee that there will be distinctive etiologies in this sense for the major psychosyndromes or that distinctive etiologies will lead to or require specific treatments. Current genetic research suggests that the same factors may predispose to different psychiatric disorders rather than specifically to manic-depressive illness or schizophrenia.[72] And even in the case of infections, the same treatment can cure quite disparate diseases.

Indeed, there is, in principle, little problem with retreating from diseases and even syndromes to symptoms (and a great deal to be gained from a research point of view). Ever since Esquirol, the leaders in the field have upbraided the profession for focusing on symptoms rather than seeking the underlying state. But delusions or hallucinations, for instance, are intriguing phenomena in their own right, and it makes perfect sense to seek out the dynamics underpinning these features, whether in attributional style or other cognitive processes, or to make them the focus of brain scan research.[73] When it comes to treatment, it is still largely symptoms like these that dictate what happens next.

Treatment commonly involves restoring function—as in cardioversion or the setting of a broken leg—rather than curing a disease. Some of the most celebrated treatments in modern medicine do just this rather than make any pretense to treat disease, as for instance in the use of Viagra for what was called impotence but is now erectile dysfunction. So, do we want cures or do we want functionality?[74] Put this way, it seems obvious—functionality will do fine. Surgeons have no problems with the philosophy of such issues, whereas physicians do—perhaps in part because aiming at functionality risks toppling over into enhancement technologies.[75]

But there is a final twist to the disease, disorder, or dysfunction controversy. Bipolar disorder was first described against the background of an approaching wave that was to lift up all these notions and wash them onto the shore of the present.

Just before Carlo Perris described bipolar disorder, another psychiatrist, Frank Fish, a German who trained in Edinburgh and later became the professor of psychiatry in Liverpool, made an extraordinary contribution that has since been written out of history. Fish was mercurial. He did more than anyone to bring German psychiatry to the English-speaking world.[76] But he was also manic-depressive, and his illness and later death by suicide in 1968 may have compromised the impact he could have made.

In 1964 Fish reported what happened when 474 schizophrenic patients classified according to Leonhard's criteria were given antipsychotics. Of those who had Leonhard's unsystematized schizophrenia, 75 percent responded to antipsychotics, whereas only 23 percent of those with systematic schizophrenia responded. Within the unsystematized group, 84 percent of the patients with affect-laden paraphrenias responded, whereas only 1 percent of patients with systematic catatonias responded.[77] This treatment difference was dramatic—much greater than any treatment difference since found between unipolar and bipolar depression. But the findings have since vanished from sight. Why this eclipse, when a much less robust distinction between bipolar and unipolar mood disorders gets adopted?

The fact that Fish, like Perris later, was himself eclipsed at a critical point probably played a part in the failure of his findings to have any impact. But the key reason there was no follow-up was that by the time the 1960s were turning into the 1970s, the clinical emphasis, under the influence of Michael Shepherd's vision of randomized trials, had moved from finding groups that responded to specific treatments to showing that drugs worked across a broad spectrum of psychotic or affective disorders.

Strapped by regulators and academics into the supposed strait-jacket of RCTs, pharmaceutical companies lost any interest in finding drugs that had major effects on particular psychiatric syndromes.[78] Why bother when statistical techniques now meant that barely beating placebo would get a company a license for all affective disorders or all psychoses, and when the rationale for subsequent treatment could be coated in the new language of neuroscience? Better again statistics proved the drugs worked, and made it all but unethical for clinicians not to give antipsychotics even to cases of schizophrenia where there was clear evidence they would be unhelpful.

This was a fork in the road. A scientific psychiatry would have followed up indications of differential treatment responsiveness—this was the reason to classify in the first instance.[79] No one noticed the growing anomaly between treatment and rhetoric before Tom Ban, a Hungarian émigré to Montreal and later Nashville, raised the issue in 1987 and subsequently, Cassandra-like, in a series of papers. Ban identified clinical trials as the Trojan Horse that brought down psychiatry. The opportunity to reclassify that was presented by the new treatments was not taken. Instead, the Kraepelinian brand was co-opted to move psychiatry into a world Kraepelin would never have recognized—a world in which diagnosing bipolar disorder could pass as Kraepelinian. In what is almost a perfect symbol of Ban's critique, the adoption of bipolar disorder, under a Kraepelinian banner, perversely inverts Kraepelin's epitaph—your name may vanish, only your work lives on.[80]

CHAPTER SIX

Branded in the USA

❋ ❋ ❋

The first use of the term *mood stabilizer* in the title or abstract of a psychiatric article, thrown up by literature search engines such as Medline, is from 1985. In that year Guy Chouinard from Montreal suggested the combined use of estrogen and progesterone might be a mood stabilizer.[1] The word crops up again in a handful of articles until 1994. Then suddenly, in 1995, the use of the term mood stabilizer explodes exponentially. By 2001 more than 100 articles a year featured it in their titles or abstracts (see figure 6.1). Everybody was talking about mood-stabilizing drugs, even though reviews written by those most in favor of the concept make it clear that no one had worked out what mood stabilization meant.[2] Everybody was acting as though it was self-evident what a mood stabilizer was. The assumption was that patients with bipolar disorders need these drugs and perhaps should be given only these and not other psychotropic drugs. Mood stabilization had rapidly become the trump suit in the psychotropic pack.

The story behind this development, perhaps better than almost any other, illustrates how science and commerce lie on differing tectonic plates that, in sliding past each other, generate a potential to buckle our familiar landscapes. We begin in Grenoble and a few miles away in Basel with two stories that remain very local for two decades until Abbott Laboratories decided to re-patent an old drug, sodium valproate, and create the mood stabilizers. We

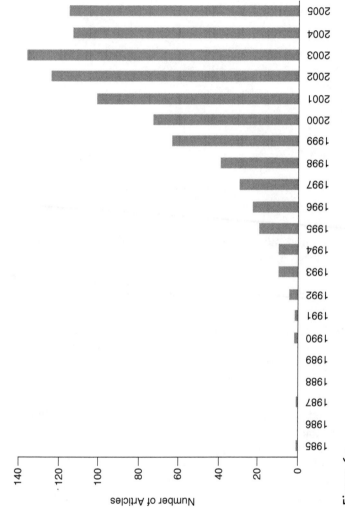

Figure 6.1
Articles Elicited by *Medline* Using the Search Term "Mood Stabilizer"

begin with examples of a set of clinical methods that depended on individuality but could overcome individual idiosyncrasy and move from there to a world in which individual insights are ever more likely to be unwelcome to corporate interests, a world in which all sorts of levers such as patents that once functioned to benefit patients no longer seem to do so. This chapter takes us from the worlds of Schou and Shepherd, Perris and Kraepelin to a new millennium in which direct-to-consumer advertising and the Internet emerge as new means of transmitting diseases.

GEORGE CARRAZ: DISCOVERER AND RECLUSE

The origin of the drug that eventually made lithium, and a range of sedatives and antipsychotics into mood stabilizers, lies in early fatty acid research. Beverly Burton synthesized one such acid in Würzburg in 1882—dipropylacetic acid, later also called α-propylpentanoic acid, or 2-propylvaleric acid. To be useful, a new compound of this sort needs to be made into a salt—that is, linked to sodium or lithium or some related ion. The salt needs to come in solid or crystalline rather than liquid form to be useful. "It forms a colorless, deliquescent mass. All attempts to obtain it in crystals were unsuccessful."[3] These difficulties a century later laid the basis for one of the most extraordinary developments in psychiatry, and in patent law.

The compound does not appear to have materialized again until the 1940s when German scientists were investigating the production of petrol and food substitutes as part of the war effort. Processes had been worked out to convert coal into hydrocarbons that could then be made into petrol or a mixture of triglycerides. The triglyceride mix was an *Ersatzbutter*. Was it safe to eat? Animals survived it and in fact did well. This led scientists at IG Farben to isolate its components, one of which was α-propylpentanoic acid, which they believed they had synthesized for the first time, and which they renamed valproic acid. Because most of this was excreted, however, its nutritional purposes were limited. But it was a useful solvent, and after the war the primary use for valproic acid was as a diluent for other drugs.[4]

In 1960 Pierre Eymard was engaged in doctoral research under the supervision of George Carraz at the University of Grenoble.

In his work on the pharmacology of khelline, a plant derivative with potential antispasmodic properties, Eymard faced a stumbling block—getting khelline to dissolve in order to administer it to animals. When he later moved to the Laboratoire Berthier in Grenoble, he found that valproic acid was often used as a diluent and was useful in dissolving khelline. When injected, the mixture produced a marked relaxation. This response was not surprising, as khelline was antispasmodic, but this relaxation was much more dramatic than expected. When told about the finding, Carraz suggested screening valproic acid for behavioral effects, including a possible anticonvulsant action.

Eymard induced convulsions with pentylenetetrazol, which valproic acid blocked in a dose-dependent way. If he had used strychnine or other agents, nothing would have been discovered. The key experiments were undertaken in February 1962 and published the following year.[5]

To be useful clinically, the liquid valproic had to be transformed into a sodium salt. Carraz undertook this task and in 1962 synthesized sodium valproate (Depakine). The conventional wisdom was that adding a nitrogen group to sodium valproate would enhance its psychotropic properties, so he also synthesized sodium valpromide (Depamide). Valpromide in fact protects animals from convulsions triggered by strychnine, whereas valproate does not. Valpromide also crosses the blood-brain barrier more readily leading to higher central nervous system concentrations than valproate.[6]

He began trials of the new compound, and in 1964 the first reports of an anticonvulsant effect of valproate in man were published.[7] To extend the trials further, Carraz approached a clinician he knew who had access to epileptic patients, Sergio Borselli, and through Borselli he came into contact with Pierre Lambert at Bassens Hospital in Rhône-Alpes.

Lambert was part of a key early psychopharmacology group based around Lyon in the Southeast of France—the Comité Lyonnais pour Recherches et Thérapeutiques en Psychiatrie.[8] This group comprised a unique collection of university neuropsychiatrists such as Jean Guyotat, pharmaceutical company representatives such as Paul Brouillot, pharmacologists such as Louis Revol, general psychiatrists such as Lambert, Paul Broussolle, and Andre Achaintre, and a group of psychoanalytically oriented early anti-psychiatrists such as André Requet, Pierre Balvet, and Jean Perrin. The group formed after the introduction of chlorpromazine and went on to collect the largest set of observations on the effects of the new psychotropic drugs of any research group in the world. Their observations on the responses of hundreds of patients to these drugs, on the clinical features that predicted response, and results for rates of relapse made them key players at early meetings outlining the new psychopharmacology.[9]

Broussolle discovered the breakthrough compound prochlor-perazine that laid the basis for the neuroleptic concept. Lambert and Revol classified the new neuroleptic drugs.[10] Lambert and Guyotat presented the first data on a new antidepressant, tri-mipramine, and indeed provided the inspiration behind its synthesis.[11] Guyotat was the first to describe the response of obses-sive-compulsive disorder to imipramine, a set of observations that led to the rediscovery of obsessive-compulsive disorder and its sensitivity to selective serotonin reuptake inhibitors (SSRIs).[12]

One of the impressive features of these researchers lay in their commitment to study the drugs collectively and to reach con-sensus on the changes they saw, including their descriptions of clinical improvements as well as their descriptions of problematic developments. They were among the first groups to describe the lack of motivation and negativity that can be caused by antipsy-chotics. They were early in the field to link suicide with the use of antipsychotics. But the group's primary claim to fame now lies in the description of the mood-stabilizing properties of the valproic acid group of drugs. Carraz's approach to Borselli meant that the primary tests of the anticonvulsant properties of both valproate and valpromide took place in Bassens Hospital, under Lambert's supervision.[13]

At that time, most large asylums in Europe had significant numbers of epileptic patients, as much as 10 percent, which pro-vided a ready population in which to try out a new anticonvul-sant. Bassens still had more than forty epileptics among its 1,000 patients. Borselli and Lambert initially found valpromide in-tensely sedative, particularly when added to other anticonvulsants such as phenobarbitone. When valpromide was finally administered on its own, however, it became clear that it had psychotropic in addition to neurotropic effects.[14] As Lambert reported, "patients felt more themselves, the mental stickiness, viscosity that had sometimes been there on older agents, was less. We saw the disappearance of tendencies to depression, sometimes even a mild euphoria."[15]

Epilepsy was then thought to induce a personality disorder. Epileptic patients were seen as importunate, manipulative, and viscous. These patients were frequently detained in hospital not because of their convulsions but because of the social disturbances they caused. They were thought to have impulse control disorders, which underlay their inability to adapt to normal social life. They were obsessional. On valpromide, these social disturbances and the characteristic importunate behavior appeared to change. Females were less likely to end up in conflicts, less likely to provoke others in their surroundings, and less likely to self-harm, leading Lambert to ask whether valpromide was antimasochistic.

Borselli meanwhile had left to go into private practice, and soon after at the age of forty-five he died from a heart attack, leaving Lambert to explore the next issue—did its psychotropic properties open up any other role for valpromide in psychiatry? The discovery of the effects of valpromide had created great enthusiasm in the hospital. This hospital was run by nuns, and they were among the most enthusiastic, talking of something close to miracles and arguing that patients looked younger—even to the point of gray hair being restored to its normal color. What was going on? Was it the case that valpromide was less behaviorally toxic than the barbiturates, or was it in fact doing something positive in its own right—was it "personality strengthening" in some way?

As lithium had fallen out of favor in France, there was a niche for an effective treatment for manic-depressive disorder. The standard management involved combining phenobarbitone for sedative purposes with antipsychotics such as chlorpromazine or levomepromazine. The sedative properties of valpromide seemed a perfect replacement for phenobarbitone and led to its use in combination with chlorpromazine for agitated and manic patients, just as phenobarbitone had been used. On recovery, patients left on valpromide alone seemed willing to take the treatment, whereas patients on chlorpromazine were much less likely to take it.

Altogether Lambert and colleagues studied the drug in approximately 250 patients and concluded that valpromide had distinct psychotropic effects that were of benefit in the treatment of both acute manic states and in the maintenance treatment of manic-depressive illness.[16] This result led to a study involving 32 patients on the impact of valpromide on rates of hospitalization before and after treatment. In line with the earlier findings of Schou for lithium, patients on valpromide appeared to experience a fall in the number of manic episodes by 50 percent and a decrease of 60 percent in the duration of hospitalization.[17]

Valpromide was not promoted by Laboratoire Berthier because valproate was selling well as an anticonvulsant both in France and abroad, and the French pharmaceutical industry was undergoing consolidation. Both valproate and valpromide moved from Berthier to Sanofi and on to Sanofi-Synthélabo in successive takeovers.[18] While these mergers happened, company eyes were focused on matters other than old drugs about to go off patent. Sodium valproate meanwhile began to creep into use for mood disorders elsewhere. In 1980 Hinderk Emrich and colleagues from the Max Planck Institute in Munich reported on its usefulness for the management of mania without knowing about the prior use of valpromide.[19]

This work was welcomed within psychopharmacology, as it appeared to open up new avenues of research. The field had been dominated by antipsychotics and antidepressants, which worked on the dopamine system and the norepinephrine system, respectively. A new group of drugs active on the serotonin system was about to emerge, but few scientists held out much hope that these would be particularly noteworthy. They were not scientifically interesting, and technical difficulties in manipulating the serotonin system seemed to stand in the way of developing the basic science necessary to further drug development.

Valproate in contrast appeared to exert its effects through the γ-aminobutyric acid (GABA) system, on which the benzodiaz-

epines also acted. The way now seemed open to search for novel
structures that might act on the GABA system. A large series of
compounds emerged—tiagabine, fengabine, progabide, and gabapentin. All of these were investigated for psychotropic, especially
mood-enhancing properties, but none bar gabapentin made it to
the marketplace.

Meanwhile Abbott Laboratories had obtained a license for
valproate as an anticonvulsant in America in 1983. It had been
known since valproic acid was first made in 1882 that making a
salt was difficult. On November 9, 1987,[20] and again January 7,
1991, Abbott filed for and was granted a patent on a new method
to produce a more stable sodium salt—semisodium valproate.[21]
The new compound, semisodium valproate, differed from the
original by one sodium ion only—as good a symbol of the vacu-
ity of current patent law as any. This difference, Abbott claimed,
was sufficient to make it more sparing of gastrointestinal function
than sodium valproate. Whereas other companies had been unable to bring a novel GABA compound onto the market, Abbott
now had the patent protection to start trials of valproate for mania, and an almost certain guarantee of success.

The first results came in 1991, when Harrison Pope and colleagues formally demonstrated the efficacy of semisodium valproate in mania.[22] Another study was run by Charles Bowden.
Bowden was born in Brownwood, Texas, in 1938 and educated
at Baylor University in Houston. He trained in psychiatry at Columbia University's Psychiatric Institute, where he had worked
in Fieve's lithium clinic. After military service at the Addiction
Research Center in Lexington, Kentucky, he moved to the new
University of Texas Medical School at San Antonio, where he participated in the National Institute of Mental Health (NIMH) collaborative study on the psychobiology of depression.

In the early 1980s, he had started using carbamazepine and
valproate to treat patients with bipolar disorders, which led to an
approach from Abbott to undertake a small study of valproate.
Persuaded that the drug would work for mania, he suggests he
encouraged Abbott to think bigger and to go for a larger-scale
study. This study was published in 1994 and formed the second

part of Abbott's submission to the Food and Drug Administration (FDA) to license valproate for mania.[23]

But while valproate clearly worked, the new compound would also be much more expensive—recently patented agents always are. Why would clinicians use semisodium valproate over the less expensive sodium valproate?

The FDA heard the license application for semisodium valproate for mania on February 6, 1995.[24] Given the lack of novelty in valproate and the financial disincentives to its use, FDA approval set the stage for an experiment in whether company marketing would have any power to influence a profession that touted its new embrace of evidence-based medicine.

Before dealing with this, we need to consider the fate of George Carraz and a sister drug to valproate, carbamazepine. By the time valproate emigrated to America, Carraz had become reclusive and paranoid. He made regular claims that he had unearthed new breakthrough molecules but that a range of forces were conspiring to deny him due credit. From being someone who could admit mistakes, he became insistent that his work went unchallenged. After retiring, he summoned Lambert, telling him that he had three novel molecules: an antisenescent agent, an anticonvulsant, and a pituitary gland stabilizer.[25] But Lambert and colleagues would have to give these to patients without knowing anything about their structure or toxicology. This they declined to do.

TERUO OKUMA: NOT INVENTED HERE

The discovery of the psychotropic effects of valproate almost exactly parallels the discovery in Japan of the psychotropic effects of another anticonvulsant, carbamazepine.[26] Carbamazepine was one of a series of tricyclic molecules stemming from the iminodibenzyl dye, summer blue, which had first been synthesized in 1898. This dye was the parent compound from which imipramine and later tricyclic antidepressants came.[27] In 1953, after the synthesis of a first carbamoyl derivative of iminodibenzyl (G-26301), Robert Domenjoz,[28] Geigy's leading pharmacologist, demonstrated that it was an anticonvulsant.[29]

In 1961 Geigy's medicinal chemist, W. Schindler, who had previously made many of the classic tricyclic antidepressants, synthesized a new series of tricyclic compounds, the dibenzazepines. One of these, 5-carbamoyl dibenzazepine (G-32283), was later named carbamazepine.[30] Theobald and Kunz reported that carbamazepine was as effective as phenobarbital against seizures induced by electric shock in rats and more potent than phenytoin. It was also effective against strychnine-induced convulsions but not against pentylenetetrazole- or picrotoxin-induced convulsions.[31]

Research on the new compound moved fast. In 1962 Hernandez-Peon reported on the effect of carbamazepine on seizures triggered by electrical stimulation in different areas of the cat brain.[32] It seemed particularly effective in the amygdaloid and hippocampal areas of the brain but not as effective in bringing cortical seizures under control, which suggested that carbamazepine might be particularly effective for temporal lobe epilepsy.

At the same conference, M. Bonduelle and colleagues reported on the use of carbamazepine for the treatment of epilepsy in eighty-nine patients, sixty-five adults and twenty-four children.[33] Of forty patients who had temporal lobe epilepsy, twenty were reported as almost completely relieved of their seizures and twelve showed improvements with eight getting worse. Of thirty-eight patients with psychological problems associated with epilepsy, thirty-two showed "a remarkable improvement." Bonduelle and colleagues attributed this improvement primarily to the reduction in barbiturate dosage and to the elimination of secondary drugs, but they speculated that carbamazepine might have some original effects.

At the time, no one knew how carbamazepine might produce these effects. Most tricyclic antidepressants have membrane-stabilizing properties and are mildly anticonvulsant. For all anyone knew, imipramine may have produced its beneficial mood effects by membrane-stabilization. Carbamazepine stabilized membranes significantly more effectively than the other tricyclics.

In 1964 Bonduelle reported on the cases of 100 patients, some of whom had been taking carbamazepine for more than three years.[34] Of these, 69 percent did well on treatment. At this stage, there was a growing hunch that carbamazepine might be particularly effective in the treatment of patients with psychomotor epilepsy and complex partial seizures. Other groups reported similar findings. Lorgé, for instance, using carbamazepine to treat 66 patients, reported that it was effective across a wide range of seizures and that it had beneficial psychotropic effects.[35]

These findings led to open studies with the drug throughout Europe and across the world. By 1974 more than 250 articles on carbamazepine had been published worldwide.[36] In the United States, however, in the wake of thalidomide, the FDA's new insistence on randomized controlled trials blocked the use of any new anticonvulsants. Carbamazepine was licensed only in 1974, after the National Institute of Neurological Disease and Stroke undertook a study on forty-five patients that confirmed it was an effective anticonvulsant. The delay meant that American investigators were almost a decade behind others in discovering the secrets of the new drug.

Carbamazepine was introduced to Japan in the mid-1960s, a difficult market to penetrate but where Geigy Pharmaceuticals had close contacts. In Japan, lithium was unavailable. In Japan, as in France, many of the patients in psychiatric hospitals were epileptic. Japanese hospitals were also in the process of institutionalizing patients following the discovery of chlorpromazine; the large increase in the hospital population there was in contrast to the reductions elsewhere.[37]

As a result, carbamazepine came into use within the asylum system. In an echo of the valpromide story, it was noted that carbamazepine made a distinctive contribution to the management of epileptic patients.[38] The availability of and sedative properties of carbamazepine on wards with both manic and epileptic patients almost inevitably led to its use in lieu of other sedative agents, such as the barbiturates for mania, where it seemed helpful.[39]

This practice set the stage for a large multicentered trial of carbamazepine for manic-depressive illness.[40] The trial happened in a series of regional centers in Japan, because at the time the Tokyo department of psychiatry was occupied by students protesting against the mind-control of biological psychiatry after visits by Thomas Szasz and Ronnie Laing.

Teruo Okuma, the professor of psychiatry at Tottori University in western Japan, organized the trial and gave a first English presentation of the results at a World Congress of Psychiatry in Hawaii in 1977.[41] The findings showed that carbamazepine was comparable to chlorpromazine in the management of mania.[42] However, the finding had a poor reception in the West. The criticism was that almost homeopathic doses of chlorpromazine had been used (250 milligrams per day) and that therefore there was no real evidence carbamazepine worked.[43] During this period, megadose regimens of neuroleptic agents were being used in the United States, in comparison with which a 250-milligram dose of chlorpromazine may well have looked indistinguishable from a placebo as a comparator. When the same protocol was later used to compare lithium and chlorpromazine, however, the lithium results were not contested.[44] Furthermore, a later Japanese study from the same trial network directly comparing carbamazepine and lithium produced similar outcomes for the two drugs.[45]

Carbamazepine did not get used widely in the West until Ballenger and Post, who were based in the National Institutes of Health (NIH), documented its psychotropic effects in 1980.[46] Many European investigators at the time suspected that NIH really stood for "not invented here." If it had not been invented in or endorsed by a senior American institution, a scientific finding did not actually exist. Previously, the Americans had played little role in biological psychiatry, but all this was now changing, and without American involvement nothing moved.

By this time, it was clear that carbamazepine had interesting psychotropic properties. It had been used in Japan to stabilize aggressive outbursts in young men with impulse control disorders, who reported that carbamazepine interposed a reflective break between them and their impulses. This result led to carbamazepine's use in the West for episodic dyscontrol syndrome.[47]

The degree of control of convulsions is not significantly better now than in the 1960s, before the joint discoveries of carbamazepine and valproate, but it is clear that epileptic patients do not end up in mental hospitals in a way that they did before the 1960s, even though a vastly greater number of and range of patients are now admitted to hospital than were admitted then. Is this outcome due to a beneficial effect of these drugs on personality and general integration that has been all but uninvestigated? Is this beneficial effect the basis for mood stabilization, or is it something else?

Such an effect on personality is all but alien to the English-speaking world and is something that regulatory authorities such as the FDA are almost precluded from dealing with. What if a disease had cleared up because the personality of the sufferer had been strengthened? What does it mean if a drug makes someone more functional: does the prior lack of function then become a disease state or risk factor for a disease state? Or do companies with drugs that enhance functioning but who are forced to sell drugs within a disease framework have to suggest that the prior lack of function or variability in function is a disease state or risk factor for a disease state, as happened with erectile dysfunction and Viagra?

A more traditional style of thinking was needed in the English-speaking world, and this was provided by Bob Post, who in so doing laid the basis for the concept of a mood stabilizer that was to explode into contemporary therapeutics and popular imagination once Abbott launched valproate in 1995.

ROBERT POST: KINDLING AND QUENCHING

Born in New Haven in 1942, Robert Post went to medical school at the University of Pennsylvania before moving to NIMH where he linked up with a group based there under William (Biff) Bunney. Bunney, who had been born in Boston in 1930, had also trained at the University of Pennsylvania, graduating in 1956. After completing a psychiatric residency at Yale, he joined the NIMH in 1960, where he became the chief of the biological psychiatry branch and helped recruit some of those who were later key players in American psychopharmacology—William Carpenter, Fred Goodwin, Dennis Murphy, Richard Wyatt, David Kupfer, and John Davies.

Post came late to this group. His first project was to give cocaine to patients who were depressed. At the time it was known that cocaine had a powerful effect on both the catecholamine and serotonin systems. The paradox was that, although cocaine is a serotonin reuptake inhibitor, it is not a good antidepressant.

However, this early work on cocaine left Post on the edges of an emerging phenomenon in substance abuse research—cocaine-induced behavioral sensitization. Animals given the same dose of cocaine on successive days typically became more active with each dose.

This effect is the opposite of the tolerance we all experience when exposed to most drugs, or to noises or novelty. Whether drugs, or passing planes or trains, the effects typically wear off with exposure—the passing train is no longer heard, and the dose of morphine has to be raised to get the same effect. But in the case of cocaine or amphetamine, exactly the opposite can happen. This sensitization probably underpins the phenomenon of craving and establishes an appetite for the drug. Post drew analogies between such sensitization and another physiological phenomenon, which leads to an amplification of behavior, called kindling. Kindling is a process whereby a stimulus that might not in its own right trigger an epileptic fit, if given successively over a period of time, can lead to a laboratory animal having spontaneous seizures in the absence of the original stimulus.

As Post describes the story, he and a colleague, Jim Ballenger, were looking at interactions between the kinds of behavioral kindling caused by cocaine and the phenomenon of electrical kindling in the amygdala of the brain, when they became aware that the newly introduced anticonvulsant, carbamazepine, was a potent suppressor of amygdala-kindled seizures.[48]

They went on to study carbamazepine in mania, and it was effective. In epilepsy, it was thought that effective treatment worked to quench the propensity to further fits. Perhaps, Post and Ballenger suggested, episodes of mood disorder needed to be seen as convulsive equivalents.[49] This suggestion hearkened back to the notion of larval epilepsy outlined by Falret in the 1860s.[50] Although Schou had talked about mood normalization almost twenty years before, Post's new proposal made a prophylactic effect seem almost inevitable, and in so doing he inaugurated a new era of mood stabilization, although the concept had still not arrived.

The new thinking had several implications. One was that mood stabilizers would be relatively disease-specific, unlike the antipsychotics and antidepressants. Consequently, the benefit of an anticonvulsant should be independent of any beneficial non-specific functional effects such agents might also have. In addition, it followed from Post's proposals that the longer the period the person was left untreated and the greater the number of episodes he had, the greater his propensity to future episodes would be. The news coming through, at just this point in time, that valproate also seemed to be a mood stabilizer appeared to endorse the kindling hypothesis. This information put a premium on investigating other anticonvulsants. Suddenly, beneficial effects on mood in patients being treated for epilepsy, echoing those previously seen with valproate and carbamazepine, were described for lamotrigine, gabapentin, vigabatrin, topiramate, and other anticonvulsants. In the late 1980s also, similar benefits were described for a new physical treatment for epilepsy, vagus nerve stimulation, which led to its use in trials for patients with mood disorders.[51]

A mania for anticonvulsants and what would soon be called mood stabilization was developing. The dimensions of this mania are best appreciated in the gabapentin story. The synthesis of gabapentin was first suggested in a memo of January 10, 1973, from Gerhard Satzinger to Johannes Hartenstein, working for Warner Lambert/Park Davies in Germany. Satzinger was a gifted medicinal chemist, with irreverent views on how pharmaceutical company management held back drug development.[52] Early work on the new compound showed that it acted on the GABA system, making it one of the first of a new generation. It was clear that it would be an anticonvulsant. Despite its novelty, however, there was little company interest in the drug. At the time, the estimated returns on an anticonvulsant were insufficient to warrant great interest, unless there was a clear route to some lucrative off-label use of the drug. Two off-label indications opened up for gabapentin: its use in neuropathic pain, a niche that later expanded with the demise of Vioxx and related pain-killers; and its use in mood stabilization.

By the late 1990s, fueled it now appears by a series of ghost-written and other articles planted by Warner Lambert personnel, or experts writing at the behest of the company, suggesting that gabapentin was effective for bipolar disorders, sales of the drug soared.[53] At one point, gabapentin was grossing $1.3 billion a year, with close to $1 billion of this coming from its off-label use as a mood stabilizer. The bubble was punctured when a randomized controlled trial demonstrated that gabapentin had little if any mood stabilizing properties.[54] A subsequent legal action unearthed details of the extensive ghostwriting and off-label promotion that had gone into making this drug one of the most prominent mood stabilizers.

It also quickly became clear that a number of anticonvulsants such as vigabatrin, tiagabine, and topiramate are not helpful or only minimally helpful for patients with mood disorders. The only anticonvulsant, aside from valproate and carbamazepine, for which there seems to be a niche is lamotrigine, and this appears to work more for recurrent depressions rather than for classical *folie circulaire*.[55]

All of this should have been enough in any rational universe to kill off the kindling hypothesis and get clinicians to go back and ask their patients just what valproate and carbamazepine were in fact doing. But by the mid-1990s, psychiatry was in a new world. No one listened to or looked at patients any more. If large randomized trials showed the drugs "worked," what was the point in talking to people? It was a new world also in which it was harder to be certain if any of the authors on these multiauthored papers could be regarded in any meaningful sense as discoverers of anything, and there was increasing doubt as to whether even the authorships were real.

Some indicators of the changing face of manic-depressive illness through this period come from figures provided by Post. In the early 1970s he estimates that 80 percent of the patients referred to the Mood Disorder Unit in the NIMH, which typically took more complex referrals, were discharged on monotherapy. By the 1990s that figure had fallen to only 25 percent of patients. The patients being seen at the NIMH were now receiving an average of three or more treatments. Patients were likely to be discharged on cocktails of mood stabilizers, lithium, and further treatments such as thyroid augmentation. Struggling with what was happening, Post wondered if the straightforward cases were being treated in primary care and therefore more complex and treatment-resistant cases were being referred to NIMH.[56]

The alternative he thought was that the illness might be getting more severe. In favor of this latter option, he noted that the patients admitted for treatment in the 1990s typically had an earlier onset of illness than patients who were admitted during the 1970s and had spent a greater period of time depressed than patients had done during the 1970s. A further factor was that they were seeing a much greater number of patients who had a rapid cycling pattern to their illness and that such patients now composed more than three-quarters of the NIMH patients and it was these patients who required treatment with combinations of lithium and mood stabilizers.

There is a third much less congenial option for mood-stabilizer enthusiasts, namely that most of the drugs in the cocktails these patients were being put on were not particularly effective. Post and others arguably seriously misinterpreted the outcomes of clinical trials, in exactly the manner outlined in chapter 4. If the outcome of a psychotropic trial is taken to mean that a drug "works," it is not unreasonable to use combinations of four, five, or six drugs that have all been shown to "work" where an individual fails to respond. But as outlined, randomized controlled trials are constructed on the basis of null hypotheses, and when they show only minimal effects on rating scales rather than substantial effects in real life, these are not results that permit claims that the drugs "work." All that has strictly been shown is that saying the drugs do nothing is just not right. If this is the case, putting people on combinations of several drugs, about which we know little more than it's just not right to say they do nothing, sounds far from rational. The new mood-stabilizing cocktails have striking resemblances to Galen's Theriac.

A further logical extension of Post's argument is to pick up patients who are thought to be prone to bipolar disorders early in life before their first episode and to start them on anticonvulsants from preschool or certainly preteen years. For the therapeutic enthusiast, the reason drugs that work fail to work, even though four or five or six of them are given together, must be because the disorder has taken too deep a root. The answer is to start treatment at the first hints of affective instability, no matter how young the child might be.

As of 2002 Post was openly advocating treating high-risk children from an early age.[57] "One would encourage major efforts at earlier recognition and treatment of this potentially incapacitating and lethal recurrent central nervous system disorder. It would be hoped that instituting such early, effective, and sustained prophylactic intervention would not only lessen illness-related morbidity over this interval, but also change the course of illness toward a better trajectory and more favorable prognosis."

The prospect of treating children with anticonvulsant drugs is not without precedent, although what has happened before and what Post seems to be advocating here are entirely different. These issues lie at the heart of the next chapter.

THE PREHISTORY OF THE MOOD STABILIZERS

In the late 1950s and early 1960s, a profusion of new and old psychotropic agents were used for a variety of indications. Although they flourished then, they are now written out of history. These compounds for the treatment of nervous problems included phenaglycodol, aspartate salts, buclizine, mephenoxalone, emylcamate, meparfynol, ectylurea, hydroxyphenamate, oxanamide, captodiame, chlormezanone, ethchlorvynol, glutethimide, benactyzine, and deanol. Most of these vanished in the 1960s in the wake of the thalidomide disaster, killed off by a drug evaluation project inaugurated by the FDA—despite good evidence that many of them may have worked as well as currently fashionable compounds.[58] While we might think that in the early twenty-first century, given developments in neuroscience, there must be a much more sophisticated arsenal of psychotropic compounds than ever before, there were in fact many more drug classes available for clinical use in the early 1960s than are available now.

In addition to a greater variety of agents, there was also a much wider range of terms in use then to describe the effects of these drugs than there are now. The terms included sedatives, tranquilizers, calmatives, ataractics, thymoleptics, mood enhancers, mood normalizers, normothymotics, vegetative stabilizers, nootropics, psyche stabilizers, and hypnotics. Few of these designations have survived other than the term hypnotic.[59]

The concept of a stabilizer once seemed almost inevitable for a psychotropic drug. While there was a profusion of new terms in the 1950s, psychotropic drugs had until then been seen as either sedatives or stimulants, all of which stabilized. Sedatives such as the barbiturates, bromides, and chloral stabilized by damping down the extremes of behavior. For more than a century, the rationale for using stimulants such as camphor and strychnine had been that these might also damp down overactivity and stabilize behavior by restoring tone.

When chlorpromazine was introduced in the early 1950s, its wide range of actions on cholinergic, sympathetic, parasympathetic, and histaminergic systems gave rise to the idea that it stabilized physiological systems against stressors—either the physical stress of surgery or the mental stress that led to breakdowns. Rhône Poulenc openly advertised it as a stabilizer.

Nevertheless, it is still something of a shock to see the words mood stabilizer in the title of a 1960 article by Harry Lichtfield, a pediatrician at Brooklyn Women's and Rockaway Beach Hospital in New York, linked to the new drug aminophenylpyridine, also known as aminophenidone,[60] one of the many meprobamate-barbiturate related compounds that appeared in the late 1950s and early 1960s. Furthermore this use of the term mood stabilizer seems to be no accident. Other authors in other articles using this drug referred to it as an emotion stabilizer[61] and either as a calmative or mood stabilizer.[62]

Aminophenidone was launched as Dornwal in April 1960 through a retail division of Wallace and Tiernan called Maltbie Laboratories. Dornwal advertisements suggested that it was effective for tension and for anxiety states and would avoid the problems of habituation and sedation linked to the barbiturates and meprobamate. This was a niche that Librium, being launched at almost exactly the same time as Dornwal, was to colonize and take over.

A few years earlier, in 1955, the overlapping introductions of meprobamate, reserpine, and chlorpromazine (Thorazine) had given rise to the notion of a tranquilizer. Although the term tranquilizer strictly speaking goes back to Benjamin Rush's wooden chair equipped with restraining straps and a head guard designed to reduce sensory input, the notion of a tranquilizer drug group was novel. There is some uncertainty over who coined this term first. The credit probably should go to Frank Berger of Carter-Wallace, who was instrumental in bringing meprobamate to the market and who in an effort to differentiate it from the older sedative barbiturates used this new term.[63]

Berger was born in 1913. After studying medicine, he became a microbiologist. He emigrated from Czechoslovakia to Britain just before World War II. During the war, he worked on one of the pressing scientific problems of the day—how to maximize the yield of penicillin, so that its antibiotic properties could be realized.[64] One of the key technical issues was to find a diluent in which penicillin would remain stable, a problem that Berger helped solve. This work brought him into contact with the series of phenylglycerol ethers, one of which was mephenesin. Penicillin had made antibiotics the hot topic, and the phenylglycerol ethers looked like they might have antibiotic properties. They did, but on injecting mephenesin into animals, Berger was much more impressed by the striking muscle paralysis it caused—the animals were left flaccid but wide-awake. When trying to describe this effect in 1946, Berger referred to it as a tranquilizing action.[65]

Previously, sedatives had both induced sleep and relaxed muscles, but mephenesin appeared to produce a greater ratio of muscle relaxation to sedative effect, opening up the possibility of a new type of agent that might block the primary peripheral manifestation of anxiety—muscular tension—without sedating. To Berger, mephenesin seemed to be an experimental proof of the James-Lange theory of emotions put forward fifty years earlier (see chapter 4). Interrupt the peripheral feedback that was linked to anxiety—in this case, muscular tension—and the anxiety vanished. A new term seemed called for to herald a new type of drug. Drugs closely related to mephenesin, the propanediols, had been reported thirty years before as being potentially useful for nerves, but while the drugs had been discovered, the idea of treating nervousness without sedation had not.[66]

Before leaving Britain for America after the war, Berger had tried mephenesin clinically—but primarily to reverse the muscle spasticity found in conditions like cerebral palsy.[67] He then moved to the University of Rochester, where he liaised with Squibb, who in 1948 brought out mephenesin, under the trade name Tolserol, as a treatment for anxiety and tension.[68] Tolserol became a big seller. Berger, who was close to penniless, felt bitter at the lack of recognition and reward. When offered the chance to outflank Squibb, he jumped at it. Carter-Wallace, then a small New Brunswick firm making shaving cream, depilatories, antiperspirants, and Carter's Little Liver Pills, approached him, wondering if there were any other mephenesins out there. There were. Berger held the patent on one of them, meprobamate, and in 1949 he joined Carter-Wallace.

The brief was to produce a better mephenesin. But mephenesin could not be improved on other than to produce a longer-acting version.[69] Finally, Wyeth came into the frame and offered to license in meprobamate, and so in 1955 the drug was launched by Wyeth as Equanil and by Carter-Wallace as Miltown.[70] Berger was hostile to marketing, but a key part of Miltown's profile was his new term—a tranquilizer. The term was the perfect advertisement—why take an older sedative when you could have a tranquilizer?

Another key to Miltown's success lay in Berger's bias against sales gimmicks. With a background in medicine, he preferred to have doctors communicate to doctors about drugs rather than have them visited by sales representatives. Wyeth took a more traditional approach and flooded the market with advertisements and detail men. But Berger in fact knew many of the key players in psychopharmacology on a personal basis and as a consequence the leaders in the field all referred to Miltown rather than Equanil. As we shall see in the next two chapters, forty years later the pharmaceutical industry caught up with Berger and started to use academics in lieu of a sales force.

Miltown scored a home run and became the Prozac of its day. It swept Tolserol aside, in part because Squibb relied on academic articles rather than intense detailing to doctors. A few years later, the growing power of marketing was brought home to Berger in stark terms when representatives from the MacAdam agency suggested he needed to take out an account with them or they would be marketing a new Roche drug, Librium, and this would be the end of Miltown. Carter-Wallace felt the price was too high—and it was the end of Miltown. It was not that Carter-Wallace didn't also advertise—it did heavily. But its account was with a general advertising agency, whereas MacAdam was a new type of agency dedicated to the sales of pharmaceuticals.

While he was the first to talk about tranquilizing, it is less clear that Berger was the first to use the actual term tranquilizer. Both chlorpromazine and reserpine helped nervousness without sedating. The effects of these two drugs were much more cerebral than those of meprobamate, as caught in later references to the effects of chlorpromazine being equivalent to those of a chemical lobotomy. These effects may have led F. F. Yonkman of Ciba, who was working on isolating reserpine from *Rauwolfia serpentina,* to the term tranquilizer in 1953.[71] Reserpine did not sedate or stimulate but rather appeared to "chill" the personality in ways that were quite different from anything that had been seen before. This response was what might now be termed an anxiolytic effect, but in the 1950s the term *anxiolytic* lay forty years in the future.

Though all were called tranquilizers, the effects of chlorpromazine and reserpine on the one hand and meprobamate and later Librium and Valium on the other were quite different. This difference led to a split in the tranquilizers, one subgroup of which including chlorpromazine and reserpine was called the major tranquilizers. These were used primarily for psychotic disorders, and the term major tranquilizer later transmuted into antipsychotic.

The minor tranquilizers, a group whose first entrant was meprobamate but which later included the benzodiazepines, became what most people regard as tranquilizers. The term tranquilizer completely supplanted notions of sedatives. It became the dominant term for psychotropic drugs in the West until the late 1980s, when the benzodiazepines became embroiled in a crisis regarding their addictive potential. As a consequence of this crisis, the notion of a tranquilizer became a dark and forbidding notion. Where once it stood for an escape from the hazards of sedatives, now it conjured up a vision of dependence, and it had to be replaced. The replacements have been two new brands—anxiolytics and mood stabilizers.

In Japan, during this period, the term tranquilizer was also applied to the benzodiazepines, which was translated into Japanese as *seishin-antai-zai,* which literally means a psyche stabilizer. The benzodiazepines have been variously called tranquilizers or psyche stabilizers in Japan and continue to be used and called psyche stabilizers, as the Japanese never had a crisis regarding benzodiazepine dependence. But where psyche stabilizer persisted in Japan, the term mood stabilizer, which seems to have functioned in the same way when applied to Dornwal in 1960, came overnight and vanished almost as quickly. What happened?

Maltbie was trying to maneuver Dornwal into a market that Miltown had made fabulously lucrative. A key tactical goal was to differentiate Dornwal from meprobamate. Although it was going to be marketed for the same conditions as Miltown, anxiety and tension, Maltbie could rebrand Dornwal as something other than a tranquilizer.[72] It is difficult to know now whether Wallace and Tiernan's efforts reflect a clear marketing strategy or whether the best way to read what happened is that what now looked like solid concepts passed through a period of greater fluidity than may seem apparent retrospectively when our awareness of the competing possibilities has vanished.

The early marketing of antidepressants reflects similar fluidity. The concept of an antidepressant now seems clear, but in the 1960s it too probably meant something close to a mood stabilizer.[73] For instance, advertisements from 1964 for Eli Lilly's new antidepressant nortriptyline, traded under the brand name Aventyl in Britain, identified it as a new wide-spectrum mood enhancer:

> When the patient is overwhelmed by normal every day stresses Aventyl often brings prompt relief. Even in the more serious behavior disturbances—whether marked by depression or anxiety, Aventyl with its unusually wide spectrum of action, broadens the doctor's power to relieve the troubled mind swiftly.
>
> "Aventyl" has an inherently beneficial effect on anxiety and hostility—it is not a combination of an antidepressant with a tranquilizer, but a *single entity* going beyond mere antidepressant action as such. Four out of five patients with symptoms

referable to anxiety and depression (including psychosomatic
disturbances) are likely to respond favorably to "Aventyl" many
of them within a week.[74]

The manner of Dornwal's disappearance may have had something to do with the disappearance of the term mood stabilizer
for a generation. Early in its career, Dornwal was linked to blood
cell suppression. Reports trickled into the company of fatalities
and other serious events. The medical director of Wallace and
Tiernan, Charles Hough, was aware of these. Echoing many drug
crises since, the company claimed that it had a duty to evaluate
these reports fully before forwarding them to the FDA.[75] Frances
Kelsey of the FDA, then sitting on a licensing application for thalidomide, was made aware through a series of accidental conver-
sations of a possible problem with Dornwal. In November 1961
she acted. Dornwal was removed from the market. Wallace and
Tiernan was subsequently indicted. After a period of huffing and
puffing, they entered a plea of no contest.

Dornwal is the lesser-known twin of a much more famous
drug. One of the early evaluations of Dornwal's use as an agent
for nervous disorders came from McGill's Hazim Azima, whose
article reporting his findings[76] was published in the *American Journal of Psychiatry* a few pages before another Azima article evaluat-
ing a new hypnotic—thalidomide.[77] Kelsey is famous for drawing
attention to the hazards of thalidomide, but she never removed it
from the market. The only drug she was responsible for removing
from use was Dornwal, and this experience may have sensitized
her to the risks of thalidomide.

When it disappeared, Dornwal took the term mood stabilizer
with it for a generation. A Dornwal success in contrast might have
established the concept of a mood stabilizer in the early 1960s.
Mood stabilizer would then have meant something closer to tranquilizer. Is this all the term really means? After all, the benzodiazepines are anticonvulsant. Benzodiazepines are also the first line
treatment for one bipolar disorder—catatonia.

THE INCOMING TIDE

As mentioned, when Guy Chouinard used the term mood stabilizer in 1985, he applied it to a combination of estrogen and
progesterone.[78] The fact that Chouinard makes no attempt to jus-
tify use of this term suggests that it was in wider use. But, on the
other hand, the idea that an estrogen-progesterone combination
might be a member of some recognized psychotropic class was
so unusual at the time that using the term in this context almost
necessarily groped toward something new.

The next use of the term mood stabilizer also came from Chouinard who in 1990 applied it to magnesium aspartate,[79] another
compound that is not traditionally seen as a psychotropic agent.

Reviewing the state of play in 1987, Leo Hollister, one of the
grandees of American psychopharmacology, noted that there were
some advocates of the term mood stabilizer but that it had not yet
come into use, and Hollister hoped that the concept would not
take hold.[80] He was doubtful that the prophylaxis that the term
implied was possible. Hollister's was the only entry for mood
stabilizer in the index of a large 1,780-page, double-column, A5-
page-sized, small-print book. Up until 1995, few books on psychotropic drugs for professionals[81] or patients[82] had any mention
of mood stabilizers.

During the period from 1985 to 1995, the term appears infrequently to describe the effects a disparate bunch of drugs. One
was flupenthixol, an antipsychotic then widely used in Europe
but not in America.[83] This antipsychotic had been cultivated by
its parent company, Lundbeck, as an antipsychotic in high doses
but an antidepressant or anxiolytic in low doses, as part of a marketing strategy to differentiate it from other antipsychotics.[84] Jonathan Cole in Boston also explored the possible mood-stabilizing
properties of the antipsychotic clozapine, when it was launched
in the United States at the end of the 1980s.[85] Finally, almost the
only other use of the term came from Les Grinspoon and Jim
Bakalar, who applied it to cannabis.[86]

All of these uses of the term mood stabilizer were far removed
from the use of the term that emerged after 1995 when Abbott
gained approval to market Depakote—for mania. Giving any

sedative to manic patients will produce a benefit on suitable rating scales, gaining a company a license. Although this result is a
long way from showing the drug is prophylactic for bipolar disorder, advertisements for Depakote still claimed that it was a mood
stabilizer. Had Abbott said Depakote is prophylactic for mood
disorders, it would have broken the law. The beauty of the term
mood stabilizer was that it had no precise meaning. It suggested
prophylaxis. What else would a mood stabilizer be if not prophylactic? And this would lead to its use, even though no controlled
trials have ever demonstrated Depakote to be prophylactic. The
term in other words, far from being a well-grounded scientific
term, was an almost perfect advertisement—as successful a brand
as the creation of the terms tranquilizer and SSRI.

Suddenly, everyone seemed to know what a mood stabilizer
was. There was an exponential increase in the number of articles
with the term mood stabilizer in their title. But now the term
was transformed from its former meaning of something close to
a tranquilizer or psyche stabilizer into a term that meant a non-
toxic equivalent of lithium. Mood stabilizers were now something
that prevented further episodes of a mood disorder by blocking
some physiological disturbances in some mood center—perhaps
blocking kindling—rather than agents, which were tranquilizers
or anxiolytics.

One of the first to use the term in this new sense was Charles
Bowden, who had been involved in the early valproate trials.[87] According to Bowden, a mood stabilizer was a drug, which would be
effective in mania, ideally also effective in depression, that would
avoid triggering switches from mania to depression or vice versa
and that would be prophylactic. Bowden suggests this definition
rules in lithium but rules out most antidepressants. But it quickly
became clear that there was little agreement on this point.[88]

The mood-stabilization tide came in with extraordinary rapidity. Valproate use had been growing in the late 1980s and early
1990s, even though the FDA had not formally approved it. By
1995 Columbia had closed its lithium clinic as most manic-depressives were now on anticonvulsants rather than lithium. By
1998, when lithium was used in 50 percent of manic-depressive
patients elsewhere in the world, and valproate in just more than

10 percent, in the United States valproate was used much more widely than lithium.[89] By 2000 graduates from training programs in Massachusetts General Hospital and elsewhere might never have used lithium and would often feel unequipped to initiate its use.[90]

A swarm of publications on mood stabilizers descended, and this coincided with increasing estimates of the prevalence of what in another successful piece of rebranding was now almost always called bipolar disorder—which advocates of mood stabilization argued affected 5 percent of the population or more.[91]

A new journal, *Bipolar Disorder,* appeared, followed in short order by the *Journal of Bipolar Disorders* and *Clinical Approaches in Bipolar Disorders,* and other journals made possible by unrestricted educational grants from pharmaceutical companies. A slew of societies and international conferences appeared—International Society for Bipolar Disorders, International Review of Bipolar Disorders, International Society for Affective Disorders, Organization for Bipolar Affective Disorders, European Bipolar Forum, Australasian Society for Bipolar Disorders, and many others. One of the features of this profusion, which we will return to in chapter 8, was its global character. Consciousness was raised about bipolar disorder globally at the same time.

The American Psychiatric Association meeting in San Francisco in 2003 provides a good example of what happened. Satellite symposia linked to the main APA meeting, as of 2000, could cost a company up to $250,000. The price of entry is too high for treatment modalities like ECT or psychotherapy. There can be up to forty such satellites per meeting. Companies will often bring hundreds of American and international delegates to the meeting in general and their satellite in particular.[92] The satellites are usually distributed across topics like depression, schizophrenia, obsessive-compulsive disorder, social phobia, anxiety, Alzheimer's dementia, and attention deficit hyperactivity disorder (ADHD), for instance.

At the San Francisco meeting, an unprecedented 35 percent of the satellites were for just one disorder—bipolar disorder.[93] These symposia have to have lecturers and a chair—all of which comes with a fee, unlike symposia on the main program. A quick tally of speakers and chairs indicates that fifty-seven senior figures in American psychiatry were involved in presenting material on bipolar disorder, not counting any other speakers on the main meeting program.

The list of speakers and chairs points to a heavy representation from Boston, which has echoes of the multiple personality disorder story and other fashions in American psychiatry that have started from Boston. However, far from all these speakers being closely linked to companies, there was something new about the bipolar story.

One of the speakers, Ross Baldessarini from McLean, has done more than anyone to put the history of bipolar disorders into the frame—articles to which he has contributed pepper the references in chapter 5. One of the key selling points for mood stabilizers has been repeated statements that if the disorder is left untreated, each relapse will trigger further relapses. Claims of this sort date from Kraepelin but are based on a simple mistake. Of course, if people have more episodes, these episodes will come closer together than episodes in those people who have fewer episodes. Indiscriminately mixing these patients will give the appearance that the natural course of the disease involves a shortening of the interepisode interval, as Jules Angst thought. But this is wrong, as Baldessarini and colleagues have pointed out, and treatment should not proceed on this basis.[94]

Baldessarini was also one of the first critics of the use of megadoses of antipsychotic medication in the 1970s and 1980s. When doses fell, there was a move instead to the cocktail regimens, exemplified by some of Bob Post's management strategies, and Baldessarini was a critic of this approach also, referring to the dynamics involved in terms of an allopathic compulsion.[95]

But this was an incoming tide that no Canute could stand against. Part of the problem was that we are in a new world in which even academics, who protest against a new fashion, or those who advocate other treatments, can be bent to a company message. As Fuller Torrey has put it, burlesque shows need a comedy straight man between the acts.[96] Few academics have caught up with the fact that jeans, informality, irreverence, and all the dissent of the counterculture has become the ultimate in consumer branding.[97] It is all but impossible to get outside the marketing universe.[98] Academics rarely realize that their presence on a meeting program may be to fill this role.[99]

Asked to account for the explosion of interest in bipolar disorder in the late 1990s, most academics find it impossible to credit that the pharmaceutical industry could be this successful. They suggest that academic institutions such as NIMH woke up to the fact that bipolar disorders were underresearched.[100]

According to Bob Post, however, in 1991 NIMH gave $6.6 million in thirty-nine grants to study schizophrenia, $4.5 million in twenty-one grants to study anxiety disorders, $4.6 million in twenty-one grants to study depression, but only $0.7 million in three grants to study bipolar illness. The reason for this lack of support was a lack of agreement about methodologies for long-term studies of bipolar illness. Bipolar disorder posed problems because of the inherent variability of its manic and depressive phases and its high rate of complication with comorbid conditions, such as alcohol or substance abuse.[101]

By the mid-1990s, Post and the kind of research that he did within NIMH were under pressure, leading him in 2000 to comment as follows on the state of affairs:

> The same critiques that have resulted in lack of funding of virtually any extramural pharmacotherapeutic study of novel agents in the last ten years in bipolar illness have now been extended to the Intramural program. Thus, no study or study design can be agreed upon as being optimal or answering as many questions as desired. Moreover negative criticism without alternative positive suggestions, personal animosity, and lack of scientific discourse have all combined to reduce substantially the resources in the Intramural program directed at bipolar illness. Groups dedicated to understanding the neurobiology and effective pharmacotherapy of bipolar illness have either disappeared (William Potter, Husseini Manji, Norman Rosenthal, and Elliot Gershon) or have been cut by more than 50 percent (Thomas Wehr, Robert Post). Younger investigators in affective disorders and other clinical research areas of psychiatry have been systematically driven from the Intramural program. A total of more than 40 junior and se-

nior investigators have left NIMH in the past ten years with only
one new recruit having been brought in from the outside.[102]

While the Stanley Foundation stepped in to replace some of
what had been funded by NIMH previously, it seems clear that
what happened cannot be readily explained in terms of a process led by academics. But the dramatic changes were not all due
to Abbott Laboratories and Depakote. Having been first discovered in 1952 when given to patients with mania, the antipsychotic
group of drugs for mania reemerged in the 1990s.

YOUR DOCTOR MAY NOT KNOW

In 1997 direct-to-consumer advertising (DTC) for medicines became legal in the United States. One of the most famous DTC
television advertisements for a drug begins with a vibrant woman
dancing late into the night. A background voice says, "Your doctor never sees you like this." The advertisement cuts to a shrunken
and glum figure, and the voice-over now says, "This is who your
doctor sees." Cutting again to the woman, in active shopping
mode, clutching bags with the latest brand names, we hear: "That
is why so many people with bipolar disorder are being treated
for depression and aren't getting any better—because depression
is only half the story." We see the woman depressed, looking at
bills that have arrived in the post before switching to seeing her
again energetically painting her apartment. "That fast talking, energetic, quick tempered, up-all-night you," says the voice-over,
"probably never shows up in the doctor's office."

No drugs are mentioned. But viewers are encouraged to log
onto bipolarawareness.com, which takes them to a Web site called
"Bipolar Help Center," sponsored by Lilly Pharmaceuticals, the
makers of olanzapine (Zyprexa). The Web site contains a "mood
disorder questionnaire."[103] In the television advertisement, we see
our heroine logging onto bipolarawareness.com and finding this
questionnaire. The voice encourages the viewer to follow her example: "Take the test you can take to your doctor, it can change
your life. Getting a correct diagnosis is the first step in helping
your doctor to help you."

This advertisement markets bipolar disorder. It can be read as a genuine attempt to reach people who may be suffering from a debilitating and serious psychiatric disease. Alternatively, it can be read as an example of disease mongering.[104] Whichever it is, it will reach beyond those suffering from a mood disorder to others who will as a consequence be more likely to see aspects of their personal experiences in a new way that will lead to medical consultations and in a way that will shape the outcome of those consultations. Advertisements that encourage "mood watching," as this one does, risk transforming variations from an emotional even keel into indicators of latent or actual bipolar disorder. This advertisement appeared in 2002. Lilly's antipsychotic Zyprexa (olanzapine) had received a license for the treatment of manic episodes in 2000. Even before licensing, it was the most commonly used drug for bipolar disorder in America.[105]

But as outlined, chlorpromazine, the first "antipsychotic," was discovered in 1952 by virtue of its dramatic effects in the treatment of mania (chapter 4).[106] It was only subsequently that it became thought of as an antischizophrenic agent. All antipsychotics essentially have since been shown to be effective for mania and for depression. There is nothing distinctive about Zyprexa—save in its marketing.

The first generation of antipsychotic drugs hit the wall in 1974 when SmithKline & French negotiated a million dollar legal settlement with plaintiffs seeking compensation for chlorpromazine-induced tardive dyskinesia. Tardive dyskinesia is a disfiguring neurological complication of treatment with high-dose antipsychotics. All antipsychotics caused the problem to a greater or lesser extent save for one—clozapine. Clozapine, however, caused a series of lethal complications, including agranulocytosis, cardiac problems, and diabetes, and it was withdrawn from most markets in 1975. The emergence of tardive dyskinesia led to a period of almost twenty years when no new antipsychotic came on the market, where there had been more than one per year on average for each of the twenty years before that.

The fact that clozapine did not cause tardive dyskinesia led a number of companies to attempt to capture the essence of what clozapine did in an effort to replicate its benefits without triggering tardive dyskinesia. There were two ways to attempt this. One was to replicate aspects of clozapine's receptor binding profile, and this replication is what lay behind the synthesis of risperidone (Risperdal) and later ziprasidone (Geodon). Another way was to tweak the molecular structure of clozapine. Lilly and Astra-Zeneca took this route. Tweaking a molecular structure risks producing all the hazards and none of the benefits of the target compound. It also produces a molecule that is by definition very similar to an already patented compound. In the 1980s the perception was that a company would need to be able to demonstrate that such a manipulation produced a significant benefit to get a patent. In the case of quetiapine (Seroquel), Astra-Zeneca demonstrated that on animal models designed to demonstrate a liability to dyskinesia, its drug did not produce dyskinesias.[107]

Lilly's first attempts to replicate clozapine began in the mid-1970s and focused on a sister compound called flumepazine. This drug was abandoned because of its toxicity. After several other compounds were tried and abandoned over a period of years, Lilly was faced with a choice of abandoning the hunt or going with one of the compounds that had been produced. On April 29, 1982, the company opted to move forward with a compound that appeared at the time to have neither novelty nor particular features to recommend it—olanzapine. Further studies were undertaken to establish a basis to patent olanzapine, and a study in which olanzapine produced less elevations of cholesterol and triglycerides in dogs than a never-marketed compound, ethyl-flumepazine, was finally put forward as a basis for its novelty and clinical importance.[108]

In 1988 Lilly moved on to clinical testing of olanzapine in psychoses.[109] The pace of development was slow, as there was not a great deal of enthusiasm for the compound. A year later in 1989, clozapine reemerged with stringent safety precautions. Despite a price tag of close to $10,000 for a year's supply, support for this drug developed on the basis of claims that it got patients better when no other drug would. It was clear that clozapine would generate huge revenues and create a new market for a second generation of antipsychotics. The development programs for Risperdal, Zyprexa, and Seroquel accelerated. The clinical trials ran from the late 1980s through to 1995.

All three drugs were licensed between 1993 and 1997—for schizophrenia. There was no need to seek a license for mania, given that there was plenty of clinical precedent to use antipsychotics in mania, and until then mania had appeared a rare disorder compared to schizophrenia. But yet, at least as early as 1995, Lilly had firmly established bipolar disorder as a target for which it would seek an indication.

By 1995 bipolar disorder was a much more interesting target than mania had been. Estimates that 50 percent of all mood disorders might be seen as bipolar disorder rather than depression meant that any drug that took even a relatively small share of this market stood to benefit handsomely. Lilly in the first instance and later the other major companies producing antipsychotics began to orient themselves toward this market. The first step was to get a drug licensed for mania. The next was to have some academics include the drug in the group of mood stabilizers.

The third was to have trials, showing a benefit in reducing further episodes. Lilly produced a trial for Zyprexa that can be read as evidence for a maintenance effect or as good evidence that it causes physical dependence and a withdrawal syndrome on discontinuation.[110] On the basis of this trial, Lilly received a license on January 14, 2004, to market Zyprexa for maintenance therapy in bipolar disorder—as the company Web site put it, "the first treatment in nearly 30 years to be recognized by the FDA."[111]

In addition to journals and symposia, Lilly, Janssen, and Astra-Zeneca were now actively courting patients—as Lilly's DTC advertisement for bipolar disorder indicates. Web site and patient support materials proliferated. Central to this effort were mood diaries, promoted to encourage subjects to monitor aspects of their behavior and rate it. This mood watching has a historical parallel in the behavior of weight watching that came with the introduction of weighing scales. The emergence of eating disorders in the 1870s coincides with the new possibilities to weight watch that weighing scales introduced. Eating disorders increased in frequency in the 1920s in parallel with a much wider availability of weighing scales and the emergence of norms for weight. These new norms had an immediate impact on our ideas of what is beautiful and healthy. In the 1960s there was a further increase in the frequency of eating disorders and again in parallel with the development of smaller bathroom scales and their migration into the home. While there are undoubtedly other social factors involved in eating disorders, it is a moot point as to whether eating disorders could have become epidemic without the development of this measurement technology. Figures, especially when stripped of context, hypnotize. The informational reductionism that mood diaries foster is almost certainly more potent that any biological reductionism within psychiatry—of which there is in fact very little.

In the case of Zyprexa, patient information books from apparently independent patient organizations such as the Manic-Depressive Fellowship in Britain state that "bipolar disorder is often a lifelong illness needing lifelong treatment; symptoms come and go, but the illness stays; people feel better because the medication is working; almost everyone who stops taking the medication will get ill again and the more episodes you have, the more difficult they are to treat."[112]

Comparable information for Risperdal states that "medicines are crucially important in the treatment of bipolar disorders. Studies over the past twenty years have shown beyond the shadow of doubt that people who receive the appropriate drugs are better off in the long term than those who receive no medicine."[113]

Far from it being the case that those on drugs are better off in the long term than those receiving no medication, all available studies on the longer-term consequences of antipsychotics indicate that they probably reduce life expectancy.[114] This is not surprising in that even in short-term placebo-controlled trials there are more dead bodies in the active treatment arms of the trials than in the placebo arms. This reduction in life expectancy may be mediated through a variety of metabolic effects. In a series of cases in 2005 and 2006, Lilly settled legal actions with plaintiffs claiming damages for Zyprexa-induced diabetes and other metabolic problems for sums of the order of $1.2 billion. The life expectancy for patients with serious mental illness is now dramatically shorter than that for the rest of us.[115]

One of the points of engagement in the set-piece battles between Shepherd and Schou in the 1960s over the feasibility of prophylactic trials of lithium in manic-depressive illness had been Schou's concern that patients randomly assigned to placebo would be at an unacceptable risk of suicide compared with those getting lithium. There is evidence that people taking lithium are at less risk of suicide than others with manic-depressive illness, although this result may reflect in part the fact that people who are treatment compliant are less likely to commit suicide.[116] In contrast, in the placebo-controlled trials of recent agents seeking licenses to claim a prophylactic effect in bipolar disorder, including Zyprexa, the rate of suicides and suicidal acts is 2.2 times higher on active agents than it is on placebo.[117]

Zyprexa produces most of the hazards of clozapine with little evidence for any compensatory benefit not present in already available compounds. Nevertheless, Lilly marketed it to the point where the company hoped it would make $6 billion per year—more than Prozac had ever done—by developing it globally and promoting it in primary care.

From 2000 it was launched in primary care where the company's intention was stated as follows: "Just as Prozac revolutionized the treatment of depression in the late 80s and throughout the 90s, so too will Zyprexa forever change the way primary care physicians view and treat bipolar disorder."[118] These physicians would be encouraged to see a variety of depressive, anxiety-laden, or irritable states, and in particular failures to respond to antidepressants, as indicators of bipolar disorder. The "change of paradigm" involved, as we shall see, a willingness to have physicians give this drug to children as young as two years old on the basis that they might be bipolar.

Aside from any specific injuries to people needlessly put on Zyprexa, this change points to a more general issue about the state of the health economy. Patents are a system put in place and supported by the public to reward innovation, on the understanding that a patent will be allowed only if the innovation brings a genuine benefit to the public.[119] The benefit proposed for Zyprexa was that it was less likely than a never-marketed compound to raise lipid levels in dogs, but it in fact appears more likely than any other available drug to raise cholesterol and triglyceride levels in humans.[120] This patent seems incompatible with a system that is supposed to deliver either benefit or novelty.

The patenting of Zyprexa and Depakote marked the start of a trend. The SSRI generation of antidepressants was followed by escitalopram and desvenlafaxine, isomers of citalopram and venlafaxine, and the first of the second generation of antipsychotics, risperidone, was followed by paliperidone, one of its metabolites. Despite vast profits, companies have been unable to produce innovative compounds that are better clinically and that by virtue of novel mechanisms of action shed further light on the neural substrates of behavior and the psychopathological constitution of mental disorders. In the 1950s and 1960s the hope had been that a flood of new agents, markedly different from each other, would help clinicians and scientists to carve nature at its joints. By 2000, in order to sell essentially identical compounds, companies have had to mine clinicians and scientists for marketing copy with which to create the appearances of difference.

Zyprexa raises further issues. Valproate and other anticonvulsants had a myth behind them—the myth they might quench kindling. Just how mythic this idea was in fact was brought out in 2005 by the results of the biggest-ever randomized trial of anticonvulsants in epilepsy. This study, which maintained 1,500 patients after their first fit in a trial for five years comparing immediate anticonvulsant treatment with placebo or deferred treatment, demonstrated that these drugs do not quench succeeding epileptic fits.[121] In fact, the quality of life of patients in whom treatment is deferred or not instituted is better than in those treated immediately.

A great deal of the use of anticonvulsants as mood stabilizers was based on an analogy with the effects of anticonvulsants in epilepsy. But the use of Zyprexa or Risperdal does not even have the fig leaf of quenching to support it. There was never any reason to think the antipsychotics would quench or otherwise reverse the disturbance at the heart of bipolar disorder.

What does it matter if the results support treatment with Zyprexa or Risperdal? Would a latter-day Paracelsus not encourage physicians to go by results rather than to prescribe on the basis of some biomythology? Would he have balked at giving these highly toxic agents to infants? Possibly not; previous therapeutic enthusiasts like Benjamin Rush have been prepared to draw blood from even their own infants. Would any older physicians have identified the frenzy to treat bipolar disorders in infants that developed in twenty-first-century America as a mania? Would it be the first global therapeutic mania? These are the questions we turn to in chapters 7 and 8.

CHAPTER SEVEN

The Latest Mania

❀ ❀ ❀

In a few short paragraphs in 2000, Karen Brooks, a reporter for Fort Worth's *Star-Telegram,* outlines the once and future dynamics of disease from ancient to modern times—the reflection on parents or family, the concerns for the future, the hope for an intervention:

> When the book *The Bipolar Child* arrived at Sheri Lee Norris' home in Hurst [in February 2000], she tore open the package with a familiar mix of emotions. Hope, skepticism, fear, guilt, shame, love. But as she read about violent rages, animal abuse, inability to feel pain, self-abuse, and erratic sleeping patterns, Norris felt something she hadn't felt in over a year. Relief. Someone finally understood. Someone, finally, knew what was wrong with her daughter . . . Within days, Heather Norris, then 2, became the youngest child in Tarrant County with a diagnosis of bipolar disorder, commonly known as manic-depression. . . .
>
> Along with insurance woes, lack of treatment options and weak support systems that plague most families with mentally ill children, parents of the very young face additional challenges. Finding the proper diagnosis and treatment is a nightmare because of scant research into childhood mental illness and the drugs that combat them. Routine child care is difficult to find. Day-care centers, worried about the effect on other children,

won't accept mentally ill children or will remove them for aggressive behavior. Few baby sitters have the expertise or the desire to handle difficult children. Parents often have no choice but to quit work or work from home. Quiet outings or family vacations are impossible dreams. . . .

A lack of public awareness means that parents are judged almost as often as their children. They're accused of being poor parents, of sexual or physical abuse, of neglect, of failing to discipline their children properly. Adding to the sense of hopelessness, parents hear stories about mentally ill adults and wonder whether the battles they and their children are fighting will go on forever.[1]

Brooks goes on to cover a set of modern and specifically American dynamics that brought Heather Norris to this point. Heather's problems began with temper tantrums at eighteen months old. Norris had a visit from the Child Protective Services. Someone she trusted had turned her in because Heather behaved abnormally. Norris was furious and felt betrayed. She brought Heather to pediatricians, play therapists, and psychiatrists, where Heather was diagnosed with attention deficit hyperactivity disorder (ADHD) and given Ritalin. This diagnosis made everything worse. Faced with this set of symptoms, a psychiatrist did not make the diagnosis of bipolar disorder because the family had no history of it—or so Norris thought. But she began asking relatives and discovered mental illness was in her family's history. She presented that information along with the book to her psychiatrist, and Heather got a diagnosis of bipolar disorder immediately.

Heather Norris's story is not unusual. The mania for diagnosing bipolar disorders in children hit the front cover of *Time* magazine in August 2002, which featured nine-year-old Ian Palmer and a cover title "Young and Bipolar," with a tag line, "Why are so many kids being diagnosed with the disorder, once known as manic-depression?"[2] *Time*'s piece and other articles stress that surveys show that 20 percent of adolescents nationwide have some form of diagnosable mental disorder. Ian Palmer, we are told, just like Heather Norris, had begun treatment early—at the age of three—but failed to respond to either Prozac or stimulants and was now on anticonvulsants. The issue of childhood bipolar disorder also hit the editorial columns of the *American Journal of Psychiatry* in 2002.[3]

The most dramatic symbol of the developing mania lies in the publication of *The Bipolar Child*.[4] Published in January 2000, by May it was in a tenth printing. It sold 70,000 hardback copies in six months in the United States. Other books followed, claiming that we were facing an epidemic of bipolar disorders in children[5] and that children needed to be treated aggressively with drugs from a young age if they were to have any hope of a normal life.[6]

A range of children's books and Web site support were also available. Parents could get *Brandon and the Bipolar Bear,* laid out in pastel colors and in fairy tale format, along with an associated coloring book from bipolarchildren.com. In this story, Dr. Samuel tells Brandon that chemicals in our brains control the way we feel, that he got bipolar disorder the way he got his eye and hair color, and that there are medicines to help people with bipolar disorder.[7] Or a *Bipolar Feeling* book, in which the protagonist, Robert, has internalized the notion that lots of kids have things wrong with their bodies, like asthma and diabetes, and they have to take medicine also.[8] The features that Brandon and Robert display that make for a diagnosis include nightmares, temper tantrums, giddiness, and sadness. At the height of the 1980s and 1990s epidemic of multiple personality disorder and recovered memories, many thought that books on these disorders were effectively coaching manuals for the condition; something similar seems to be happening in the children's domain now.

In common with the mood-watching questionnaires for adults, distributed widely by companies and patient organizations, the Juvenile Bipolar Research Foundation, linked to *The Bipolar Child* book, had a sixty-five-item Child Bipolar Questionnaire on the Internet, also featured in the *Time* article mentioned earlier, on which most normal children would show some indicators of bipolarity—particularly if left to answer the questions themselves as the instructions suggest.[9] The foundation notes that bipolar disorder in children simply does not look like bipolar disorder in adults, because children's moods swing several times a day—they do not show the several weeks or months of elevated mood found in adults. "The *DSM* needs to be updated to reflect what the illness looks like in childhood."[10]

The Juvenile Bipolar Research Foundation also notes that the disorder is being diagnosed in very young children now where it would not have been diagnosed before. How young? Papolos and Papolos in *The Bipolar Child* indicate that many of the mothers they interviewed remembered their baby's excessive activity in utero, and they seem happy to draw continuities between this and later bipolar disorder. The excessive activity amounts to hard kicking, rolling and tumbling, and then keeping the nursery awake with screaming when born. Or in some instances the mothers were told by the sonographer and obstetrician that it was difficult to get a picture of the baby's face or to sample the amniotic fluid because of constant, unpredictable activity.[11] It is not unusual to meet clinicians who take such reports seriously.

We are in a world here of diagnosis by proxy. Clinicians making these diagnoses are as far as it is possible to be from Greek physicians making diagnoses based on publicly visible signs. Even with medicine's technological advances in the late nineteenth and early twentieth centuries, which opened up the body's interior, diagnosis was still something physicians and others could agree on by looking at cultures of bacteria or distorted shapes on x-ray. Psychiatry in the twentieth century took medicine into a world of diagnosis based on what patients said—often in the absence of any visible signs. But now the process has moved one further step to diagnosis based on the words of a third party, such as a parent or teacher, without apparently any method to assess the range of influences that might trigger such words.[12]

In 1980 *DSM-III* attempted to solve the diagnostic problems psychiatry had then by introducing operational criteria—if a patient had five of the nine features of depression, they could be said to meet criteria for the illness. The hope was that such criteria would obviate the need for clinical judgment. No one then appears to have foreseen the possibility that patients with influenza or women who are pregnant might be declared depressed on the basis that they commonly meet criteria for depression. The expectation was that operational criteria would on the one hand constrain those who were psychoanalytically oriented but that clinical judgment would still apply so that nothing so ludicrous as making an automatic diagnosis of depression in the case of a pregnant woman would happen. But now criteria of all sorts have proliferated and can be readily accessed on the Internet, so that we can all readily find we meet criteria for a disorder, and that our children have ADHD, bipolar disorder, Asperger's syndrome, or autistic spectrum disorder and sometimes several of these disorders simultaneously, and nobody has the authority to gainsay us.

The criteria involved are so vague that, in the absence of judgment, this exercise differs little from reading a horoscope. None of this might count for much more than reading a horoscope but for the fact that meeting criteria for a disease now brings with it a need for and indeed expectation of treatment.

ACADEMIC BROKERAGE

The possibility of manic-depressive illness in childhood had been recognized from the early years of the twentieth century. Theodore Ziehen, who trained with Kahlbaum, was the first to tackle the issue. Kahlbaum had been the first to provide sanatorium access to children. Ziehen argued that manic-depressive illness could happen in children—in early adolescence or after the onset of puberty.[13] This became the dominant clinical view worldwide—until the late 1990s in the United States.

Far from academia or research bringing a skeptical note to bear on the speculative bubble of *The Bipolar Child*, as it would have done at any point from the 1950s through to the 1980s, the American academic establishment of the 1990s appears to have fueled the fire. Institutions that might once have been thought of as sober, like Massachusetts General Hospital (MGH), have run trials of Zyprexa and Risperdal on children with a mean age of four years old.[14] MGH recruited juvenile subjects for these trials by running its own DTC advertisements alerting parents to the fact that difficult and aggressive behavior in children aged 4 and up might stem from bipolar disorder. Given that it is all but impossible for a short-term trial of sedative agents in pediatric states characterized by overactivity not to show some rating scale changes that can be regarded as beneficial, the research can only cement the apparent reality of juvenile bipolar disorder into place.

As of 1991, there had been isolated suggestions that mania might occur before puberty, although such suggestions had concerned the preteen rather than preschool years and involved questioning whether some severe disorders presenting as early-onset schizophrenia might not in fact be better seen as manic-depressive illness.[15] In response, Barbara Geller and colleagues in St. Louis framed the first set of criteria for possible bipolar disorder in children in 1996 as part of an NIMH-funded study.[16] Using these criteria the first studies reporting in 2002 suggested that essentially very little was known about the condition. There were children who might meet the criteria, but these had a very severe condition that in other circumstances might have been diagnosed as childhood schizophrenia or else they displayed patterns of overactivity against a background of mental retardation.[17]

The course of this study and the entire debate, however, had been derailed by the time the Geller study was reported. Starting in 1996, a succession of papers from a group linked to Joseph Biederman, based at Massachusetts General Hospital, whose previous work had been primarily on ADHD, suggested there were patients who might appear to have ADHD who in fact had what this group termed juvenile mania or bipolar disorder.[18] This study had used lay raters, did not interview the children about themselves, did not use prepubertal age-specific mania items, and used an instrument designed for studying the epidemiology of ADHD. Nevertheless, the message stuck. Cases of bipolar disorder were being misdiagnosed as ADHD. Given the many children diagnosed with ADHD who do not respond to stimulants, and who are already in the treatment system, this was a potent message for clinicians casting round for some other option.

A further study by Lewinsohn and colleagues in 2000 added fuel to the fire.[19] Even though this study primarily involved adolescents and pointed toward ill-defined overactivity rather than proper bipolar disorder, the message that came out was that there was a greater frequency of bipolar disorder in minors than had been previously suspected.

These developments led in 2001 to an NIMH roundtable meeting on prepubertal bipolar disorder to discuss the issues further.[20] But, by then, any meeting or publication, even one skeptical in tone, was likely to add fuel to the fire. Simply talking about pediatric bipolar disorder endorsed it.

Also endorsed was the assumption that a diagnosis required vigorous efforts at mood stabilization. Children as young as one and two years old—such as Alex, whom we met in the preface—were put on antipsychotics and anticonvulsants, with their clinicians apparently unable to see the very visible weight gain, tardive dyskinesia, and diabetes that resulted and adjust tack accordingly.[21]

The Child and Adolescent Bipolar Foundation convened a meeting and treatment guideline process in July 2003 that was supported by unrestricted educational grants from Abbott, Astra-Zeneca, Eli Lilly, Forrest, Janssen, Novartis, and Pfizer. This process assumed the widespread existence of pediatric bipolar disorder and the need to map out treatment algorithms involving cocktails of multiple drugs.[22]

There are many ambiguities here. First is the willingness, it seems, of all parties to set aside evidence from adult manic-depressive illness, which involves mood states that persist for weeks or months, and argue that children's moods may oscillate rapidly, up to several times per day, while still holding the position that this disorder is in some way continuous with the adult illness and therefore, by extrapolation, should be treated with the drugs used for adults.

There is another ambiguity that the framers of the American position fail to consider. Advocates of pediatric bipolar disorder repeatedly point to problems with *DSM-IV* that hold them back from making diagnoses. But in fact, *DSM-IV* requires a diagnosis of bipolar disorder following a manic episode—in practice any sustained episode of overactivity. The International Classification of Disease, in contrast, allows several manic episodes to be diagnosed without a commitment to the diagnosis of bipolar disorder. The rest of the world believes it does not know enough even about the relatively well understood adult illness to achieve diagnostic consistency worldwide. *DSM-IV* therefore makes it easier than any other classification system to diagnose bipolar disorder, but therapeutic enthusiasts want an even further loosening of these already lax criteria.

Elsewhere in the world, as of 2006, it was rare for clinicians to diagnose manic-depressive illness before the mid- to late teens. Some of those responsible for early suggestions that there might be a preteen onset of manic-depressive disorder found the rush to diagnose infants as having bipolar disorder quite bizarre.[23] But a bandwagon had begun to roll and between 1996 and 2001, in America, there was a fivefold increase in the use of drugs like Zyprexa and Risperdal in preschoolers and preteens with little questioning of this development.[24] Far from producing benefits, between 1996 and 2004, there was also a fivefold increase in the rate of hospitalization among children for bipolar disorder.[25] Several studies outlined an up-to-fortyfold increase in the rate of outpatient diagnosis of bipolar disorder in children.[26]

When Dr. Jennifer Harris from Boston did question what was going on in 2005, asking whether clinicians were taking into account the range of influences that might trigger parents or teachers to seek a diagnosis—the range of influences brought out vividly by Karen Brooks in her *Star-Telegram* articles[27]—the response was aggressively dismissive. "Mood need not be elevated, irritable etc for a week to fulfill criteria. . . . A period of 4 days suffices for hypomania. This is . . . itself an arbitrary figure under scrutiny. . . . There are still those who will not accept that children commonly suffer from bipolar illness regardless of how weighty the evidence. One cannot help but wonder whether there are not political and economic reasons for this stubborn refusal to allow the outmoded way of thought articulated by Dr. Harris to die a peaceful death."[28]

The sales of the drugs were rocketing in tandem with the increase in diagnoses. But none of the drugs involved was licensed for bipolar disorder in children. In part, the usage stemmed from usage with adults. But pharmaceutical companies were doing more than creating a culture in the adult domain that resonated in the pediatric domain. At least as early as 1997, when mapping out how to make Zyprexa into a $6 billion product, Lilly had scheduled studies to be undertaken in juvenile mania—a term linked to the MGH group of researchers.[29]

The following year an article appeared reporting on the effects of giving Zyprexa to five children, six to eleven years old.[30] The outcomes were poor. The children all dropped out of treatment within weeks—something that the three- and four-year-olds in the later MGH study were unlikely to be able to do. While pharmaceutical companies conduct studies to their own specifications, and suppress inconvenient data from these studies or entire studies if need be, one of their most potent means of influence lies in their ability to select and distribute research that suits their interests—especially apparently independent research. Articles claiming benefits for Zyprexa in children will travel further than any articles describing problems.

At the San Francisco American Psychiatric Association meeting in 2003, mentioned in the preceding chapter, dominated by bipolar disorder satellite symposia, one of the symposia was a first-ever symposium on juvenile bipolar disorder at a major academic meeting. This was supported by a pharmaceutical company's unrestricted educational grant. It featured a series of four lectures from the MGH group of researchers.

Studies run by academics that apparently display some benefits for a compound have possibly become even more attractive to pharmaceutical companies than submitting the data to the FDA in order to seek a license for the treatment of children. Companies can rely on clinicians to follow a lead given by academics speaking on meeting platforms or writing in published articles. None of the speakers at the APA symposium will have been asked to say anything other than what they would have said in any event. The power of companies does not lie in dictating what a speaker will say but in providing platforms for particular views. If significant numbers of clinicians in the audience are persuaded by what distinguished experts say, companies may not need to submit data to the FDA and risk having lawyers or others pry through their archives to see what the actual results of studies look like. This was a world that appeared to conform to the one Frank Berger hoped for in the 1950s where doctors would take up new drugs on the basis of informed discussions with other doctors (chapter 6), but one can only suspect that, if faced with the reality, Berger would have a Macbeth moment and would wonder about juggling fiends that palter with us in a double sense, that keep the word of promise to our ears but break it to our hopes. As an additional benefit for the companies, academics come a lot cheaper than putting a sales force in the field.

It would seem only a matter of time before this American trend to diagnose bipolar disorder in children and infants spreads to the rest of the world. In a set of guidelines on bipolar disorder issued in 2006, Britain's National Institute of Health and Clinical Excellence (NICE), which is widely regarded as being completely independent of the pharmaceutical industry, has a section on bipolar disorder in children.[31] The guideline contains this section because if there are treatment studies on a topic, NICE has to perforce consider them; it cannot make the point that hitherto unanimous clinical opinion has held that bipolar disorders do not start in childhood. By considering the treatment for bipolar disorders in childhood, however, NICE effectively brings it into existence. And, again, the need for a company to seek an indication for treatment in children recedes if influential guidelines tacitly endorse such treatment.

As with so many trends in American medicine, Boston has arguably been the birthplace of this mania. Ironically, there is a real sense here that Boston physicians were returning to the Greek roots of the word mania and were making the diagnosis based on nonspecific overactivity rather than anything else. The other sense of mania to which the field had returned was in the sense of a full-blown speculative mania.

The contrast between the developing situation and the historical record is striking. The records of all admissions to the asylum in North Wales from North West Wales for the fifty years from 1875 to 1924 show that close to 3,500 individuals were admitted, from a population base of slightly more than a quarter of a million per annum (12,500,000 person years). Of these, only 123 individuals were admitted for what we would now call manic-depressive disease or bipolar disorder. The youngest admission for manic-depression was aged seventeen. The youngest age of onset may have been EJ, who was first admitted in 1921 at the age of twenty-six, but whose admission record notes that she "has had several slight attacks in the last 12 years, since 13 years of age." All told there were twelve individuals in fifty years with a clear onset of illness under the age of twenty. But it would seem almost inevitable that there will be a greater frequency of hospital admissions for juveniles in the future diagnosed with bipolar disorder. This admissions pattern is not what ordinarily happens when medical treatments work.

BIPOLAR CHILDREN?

While there are many things that seem novel about the current use of drugs for children, treating teenagers and preteenagers with psychotropic drugs did not begin in the 1990s. One of the problems in seeing what has happened was that in America until the mid-1980s there was a professional perception that giving psychotropic drugs to children for behavior disorders was wrong or a confession of failure.[32] The appropriate treatment would be psychotherapeutic. In Europe, there was a similar perception, although held less strenuously than in the United States. While not held with such rigidity in Europe, these perceptions were more enduring than in the United States, so that by the mid-1990s, when psychotropic prescribing in the United States was rocketing, it was still the proud boast of many British child psychiatrists that they had rarely prescribed a psychotropic drug.

This perception, however, is at odds with the fact that in the *British Journal of Psychiatry*, as in other major psychiatric journals, through the 1960s and 1970s there were regular advertisements for drugs such as sulthiame and beclamide and diphenylhydantoin, which portrayed these compounds as useful drugs to manage disturbed behavior in children. The behavioral disturbances to which the text of these advertisements referred involved "hyperactivity, conduct problems, and oppositional behavior." This was before *DSM-III* had codified ADHD and conduct disorder.

Sulthiame, beclamide, and diphenylhydantoin were anticonvulsants rather than stimulants. The interesting feature here is that this use of anticonvulsants for behavioral purposes could emerge without anyone coming up with a mood-stabilizer hypothesis, although it happened at exactly the same time that carbamazepine in Japan and valpromide in France came into use for manic-depressive illness. Why did the use of these anticonvulsants not lead to the concept of a mood stabilizer or to the recognition of bipolar disorders in children?

The question brings us back to the intersecting themes of biological and informational reductionism, outlined in chapter 4, and back to Cesare Lombroso's *L'uomo deliquente*, discussed in chapter 2.

By introducing the notion of personalities and the scientific study of personalities, Lombroso set up an alternative framework to the disease model, at least the bacterial disease model. Carl Jung in 1909 was the first to develop Lombroso's theme of inherited personality types when he outlined the introversion-extraversion dimension of personality.[33] While introversion and extraversion later seeped into lay language to refer to quiet, shy types and noisy, gregarious types, respectively, what Jung had in mind was quite different. Introverts internalized their problems, which made them prone to phobias and obsessions. Extraverts acted out their problems in interpersonal space, which made them prone to hysteria and to the psychopathic behavior outlined by Lombroso.

Pavlov elaborated on this idea after the river Neva in Leningrad overflowed in 1924, flooding his laboratories. Pavlov had famously conditioned dogs so that they would salivate at the sound of a bell.[34] The floods came close to killing many of the dogs and made their prior training worthless. They had what Pavlov termed a traumatic neurosis.

Pavlov felt he could have predicted which dogs were most vulnerable to neurosis on the basis of temperament. Some he classified as extraverts and some as introverts. This classification led him to set up an experimental paradigm, which in modified forms has been followed ever since, aimed at teasing out what makes for vulnerability to stress and what for resilience. These dogs could also be treated, and it seemed that some traumatized dogs reliably responded to stimulants, where others responded to sedatives.

Jung's and Pavlov's observations were picked up by Hans Eysenck in the 1940s. Eysenck was unremittingly hostile to psychoanalytic ideas. His adoption of these Jungian terms was on the basis that these variations in personalities were biologically determined rather than the product of upbringing. He argued that introversion and extraversion had a basis in inhibiting and activating brain systems.[35] At just the same time, Morruzzi and Magoun were describing a new brain system, the reticular activating system, which is a network of small nerve cells that runs up through the brain stem and midbrain from where it inhibits and activates the cortex and other brain areas.

From the start, the reticular activating system was explored in terms of its functions, in part because physiology rather than biochemistry was still the dominant neuroscience and specifically because neurotransmitters had not at this point been discovered. W. R. Hess, the most famous Swiss physiologist, split the reticular activating system into an ergotrophic or work-oriented system and a trophotrophic or vegetative system. In the late 1960s, it became clear that these systems map onto the catecholamine and serotonergic pathways in the brain. Following this discovery, the research focus slipped from questions of function to establishing variations in neurotransmitters that might be the basis of a pathological disorder.

Some of the pioneering generation of psychopharmacologists recognized the risk in this change in focus. As Fridolin Sulser noted in 1998,

> Hess explained to his students that single facts mean nothing for CNS physiology unless they are "leistungsbezogen," that is, related to function or to the biological goals of the behavior. For example, when in vitro experiments were conducted in tissue culture, Hess would come by and comment "'you are studying monolayers of cells; how do you think you will learn from such studies why you fall in love with a girl or why you can't remember the name of your grandmother?'" Very sarcastic, but he had a point you know. He contrasted his systems-oriented physiology with the fact-oriented British physiology.
>
> I think, we need somebody like him today when the momentum of molecular biology threatens to neglect the very functions so dear to him. Molecular biology operating in a functional vacuum will not contribute substantially to our understanding of emotional and cognitive functions of the brain. I think it is very important to get this philosophy across and I hope someone like Hess would emerge in the next few years. Otherwise I am afraid we just become technocrats. It worries me when I see today's

students. They don't know Hess, they don't know the history of Science.[36]

Eysenck constructed the Eysenck personality questionnaire and used a range of psychological tests including some pioneered by Wundt, and later used by Kraepelin when testing for the effects of various drugs, as a means of tapping into the domain of personality variation. On these tests, it was shown that introverts and extraverts performed quite differently. Introverts were harder to sedate than extraverts. Extraverts in contrast would respond better to stimulants. And, indeed, the questionnaire can be used to predict how much anesthesia it takes to put someone to sleep for surgery—a scientific finding that would have impressed Kraepelin.

The notion of constitutional types became the dominant view within biological psychiatry. Psychiatric textbooks were filled with photographic plates showing naked men, women, and children aimed at illustrating the features of different body builds. Europe accepted Kretschmer's categorization of constitutional types into endomorphs, mesomorphs, and ectomorphs.[37] America followed Sheldon's differentiation between schizothymes and cyclothymes.[38] Tall angular constitutions supposedly predisposed individuals to schizophrenia, whereas manic-depressives were short and squat.

Biological psychiatry followed Lombroso into anthropometry. A huge array of techniques was pressed into use, aimed at measuring all sorts of physical dimensions from body fat and its distribution around the body to ratios between leg and arm lengths in an attempt to determine whether there were any visible physical predictors for illness.[39] X-rays and other technologies as they became available were similarly employed to construct a variety of indexes. Loosely, the idea was that the genetic factors controlling for these bodily characteristics were also responsible for major psychiatric disorders. More generally, the notion of disease during this period was different. There was no sense that psychiatric illnesses involved a chemical lesion or imbalance that would be corrected by a psychoantibiotic.

Eysenck's theory gave rise to a psychology of individual differ-

ences.[40] This approach was oriented toward dissecting constitutional types by a variety of experimental means, including the use
of drugs. Whereas the assumption now is that all cases of social
phobia will respond to paroxetine just as all staphylococcal bacteria respond to penicillin, the psychology of individual differences
predicts that people will react quite differently to drugs from Prozac and reserpine to lithium.

Eysenck's work smacks right into a key debate in the history
of diseases. For historians, the issue has been whether to focus
on the abstract idea of a pure disease entity that may be manifest
variously in individuals, or whether the focus should be on people
who are dis-eased. Has manic-depressive disease in fact existed in
unchanged form since the Greeks and is the primary historical
issue to catalog the series of failures to recognize the "real" illness that is only now being managed properly? Or is this view of
what happens in history completely inadequate? Owsei Temkin
brought out the dialectical interplay between these two poles as
an issue for historians.[41]

This dialectic is playing out in the lives of and being funneled
into the bodies of American children at the moment. In addition
to Heather Norris and Ian Palmer, thousands of children are having adverse reactions to stimulants and antidepressants, and the
response has commonly been that this reaction proves they were
in fact bipolar. The bare facts are that some children are helped
by stimulants, and of those that are not, some are helped by sedatives—albeit called mood stabilizers or antipsychotics. But there
is no hint now that fifty years ago there was quite another way to
frame these responses. An entire field of study and its key figures
from Lombroso to Eysenck has been written out of history.

In February 2007 Rebecca Riley, a four-year-old being treated
for bipolar disorder, with a cocktail of antipsychotics, mood stabilizers, and other drugs, dropped dead in Boston. She had been diagnosed bipolar at the age of two. Her death caught the attention
of the media, who turned to MGH for an explanation of why
someone as young as two years old would be diagnosed in this
way. Janet Wozniak of the MGH group said early diagnosis and
treatment was important because the disorder brings reckless and
impulsive behaviors here and now and in the longer term a risk

for suicide, drug abuse, and crime.[42] The specter of drug abuse and crime brings us back to themes first developed by Lombroso in the 1870s that were later elaborated by Eysenck.

But Lombroso's and Eysenck's biology was very different from that of MGH. Few people would deny that children differ in their temperaments. This view has been generally accepted for centuries, perhaps millennia, maybe forever. While clinicians may be able to offer greater precision in the delineation of temperaments than members of the public, the broad differences are publicly available in a way that ADHD and juvenile bipolar disorder are not. Furthermore, an acceptance that there are differences in temperaments does not bring with it an expectation of drug treatment in the way that ADHD and bipolar disorder do, with their "chemical imbalances" that stem from "genetic sources" and can be put right only by pharmacological means. Temperament calls for management—it gives parents and others something they can understand and work with; in contrast bipolar disorder calls for correction or even extirpation by an expert.

While I have made these points, my purpose in raising this issue is not to suggest that modern clinical practice has it wrong and clinicians should return to Eysenck. Rather, it is to illustrate that there is nothing inevitable about the current situation. There are quite different, equally coherent, ways in which the issues could be framed. If the currently dominant views were the only option, there would be little for a history to do except to recognize the contributions of great women, men, or institutions that have led us to this point. But if there is a reasonable alternative, we can ask what forces led us one way rather than the other and wonder whether the key players have had figurehead status thrust upon them.

The issue is deserving of scrutiny for more than just this reason. These two different biological options, one seeking out individual differences and the other discounting such differences and trumping biology with an informational reductionism, played a largely unrecognized part in an international scientific crisis that contributed to interest in bipolar disorder.

In 2004 concern focused on the question of whether SSRI antidepressants could trigger the risk of suicide in children. The response from many in the psychiatric community was to discount the possibility that drugs that worked for some might have quite contrary effects for others. One response was to argue that there had been a failure of diagnosis, and the problem stemmed from bipolar children being inappropriately treated with antidepressants. Eysenck's framework, in contrast, indicates that expecting all children to react the same way was biologically implausible. If there are disease processes, they nevertheless play out in different constitutions, and just like Pavlov's dogs, children who might be indistinguishably overactive or nervous might respond quite differently when given sedatives or stimulants.

On the face of it, two competing scientific visions come to a clear point of difference here, and it should be a relatively simple matter to determine which is correct on the basis of this natural experiment. But there is another aspect to the SSRI story that shows that the crisis has little to do with science or medicine, and a great deal to do with another set of dynamics. It is at present uncontested that in the case of SSRI drugs being given to children, we have an unprecedented divide between what the scientific literature says on the one hand and what the scientific data says on the other.[43] A divide at such odds with the rhetoric of evidence-based practice cannot be left unexplored.

THE GREATEST DIVIDE IN MEDICINE

As of the late 1990s, there was awareness that it had been difficult to show in clinical trials that older antidepressants offer benefits to depressed children. Despite this awareness, there were grounds for using antidepressants for children, and guidelines on the treatment of depressed children endorsed such usage.[44] The advent of the SSRI antidepressants offered hope that these agents might be effective for children where older agents had failed.

From the late 1980s, regulators approved fluoxetine (Prozac), paroxetine (Paxil), sertraline (Zoloft), citalopram (Celexa), and venlafaxine (Effexor) for depression in adults. The standard letters of approval to companies noted that, because these drugs were likely to be used for children, studies to establish the safety of the drugs in children would be helpful. A series of studies of SSRIs in children began in the early 1990s. A further incentive was put in place in 1998 with an FDA Modernization Act,[45] which offered six months' patent extension on the basis of testing for safety in children. If its drug showed a hazard, the company still got patent extension but had to incorporate the information in the label. As of 2004, such an extension was worth a billion dollars for the makers of antidepressants and antipsychotics.

Altogether fifteen randomized controlled trials (RCTs) were done in children who were depressed and a further ten in children with anxiety disorders. These twenty-five studies had led to six articles and three abstracts at the time the crisis blew up in 2004. In addition, there were approximately seventy publications of open studies with Celexa, Prozac, Paxil, Zoloft, and Effexor. The open studies and published RCTs appeared to be authored by many of the most senior figures in the field, and all portrayed these drugs with metronomic regularity as safe, well-tolerated, and effective when given to children.

In 2002 an issue of *Newsweek* coinciding with World Mental Health Day carried a cover feature of a depressed teenage girl.[46] Articles like this are common just before the launch of a new drug. The inside story outlined that there were 3 million depressed teenagers in the United States, and that if they were left untreated, the result would be a high toll in substance abuse, failed marriages and careers, and deaths from suicide. The article noted that new antidepressants, such as Paxil, Zoloft, and Prozac, could help. The expectation was that a number of SSRIs would soon have a license to treat teenage depression.

It is important to understand what licensing means in this context. It does not mean that physicians are thereafter enabled to treat depressed children in a way that they had been unable to do before. It means rather that the major pharmaceutical companies are enabled to convert the vicissitudes of teenage angst into an illness, one supposedly stemming from a chemical imbalance, and one that it was appropriate, indeed almost morally necessary, to detect and treat.

But fate and the media intervened.[47] As a result of media scrutiny, when GlaxoSmithKline submitted the raw data from its clinical trials in children to a number of national regulators, the British regulators, within a fortnight of seeing the data in May

2003, issued a warning against the use of Paxil for minors, and later raised doubts about the use of all these drugs in children.

These developments led to a projected FDA hearing on February 2, 2004. Ten days before this hearing, a task force of the American College of Neuropsychopharmacology, the most distinguished scientific body in the field, issued a report stating that, after reviewing the evidence, it was the task force's view that SSRI drugs were safe and effective and well tolerated by children.[48] Many of the authors of this report had been authors on the published RCTs on SSRIs given to children.

Nevertheless, the FDA hearing on the use of psychotropic drugs for children strengthened the warnings on these drugs, against a background of regulatory assessments that at least thirteen of the fifteen depression studies failed to show efficacy for the drug,[49] and panel views that there appeared to be an activation syndrome due to these drugs that might account for a doubling of the rate of suicide attempts on active treatment compared to the rate on placebo.[50]

In a marvelous symbol of the new world into which psychopharmacology had moved, it seems that the apparently independent task force's report was prepared by GYMR, a Washington-based public relations company, whose Web site states it was

> founded in 1998 by a team of experts in healthcare and social change. . . . [GYMR] offers clients marketing and communications expertise that strategically support public policy goals . . . [clients] include many of the nation's most respected associations, government agencies, pharmaceutical companies, philanthropic organizations and health initiatives. . . . Whether it's provoking action on a national health issue or crafting an organizational image that appeals to internal and external audiences, GYMR excels at designing and implementing issue and image campaigns. . . . Our media events are successful because we have a nose for news. We know how to take the language of science and medicine and transform it into the more understandable language of health. We advise clients of the best dissemination strategy for their news and make sure that the message they deliver is com-

pelling, documented and contributes to other national dialogues in a real and meaningful way.[51]

But the best symbol of the new world lies in GlaxoSmithKline's study 329. The huge authorship line of this study, when published in 2001,[52] contained a galaxy of North American psychopharmacological stars. The study had in fact been completed by 1997, when internal assessments indicated the company view that Paxil did not work for depressed children, but that the data would not be submitted to the regulators, as acknowledging that the drug had not worked for children would have a negative commercial impact.[53] Selected positive data, however, would be progressed to publication. This ghostwritten publication offers a landmark for the point at which clinical trials transmuted from scientific exercises into marketing exercises in which doctors would be used to persuade doctors.

The contrast between what can now be seen to be fifteen negative randomized trials and seventy positive open trials is as powerful a demonstration as there is in medicine of the value of RCTs. Had they been published as they happened, these trials would once have brought the therapeutic bandwagon aimed at treating childhood "depression" to a halt. In company hands, though, the RCTs, presented by leading academics at major meetings, and in ghostwritten articles, instead helped change the climate in favor of treating children with psychotropic drugs.

When the glitch that was the possibility of antidepressant-induced suicide struck, it was finessed into an opportunity to market bipolar disorder for both adults and children as an answer to a need clinicians had, now that antidepressant use had become more complex.

This crisis spotlights the forces currently shaping medical culture. Among these are the interactions between business patents and medical practice, as well as between expert clinicians and company marketing departments. In chapter 1, the continuities over time of both disease entities and medical commerce were emphasized. The continuity of manic-depressive disease or lack of it has been explicit in all chapters since then. The medical commerce theme went underground, before resurfacing in chapter 4 with Mogens Schou. In chapter 6 we traced a number of tributaries leading to the commercialization of bipolar disorder that in this chapter have merged into a flood that has broken through the banks of medical restraints that had hitherto contained it. Chapter 8 lays out the new landscape of the floodplain.

CHAPTER EIGHT

The Engineers
of Human Souls

❋ ❋ ❋

There are great arguments about whether diseases have a real essence that transcends the lived experiences of affected individuals. Insofar as diseases must be expressed through a lived experience, given that these experiences are shaped by circumstances and culture, some doubt about the continuity of diseases over time is inevitable. Whether a sweep through two millennia of history can shed light on diseases in general or, in this case, on manic-depressive disease in particular is a moot point. But at least some of the biases of the past seven chapters can be laid bare, leaving readers better placed to judge what if anything is left.

The events selected attest to the reality of mental illness, if by mental illnesses are meant brain disorders or dysfunctions that give rise to behavioral disturbances, and also to continuities that stretch from the Greeks to us. While the mania afflicting the Greeks for the most part stemmed from delirium, it seems highly likely that mixed with these febrile, toxic, and other metabolic states were a number of what would now be termed psychotic disorders, among which were both manic and melancholic states. These latter disorders were comparatively rare then and are hard from this distance to disentangle from the frenzy of delirium. The signal from these nonfebrile mental disorders, and in particular the signal from the mood disorders, grew stronger for a century from about 1880 to 1980. But recently it has begun to fade into a background of static from another source.

Thus, this story leans toward according diseases a reality in their own right, but the encounter with disease brings another contingent factor into play—the dynamics and logic of care.[1] In the face of infections, cancers, and diabetes, doctors and others involved in caring have endured with their patients, sometimes mutely in the face of disorders that cannot be remedied, sometimes trying heroic measures in the face of the odds. As our technical capacities have evolved, both caregivers and those cared for have been given chances to juggle with drugs and other measures to ameliorate the lot of those suffering, opening new domains of patienthood.

Aside from a possibly real disease, and the changing experience of that disease as doctor and patient adapt to emerging possibilities under the thundercloud of a common culture, however, the lived experience of a disease comes with a mental shadow, a ghost in the machinery of disease, now commonly referred to as illness behavior. Our very anxieties in the face of changes in our bodies can give rise to symptoms. Sometimes our distress can come to dominate the clinical picture. This possibility has in one sense been obvious since the Greeks, who noted that the effect of the passions on the body can be so profound that it did not seem unreasonable to wonder if some diseases might be caused by disordered passions.

All health care copes with such shadows—up to a certain point. There is a limit, beyond which illness behavior becomes a disorder in its own right and leads to a psychiatric referral. Psychiatrists are called in to deal not just with a patient who is unduly anxious but with a shadow that has morphed into something closer to the grin of the Cheshire cat, something that can have a life of its own in the absence of a disease. Being ill is a ticket to care in the face of life's terrors and dissatisfactions, a way out of the here and now—if we can fool the doctor.

There is a constant pressure toward illness. Within the mental illness domain, the scope for illness behavior is even greater because the boundaries are much less distinct between behaviors of various sorts than they are between behaviors and urinary ketones or bacteria-laden sputum. Indurated breast lumps cannot be simulated, but even convulsive behaviors can.

Psychiatry brings another boundary into play. Quite aside from variations in their causes, different diseases pose different dilemmas and choices for those they afflict. A lethal infection poses different problems from cancer, which in turn is different from living with diabetes. But it is the sufferer who faces her illness and does the choosing. In addition to the problems that living with a mental disease poses, psychiatric patients have faced the prospect of an incarceration, and forced treatment, which for the better part of the past 150 years would have given them fewer rights and less access to due process than they would have had were they charged with homicide.

Given these various dynamics, it is clear that even if mental illnesses can be real, abstracting a real entity from the experience of a disease sets up something of a fiction. But this fiction and the dialectic between a central signal and surrounding static are not unique to medicine. They overlap distinctions made in commercial circles between real needs and wants. And it is to the interaction between these distinctions we now turn, because the dynamic behind these interactions increasingly drives events forward within all areas of medicine, giving rise to a new source of static around the signals from disease entities. The dynamic is important because while caring has always involved elements of business or commerce, it is not clear that the industrialization of medicine is compatible with the logic of care, which comes much closer to parenting than it does to a contracted relationship. Indeed, pushed the whole way, we can ask whether modern economic practices should provide the model for medical care or whether traditional medical care provides a better model on which to build an economy that would look after its citizens, and its resources.

UNMET NEED: CONSTRUCTING THE PSYCHIATRIC MARKETPLACE

In the midst of the SSRI and suicide crisis, outlined in chapter 7, an article appeared: "Depression and Bipolar Support Alliance Consensus Statement on the Unmet Needs in Diagnosis and

Treatment of Mood Disorders in Children and Adolescents."[2]
Here in one article title and authorship line are some of the most
distinguished academics in the field, from our leading institutions, along with patient groups, and companies, and the issues
are framed in terms of the marketing or commercial concept of
unmet needs.[3] The language of marketing is used to map out a
medical landscape as though it was the most normal thing in the
world. How did we get to this landmark point?

Western corporations faced a crisis around 1900. The production of goods had been mechanized and automated to a point
where commodities could be produced ever more cheaply. At the
same time wage costs were falling. This combination of factors
raised the specter that more goods might be produced than individuals could consume.

One of the methods of supporting prices in the nineteenth
century, when this problem first emerged, involved cartels. Competition between companies is expected to drive prices down in
an open market, but agreement between companies can produce
an effective monopoly. The chemical industry was among the
more famous for its cartels, and these were often set up to protect
emerging pharmaceutical products. Legal and political action at
the end of the nineteenth century curtailed cartels and made the
marketplace more democratic.

With the demise of cartels, companies revisited patents. Patents had been introduced in sixteenth-century Britain as a re-
striction on trade aimed at boosting the domestic production of
commodities in short supply. It was hoped that greater returns
on investment might lure producers to Britain.[4] Copyrights were
introduced at the same time. Patents and copyrights went hand
in hand with a developing notion of piracy, an issue that now
confronts everyone who watches a movie. It was difficult, however, to enforce patents or copyrights outside a national territory.
The Americans in the nineteenth century mass-printed Charles
Dickens and Victor Hugo, ignoring issues of copyright, and India throughout the twentieth century copied Western books and
drugs with impunity.

The renewed interest in patents also stemmed from an awareness, led by the success of the German chemical industry, that the

emerging electrical and chemical companies would make their profits through research conducted on a new scale. The new focus on research made these companies an obvious place for the increasing stream of graduates from universities to seek work.[5] And so where neuroscientists from Willis onward had for 300 years been largely independent of industry, the overwhelming majority of them now work in industry.

Pharmaceuticals meanwhile began to play an ever-bigger role in medicine following Paracelsus. The new chemical doctors turned to either concoctions or pure ingredients, whether herbal or chemical. The sale of pure ingredients was primarily to doctors, and this fact later formed the basis for distinctions between prescription medicines, or ethical drugs as they were also called, and concoctions or patent medicines. Ethical drugs were produced for physicians and not for the public, whereas proprietary medicines were sold directly to the public and their ingredients were a patented secret.[6]

When the first research-based ethical drugs began to appear in the mid-nineteenth century, the proprietary medicines' industry was already booming. Many of the principles of modern advertising were worked out in the context of selling these compounds that aimed at balancing humors through sedation, diuresis, and the purging of bowels, or selling them as tonics. These were agents that managed problems that lay as close to beauty as to health, agents that promised what might now be seen as enhancement rather than treatment. Remedies for halitosis and fatigue, for instance, were among the biggest sellers.

Just as the first research-based drugs that warranted protection under proper patents were synthesized, there was another development—the creation of brands. Unable to take out a process patent on acetanilide, a new antipyretic agent, the German company Kalle took out a copyright on its trade name, Antifebrin. Bayer followed by registering Aspirin and Heroin—names with far more resonance even a century later than their real-life names. This development came from the ethical pharmaceutical industry rather than the patent medicines industry. It pointed a way for research-based companies to monopolize the market—a model that Hoover later adopted to monopolize the vacuum cleaner market.

While other industries might aim at wallets, the pharmaceutical companies aimed at the minds of their physician consumers.

The spirit of the patent laws at this time aimed at providing a period of exclusivity in return for novelty that would be beneficial to the public. The notion of benefit to the community, however, has receded, while an ever-greater premium has been placed on novelty. This shift has raised the prospect, arguably now realized, that in due course companies might be awarded patents for trivial variations on a parent compound that did not clearly confer any benefit in terms of health or other public value. Any country wishing to build up its pharmaceutical sector would drift this way—as the United States has done.

In the wake of World War II, companies lobbied for stronger patent protection and ultimately for a switch from patents on processes to patents on compounds. Previously, if a company could find another way to make a best-selling drug, it could have its version of the drug—and, as a result, there were often several different versions of ethical drugs on the market at the same time. But with this change in the law, in the 1960s, there could be only one Prozac or Zyprexa.[7] This opened the way for an increasing focus on brand.

The scene was set for a shift in pharmaceutical medicine, from "thinking about medicine and molecules along a scientific continuum, to seeing molecules as pawns in a game of capturing market niches. The shift is so subtle as to be almost imperceptible from the outside, but to the industrial actors involved and their clinical consultants, it is the very source of their motivation."[8]

The concept around which everything else circled was the concept of unmet need. Faced from 1920 onward with the prospect of being able to meet peoples' basic needs with capacity to spare, in a manner that could only drive prices down, companies turned to the question of how to move beyond the satisfaction of basic needs and tap into what people might be persuaded they wanted.[9] Within medicine, this point was reached with the elimination of unnecessary deaths from infectious diseases, diabetes, and malignant hypertension.

The 1920s saw the emergence of the first marketing departments within industrial companies and the first university courses on marketing as opposed to commercial courses on sales or distribution.[10] The role of marketing was to establish the wants consumers might have beyond their basic needs, wants of which they might be unaware. This change led to a focus on segmentation of the market, so that rather than simply producing running shoes, companies might produce different running shoes for women and men and different shoes for younger and older runners.

The increase in the number of disorders in psychiatric classification systems from *DSM-I* to *DSM-IV* is a good example of a potentially useful segmentation of the market from a marketing point of view. The skill in marketing lies in understanding the market and then positioning the compound to capture the marketplace. Branded products, branded companies, and disorders that can be sold (as opposed to real disease entities), of which psychiatry has more than any other area of medicine, are the keys to capturing the market.

If we look at knowledge-based brands and ask the question where the knowledge comes from, it becomes clear that while the pharmaceutical company may manufacture the raw ingredient of a pill, it does not manufacture the knowledge that goes into the brand. Very little therapeutic research is in fact done with the pill. But a great deal of "anthropological" research goes into establishing the mind-set of clinicians at the time of launch.[11] The huge research and development budgets needed to bring a drug to market today are devoted primarily to this latter research rather than to the therapeutic studies most people assume are the research activities of modern research-based companies.

In psychiatry, branding depends heavily on neuroscientific research funded by government and research-granting bodies. Without this research, there would be very little understanding of what the pill does in the brain and, as a result, very little language available with which to describe the effects of the drugs for marketing purposes. From the point of view of marketing, the advantage in a flourishing neuroscience is not that it might lead to better drugs, or a better understanding of how brains work, but rather than it provides concepts and languages for marketers to use. For this reason, when the first psychotropic drugs emerged in the 1950s, the pharmaceutical industry had little option but to bankroll "academic" organizations to help grow the necessary language. When in the 1990s neuroscience threw up colorful images of the brain, marketers found these invaluable for purportedly showing the cleaner effects of SSRIs compared to older antidepressants. There was little neuroscientific value to the images—but they provided wonderful marketing copy.

This marketing process stands the science of psychopharmacology on its head. Tom Ban first noted in the 1980s the increasing gap between the former hope that new psychotropic drugs would help carve nature at its joints and the reality of psychiatric practice, which was that the neuroleptic drugs had become antipsychotic agents that it was impossible not to give to all psychotic patients despite good evidence that many would not benefit (chapter 5). We have now arrived at a point that is almost the precise inverse of the original hope. Rather than drugs being used to carve nature at its joints, nature instead is being used to differentiate drugs whose differences are essentially trivial.[12] A psychopharmacology of this sort will inevitably be sterile and is capable of rescue only by serendipity.

The ultimate symbol of this trend has been the notion of a chemical imbalance. Early psychopharmacological research led to the identification of neurotransmitters in the brain in the early 1960s. In 1965 this research led to catecholamine and serotonin hypotheses, which posited a lowering of neurotransmitters that treatment corrected. By 1970 the science in psychopharmacology had abandoned these hypotheses.[13] But the serotonin hypothesis was resurrected within the marketing departments of SSRI companies, because it was marketing copy par excellence. It enabled physicians to communicate simply with patients and, as there is something of an obligation on us to correct things that are abnormal, it put the onus on patients to take a treatment of which they might otherwise have been wary. And this notion made the SSRI drugs among the most profitable income streams for the pharmaceutical industry from 1990 onward.

But companies do not just use neuroscientific copy; they also use clinical copy. One of the clearest strategies has been to market diseases in the expectation that sales of the pills will follow. This strategy was first used in 1960 in the case of treating depression, when Merck commissioned 50,000 copies of Frank Ayd's book *Recognizing the Depressed Patient*, realizing that clinicians had to be educated to recognize this illness if they were going to use the new treatment Merck was offering them—amitriptyline. In the course of the 1970s, 1980s, and 1990s, obsessive-compulsive disorder, social phobia, panic disorder, and even compulsive shopping disorder have been marketed in the expectation that sales of the SSRIs or of tranquilizers such as alprazolam would follow.[14]

Marketing is now all but completely dominant. This was the reason to note in chapter 7 that the important thing now about achieving an indication for a drug is not that pharmaceutical companies get the rights to sell a drug, so much as that they get the power to sell the condition. Capturing the marketplace in this sense is quite different from selling pills. The marketeer aims to convert people from thinking that childhood has its vicissitudes and developmental stages and that most distress is transient to thinking in terms of diseases and chemical imbalances. Adolescence has been easy to deal with because until fairly recently it was all but standard to view adolescence as a time of semipsychosis, when suicidal ideation or erratic behavior was common. But this period of turmoil was also seen as a necessary development phase that often laid the basis of later creative genius or other accomplishments. It is not clear what we might lose if marketing departments capture our views of adolescence. Many of the pioneers of psychopharmacology had significant depressions in adolescence.

A further reason to medicalize distress in this way lies in the fact that until recently sales of the product have not been to consumers in the street but rather to clinicians, who, operating within a medical model, have been much more comfortable with prescribing for disease entities rather than to modify dispositions or even alleviate distress. Clinicians find ADHD and bipolar disorder more comfortable notions than introversion and extraversion. There is a moral force to eradicating infections or restoring people to "normal" by correcting deficiencies, not found in notions of adjusting people along a dimension of functionality.

If, in seeking to meet unmet needs, companies produced treatments for diseases for which the public clamored, and were raising awareness of diseases that could now be eliminated, it would be reasonable to celebrate this industry. But companies do not do this anymore. This point came through dramatically in the marketing of the SSRIs. A handful of cases is all it takes to show that the drugs work for premature ejaculation, while hundreds need to be recruited to controlled trials to suggest a possible benefit in depression. The decision to market these minimally effective drugs for depression rather than premature ejaculation was a business rather than a scientific decision. Marketing in the 1980s decided that it would not then have been culturally possible to promote a drug to improve sexual functioning to physicians.[15] The actual effects of the drugs, and the science behind them, were not the driving force in the drugs' promotion but something to be circumvented.

Taken to its extreme, the new marketing mandates an all-but-exclusive focus on agents to manage Western life-styles—or illness behaviors—rather than agents for serious diseases that affect a few or diseases that affect multitudes living in parts of the world who are too poor to pay. Within the life-style domain, modern patent laws create the possibility of blockbuster drugs—drugs that earn billions per year. But even in the current patent framework, conventional medications will not do this. For some time, it has been a matter of common knowledge that companies no longer develop drugs for real illnesses in the Third World, such as AIDS, or make them available, owing to the lack of returns on such products. What is less well known is that many companies regard it as no longer economic for them to produce drugs for major illnesses in the West, such as multiple sclerosis or epilepsy, unless these drugs can be sold off-license for other indications. The off-label use of gabapentin for bipolar disorder, outlined in chapter 6, brings this point out.

Allied to marketing, however, is a professional failure. The knowledge needed to construct a blockbuster brand is derived almost entirely from the physicians to whom the product is being sold. The careers of Prozac, Paxil, and other SSRIs, and now Zyprexa and Depakote, make it clear that it has been marketing departments that have distinguished often barely distinguishable drugs from each other in the minds of their physician consumers rather than clear product differences that have created these brands. The value lies in the minds of the consumer rather than in the product, and the role of marketing is to establish this value.

In just the same way that marketing tries to understand how individuals of different ages might have different perceptions as to what they require from a sports car or a soap powder, so also most clinicians will have found themselves phoned by market researchers interested to know what characteristics of a mood stabilizer or other psychotropic drug would be of greatest value to the prescriber.

In the case of the SSRIs, calcium channel blockers, or statins, and now mood stabilizers, just as in domains like running shoes, companies will often cooperate to make a market. Once the marketing need has been identified, marketing builds a consensus by means of scientific symposia and also articles and opinion-leader educational initiatives. Public relations firms place stories in the media and help sponsor books such as *Listening to Prozac*. Increasingly, as in other industries, marketers utilize Internet sites where patients can go and diagnose themselves and take the resulting information back to their doctors.

Psychiatry and medicine have nothing so crude as "focus groups," but opinion-leader panels are convened to see what the consumer wants. The consumers in this case are nonacademic clinicians, and the process is aimed at guessing how these clinicians can be influenced rather than working out what works best or what costs least. The new role of medical academics is to broker this exchange. The key issue is what prescribers can be made to want rather than what is best for the patient. Thus, when cognitive function became an issue, the marketing of antipsychotics concentrated on this even though there was nothing to recommend the new products in terms of enhancement of cognitive function compared with older products. The appearances of scientific support can always be manufactured. On the question of whether psychiatrists are responsive to marketing of this type, the answer is clearly yes.

But we must note that the marketplace is no longer determined by the unmet needs of psychiatrists alone. Since the 1960s consumer input to medicine has played an increasing part. Amer-

230 Mania

ican and European consumers have differed significantly. In the United States, the market for psychotropics has been an enhancement market, whereas in Europe the greatest usage of psychotropics is often in areas of social deprivation and the pills are viewed as dulling the pain of a harsh reality rather than as enhancement agents. Differences between America and Europe in some of these areas have been commented on for more than fifty years. In 1955 Henri Ellenberger noted that Europeans have diseases, whereas Americans have problems and reactions.[16] The role of the physician has also been different, with American physicians being called upon to be problem solvers or enabling the individual to problem solve, whereas Europeans diagnose disease entities with which people have to live.[17]

But while different national traditions may lead to certain issues coming to a head in one place before another, persisting differences between Europe and America are increasingly out of date in a globalizing market. The new psychiatry aims at replacing class and social divisions with life-styles. The objects we consume become our badge of identity rather than our background in place or time. This consumption is driven not by our need for objects so much as our want for the kinds of difference that offer social meaning. In terms of medicine, one can see an ultimate horizon here in enhancement technologies rather than in disease relief.

While marketed under the category of disease, arguably conditions like ADHD are better seen as opportunities in which parents or others can deploy enhancement technologies rather than treatments. This approach is particularly the case with adult ADHD, where use of these drugs, which either enhance performance or give the subjective impression of enhanced performance, is legitimized under the heading of a disease entity. Diseases have all but become commodities and are as subject to fashions as other commodities, with the main determinant of the fashion cycle being the patent life of a drug. In this sense, it is arresting to find at present so many Americans saying "I am bipolar" rather than I have bipolar disorder.

For all these reasons an article on "Unmet Needs in Diagnosis and Treatment of Mood Disorders in Children and Adolescents," apparently authored by the most distinguished figures in psychiatry, as well as patient group representatives, is a landmark.[18] But it surely takes more than trips to a plush consensus conference venue and the creation of an apparent common interest to treat a disease to get the leaders of a field to sign up to such a statement. How did we get there?

THE APPEARANCES OF SCIENCE

The key unmet needs of psychiatrists are to think their field is scientific and that they are not influenced by commerce. Controlled trials were put in place in the mid-1960s as a means to meet both these needs. They would force the financial camel that was the pharmaceutical industry through the eye of a scientific needle. And, as long as clinicians practiced in accordance with the evidence from controlled trials, many thought that any gifts or educational support from industry were irrelevant. It was aspirations of this sort that underpinned the ferocity of Michael Shepherd's attack on Mogens Schou.

Guiding Clinicians

If randomized controlled trials (RCTs) are designed to achieve this end, what could be wrong with combining trials and seeking consensus? Consensus conferences aimed at producing guidelines for clinical practice based on RCT data began in the late 1980s. A range of scientific bodies took up this development, which in the first instance appeared to be a means for academia to rein in the continuing excesses of marketing departments. But the first consensus conferences were aimed at telling physicians what they should not be doing—they should not be stripping varicose veins—rather than what they should be doing. A simple switch of emphasis enabled companies to get control of the marketplace.

That companies had begun to move in on this area was obvious to some at least by the early 1990s.[19] But for anyone alert to the risk that companies might commandeer this terrain, there was a puzzle. It might have been expected that company-sponsored guidelines would clearly differ from independent guidelines. However, company-sponsored and independent guidelines on the treatment of conditions from depression and bipolar disorder to schizophrenia appear indistinguishable. A good example lies in a comparison between the Texas Medication Algorithm Project (TMAP) guidelines and those from Britain's National Institute of Clinical Excellence (NICE).

Following the launch of the second generation antipsychotic risperidone in 1994, TMAP was instituted in 1995, initially funded by Janssen Pharmaceuticals, the makers of risperidone, and soon afterward by all major companies. TMAP drew up a panel of consultants to produce an expert consensus on the use of antipsychotics and later on the use of antidepressants and mood stabilizers.[20] A panel of child psychiatrists formulated guidelines recommending new antipsychotics and antidepressants for the management of children's problems.[21]

In a number of U.S. states, legislators have the powers to rule that algorithms and guidelines such as these must be applied in the care of any patients receiving treatment in public facilities. If evidence-based guidelines really do reflect reality, then adopting them is logical and can be expected to be cost-effective over time. TMAP was administratively endorsed in Texas, and as a result state hospital doctors were required to follow its algorithms and use these newer drugs first.

The TMAP algorithms and guidelines were subsequently marketed to other states.[22] In this way a very few people effectively produced a situation in which a growing cohort of patients treated in the public sector end up being put on and maintained on a set of more costly drugs.

These guidelines have helped companies defy the laws of commercial gravity. On the launch of Risperdal and Zyprexa, for instance, the FDA ruled that it would be effectively illegal for the advertisements for these agents to state that they were superior to older drugs in the field.[23] Given this, and the fact that the new compounds cost forty times more than chlorpromazine or haloperidol, one might have thought that managed care and hospital formularies, set up in part to get value for money, would have refused to endorse these new compounds.

But the FDA does not regulate what academics say. In this context, the evolution of expert panels, which manage to endorse only patented drugs over older unpatented products and successively replace off-patent drugs with newer patented agents, is almost the perfect mechanism to retain market share.

It would be a mistake to put the outcomes of TMAP down to the conflicts of interest of any experts involved in the process. Senior academics risk losing credibility if it is shown that their opinions were bought. These experts almost certainly had no pressure put on them to come to a particular point of view. All of the publications of clinical trial data for antipsychotic drugs will have been available to them, and they will have been encouraged to be evidence-based.

The power of the system comes through by looking at the NICE guidelines in Britain. Around the same time as TMAP, the National Institute of Clinical Excellence was set up in Britain with a brief to make recommendations on cost-effective treatments. NICE guidelines are a similar creation to TMAP: a consensus of expert views rather than evidence-based views. The process involves psychiatrists, psychologists, and other stakeholders in mental health collating evidence and sending draft reports to selected experts for comments. Decisions are reached not by experiment or evidence but by agreement. They are independent of industry, but the upshot in the case of psychotropic drugs has been a set of guidelines indistinguishable from TMAP, or explicitly company-sponsored guideline groups.[24] Just as in Texas, the medical directors of hospitals within the NHS in Britain will want all their clinicians to adhere to NICE guidelines. To practice otherwise would be to fly in the face of the evidence and would be legally indefensible should things go wrong.

Producing Evidence

Two critical developments play a part in enabling companies to achieve the outcomes outlined here. One was getting control over clinical trials and the other was control over the reporting of those trials. Control of trials was gained through the setting up of Clinical Research Organizations (CROs). Control of the reporting of trials was gained by means of ghostwriting.

Most pharmaceutical companies restructured in the mid- to late 1960s, in response to new management and marketing practices.[25] This restructuring led to an outsourcing of functions, including clinical trial management and medical writing. Previously companies had supported RCTs initiated by academics who held the resulting trial data. In the 1970s, RCTs became multi-centered and multinational, and the former clinical trials units within companies, now set up as independent companies, began to run them. The new companies included Quintiles Transnational, established in 1982, Parexel International set up in 1983, and Covance in 1987.

As of 2000, CROs ran more than two-thirds of clinical projects undertaken by the pharmaceutical industry.[26] Industry spending on RCTs grew from $2 billion in 1980 to more than $30 billion in 2001. The new companies offered banks of clinicians as potential trialists. They were more flexible in looking at non-academic health centers such as general practice networks. And CROs could police trials without compromising the "friendships" built up between companies and their academic supporters, who would be needed for subsequent educational exercises and market development.

Industry portrays CROs as a response to cost and efficiency requirements. But privatized research of this sort is profoundly different from previous clinical research. The trials run by CROs are geared exclusively to the marketing interests of pharmaceutical companies rather than to answering scientific questions. CROs have restructured controls of disclosure and confidentiality and managed intellectual property in an entirely new way. RCT data are now held exclusively within the company in a way they had not been when federations of academic centers conducted such trials.

It is now clear that some of these organizations have run trials on drugs featured prominently in this history that have included bogus patients, for which investigators and others have ended up in jail.[27] CROs, in addition, now provide a privatized institutional review board (IRB) system that grants ethical approval to company studies,[28] and they have made it possible to move clinical trials on drugs for Western markets out of America and Europe into Eastern Europe, Asia, or Africa, in a way that university departments could not have done.[29]

In part, this change in character has arisen simply by accident, in that, once trials are multinational, having one organization run them makes sense. Data from different centers also need to be brought together for analysis, and CROs do this. Thus, the growing scale of the exercise in its own right would tend to prize control out of the hands of academics. But whatever accidents of history need to be factored in, there was also a concerted move by companies in the 1980s to redefine intellectual property in a manner that sidelined academics.[30] And there is a small detail to note, which is that large multicentered trials are not needed for drugs that really work.

As involvement in the initiation of research in psychopharmacology slipped out of academic hands in the 1970s, so also control of research publications slipped away in the 1980s. While companies since the 1950s authored medical pieces, often using a clinician's name, this practice had a disreputable air to it. The clinicians were not the leaders of the field, and the publications appeared in obscure journals or later in journal supplements. But, as companies outsourced their medical writing to newly professional writing agencies, all this changed.

The changes were first noticed by leading journals in the mid-1990s.[31] In response, journals tightened up their authorship criteria. There was still at the time no hint that the great majority of company trials appearing in major journals might be ghostwritten. But by 2000, 75 percent of the RCTs appearing in major journals like *JAMA, NEJM,* and the *Lancet* were sponsored by pharmaceutical companies, and it now seems unlikely that companies would have been prepared to leave the preparation of any sizable proportion of these key marketing tools in academic hands. The picture that emerges is of an academic medicine transformed from what it had been during the 1960s.

Still, academia has gone through many transformations. Is this not just a necessary evolution, if the reach of science is to extend fully? This question returns us to the real significance of the crisis about antidepressants in children. The SSRI crisis pointed to a comprehensive divide between the statements appearing in the scientific literature and the raw data that those statements purported to represent. Many, possibly all, of these articles were ghostwritten.

As a result, independent agencies like NICE come up with the same answers as company-sponsored guidelines. Both company-sponsored and independent experts work from the published articles, and these stem from trials run by CROs that are written up by writing agencies before being topped off with the names of some of the most distinguished experts in the field.

The academic hierarchy seems unaware of being enmeshed in the problem. Its lack of awareness must stem in part from the fact that this process crept up unobtrusively on experts and journals. Experts until recently had little reason to believe that there might be a systematic difference between the material presented to them for endorsement and the actual trial data.

One of the upshots of the process has been that clinical trials, which had once been exercises designed to investigate the scientific character of new products, have become instead a set of methods designed to smooth the development cycle of new pharmaceuticals. As such, it is not clear how such trials should feature in a history of "science." If they do feature, we need to acknowledge that the apparent consensus of senior figures in a field around a new view, which is often called a paradigm, may now arise from a marketing process that adds the authority of distinguished names to a new view for the purposes of verisimilitude. It would make more sense, though, to concede that most of what is happening belongs to the domain of commerce rather the domain of science, whatever about medicine.

Unmet Global Needs

Emil Kraepelin was perhaps the first psychiatrist to take a global perspective. He was a regular traveler, heading as far as Indonesia to see whether patients there displayed comparable mental illnesses to those found in Germany and using his observations from far-flung places as support for his classification system.[32] Today, in contrast, the force driving globalization within psychiatry is not any recognition of common disorders across cultures but rather the marketing of diseases and their treatments.

The data from RCTs are central to this globalization. The universalization claimed for scientific methods and for the resulting data mean that the results of trials conducted in what may be a small subset of volunteers recruited by advertisement are held to apply in Japan as well as America, for children as well as adults, and for all ethnic groups, ages, and sexes. Guidelines such as TMAP should be equally valid in Japan, Afghanistan, and Texas.

This claim leads both to globalization and to the conversion of all experiences from cradle to grave into potential life-style pathologies. The same mechanisms that have been employed to transform the innermost and intimate experiences of many westerners can be expected to lead to a homogenization of experiences on a global scale. In this way, the boundary between disease and its experience blurs.

Life-style means two things in this context. The first meaning is linked to the concept of reliability. From an industrial point of view, quality products are ones that are reliable in the way that Big Mac hamburgers are—they offer the same return every time. When drugs become quality products in this sense, companies appear happy to drop the medical or disease framework. In the case of Viagra, companies talk openly about life-style products for this reason as much as for its effects on sexual functioning.

The second meaning of the notion of a life-style drug marries reliability and risk.[33] The best-selling drugs in the marketplace have for the past twenty years been drugs that act on risk factors for diseases, such as elevated blood pressure or elevated lipid levels, rather than on core diseases—strokes or heart attacks.

There are a huge number of incentives to companies to think in terms of treating risks. It is much easier to alter risks such as elevated blood pressure or lipid levels reliably than it is to cure a disease. While antihypertensives reliably lower blood pressure, they may have little impact on the wider state of the health of the population. Agents targeted at risks are more likely to meet industrial criteria for quality.

A second attraction is that if 1 person per 100 has a disease, at least 10 per 100 can be expected to carry a risk factor for this disease. Traditional medicine mandates the treatment of the 1 diseased individual, whereas the new emphasis on risk mandates the treatment of all 10 who are at risk. A further attraction is that whereas the treatment of a disease comes to a full stop when the patient is cured, the predisposing risk and the risk of relapse may go on forever.[34]

Finally, when it comes to treating risks, drugs that do so are often life-style agents in the further sense that many of these treatments act to reverse the effects of life-style options. Lipid-lowering drugs are often deployed to reverse the effects of a diet chronically high in lipids. Antihypertensives may be acting to reverse the effects of a sedentary life-style laced with too much alcohol. In many ways, we seem to have come back to the *Tacuinum Sanitatis* and other medieval health handbooks that endorsed dietary and other manipulations to forestall the emergence of diseases that could not be treated.

The clinical trial process feeds figures on the effects of drugs on risks into the marketplace. Quite aside from the sequestration of data and ghostwriting in modern trials, another problem for both patients and physicians lies in the selection process that controls what figures appear in academic and lay markets. In addition to figures that demonstrate a lowering of blood pressure, the same trials yield figures that can tell us how many people need to be treated in order to save a life. Knowing that it might take 800 people to be treated with antihypertensives to save one life would influence many of us, when it comes to contemplating whether to take a drug that might wipe out our sex life or otherwise impair our quality of life. But these figures are usually concealed. And, the marketing of the past decade has blurred the boundaries between risks and diseases so that physicians increasingly fail to see that there is a world of a difference between not treating a mild hypertension and not treating a fulminant pneumonia.

The rhetoric of marketing similarly equates those who can be conceived as being at some theoretical risk of suicide with those who have tried to commit suicide. This equation contributed to the competing perceptions that fueled the SSRI and suicide crisis. Some physicians saw children at risk of suicide who were now being denied treatment, while others saw children at little risk of suicide being put at risk.

THE WOUNDED HEALER

The market in psychotropic drugs functions in almost exactly the same way as any other market. It is critically dependent on sensitive sales data. Most readers will have noticed the developing capacities of supermarkets like Wal-Mart or Safeway to monitor what we buy in order to better match its produce and its layout to our needs. However the market information-gathering capacities of supermarket chains are decades behind those of pharmaceutical companies and organizations such as IMS Health.

Good businesses should have good information-gathering capacities. But the other businesses involved in health care, from HMOs through to the NHS in Britain, lack even the basic data that one might think would be needed to ensure their survival in a hard-nosed business world. As scientists, data should be central for clinicians also. But clinicians have no data on the numbers of people prescribed various drugs or the trajectory of their exposure to these drugs.

When this fact is allied to the fact that physicians report serious adverse events on treatment to regulators in no more than 1 case per 100, and these are hardly ever reported in journals, which are reluctant to take "anecdotes," a picture emerges in which we track the fate of parcels put in the post 100 times more accurately than we track the occurrence of adverse events in people put on treatments.

Two issues emerge from these figures. First, not only have journals and academics sacrificed descriptions of individual patients to reports of controlled trials, but they have helped create a situation in which, as outlined in chapter 4, the data from 90 percent of the recipients of treatment are consigned to the waste bin of history.

Second, both physicians and the public have been conditioned to believe that psychotropic drugs are as effective as penicillin. Americans in particular believe in science and progress, and they clamor for agents that help solve their most pressing problem— that messy and risky common endeavor we call life. Companies have made a huge contribution to creating this need by wheeling out experts to assure people that answers to that most pressing of problems, the future safety and well being of their child, are at hand. This expectation has fueled the extraordinary sales of *The Bipolar Child*. Getting the diagnosis confers access to something close to sacramental.

When we arrive at a situation in which the mental sets of clinicians have been captured so that it is difficult for them to conceive of alternatives to those being sold to them, there are reasonable grounds to state that such a field is no longer scientific. When there is almost no possibility of discrepant data emerging to trigger a thought that might be unwelcome to the marketing department of a pharmaceutical company, these marketing capabilities would seem appropriately described as totalitarian.

At this point a fundamental opposition between science and marketing becomes apparent. Whereas the goal of marketing is to build a consensus, and in the domain of therapeutics to build an expert consensus, the goal of science according to many philosophies of sciences is to fracture consensus. Science is supposed to thrive on the registration of discrepant observations or discordant incidents, which lead on to a refutation of previous conjectures or consensus. Even drug companies should benefit from this process, in that the major source of discovery of new drugs still comes from someone recognizing that a drug is doing something other than what it was supposed to do—as with Viagra.

If discrepant observations fail to register, is there any hope of progress? Theriac, which can retrospectively be seen as the ultimate brand medicine, after all lasted for more than a millennium. Two points offer some hope. One is that a great deal of our current predicament stems from a gross failure by academics and clinicians to understand statistics.[35] Hitherto, I have used the term *informational reductionism* throughout this text rather than statistics, as it is far from inevitable that taking statistical approaches should reduce individual variability to aggregate uniformity in the manner that is so obvious in current psychiatry. At some point, we are likely to come to grips with these issues.

A second hope lies in the role of physicians. The mundane side to all this is that the processes outlined here have made the experience of many psychiatrists truly awful. Thomas Bittker nearly three decades ago predicted that these industrial processes, applied to health care organizations, would impinge on the life of physicians.[36] He outlined a world in which clinical care would be restructured just as pharmaceutical companies had been a decade before. The clinical encounter would be dissembled into its component parts and reassembled in a way that would enable managers, who clearly cannot alter the course of disease, to get as close to quality outcomes (in the industrial sense of quality) as they could by managing their physician resource. All predictions have come true, so that physicians now practice in terms of strictly defined brief medication management sessions with patients.

Combining these brief visits where there is no chance to find out anything about the person who might have a disease, with a set of categorical disease criteria with which many psychiatrists fundamentally disagree, and sets of algorithms that dictate treatments with drugs that many think may well be inferior, produces a profoundly dispiriting situation for many psychiatrists.[37]

The fact that the lot of a physician has become something of a factory or office job will not cut much mustard with anyone who has always had to work in a factory or office, and this transformation in itself does not offer much hope for change. But there is one aspect to what has happened to physicians that puts them in a position to perhaps finally fill a role carved out for them when ethical drugs were made available on prescription-only status. There is a sizable literature on the wounded healer and how the sickness of a physician can transform his practice of medicine. Where once there was an occasional wounded healer, and he shared the patient's situation by virtue of suffering from a disease, the current situation has made all physicians vulnerable in ways that only patients have been hitherto vulnerable.

In the 1960s the emergence of clinical trial data grounded the modern notion of informed consent.[38] Prior to this, patients who dared to challenge the authority of a physician were likely to be dismissed with the suggestion that their views might be entertained if they qualified in medicine. RCTs, however, made a mass of data on the outcomes of treatment available, to which patients could appeal and against which physicians could be held to account.

Drugs were made available on prescription-only status because it was thought that patients in the 1950s and 1960s simply did not know enough to understand the data and the issues. Physicians, however, would be able to prize relevant data out of drug companies where this was needed and would be able to assess the potential for risks and benefits in new and potent therapies.

But both patients and physicians now face a new and common problem, which is the lack of access to data. The publicly available data are close to worthless. If the physician or her relatives get ill, there is nothing to depend upon. They are as vulnerable now as any patient ever was, and the only way forward lies in common cause with patients to ensure that the consent of both is informed. Survival and safety are needs—not just wants—that the pharmaceutical industry is moving ever further from meeting.

Meeting this need would do far more than simply make individual therapeutic encounters safer. If the data on the true benefits and hazards of treatment were available, the exuberance that companies can engender by apparently marketing agents of extraordinary efficacy and almost no risks would be curbed, and if curbed, the vast profits that now support the most sophisticated marketing on the planet, a marketing that conjures diseases out of vicissitudes, would be limited. And if this happened, medical practice might return to something recognizably closer to what it once was.

THE PIED PIPER

Manic-depressive illness provides a compelling symbol of the current problems of medicine. Its dominant therapies are classified under an advertising rubric—mood stabilization. The core illness has been rebranded in a way that is all but meaningless. The basis on which its leading drugs were patented appears to make a mockery of the patent system, in terms of the goals of both novelty and public utility that the system is supposed to serve.

In the past, Stalin earned the epithet of The Engineer of Human Souls on the basis of his ability to shape the way people thought; now the market leads patients to queue up to confess their bipolarity or whatever is au courant. The market also arranges for the formerly independent voices of physicians to be silenced by the *una duce, una voce* process of guidelines. The market arranges for critics of current products to be marginalized or silenced in a style that conjures up the notion of brand fascism.

And just as everything was crumbling behind the rhetoric of Stalinism, so also there is good evidence that outcomes within mental health are deteriorating. While the absolute numbers of patients occupying beds in asylums began to fall in the 1950s, the numbers of both voluntary and involuntary admissions per annum has been rising steadily since then. In North Wales, there has been a fifteenfold rise in admissions.[39] Rates of suicide for patients with schizophrenia have increased more than tenfold.[40] Uniquely among major illnesses in the Western world, the life expectancy for patients with serious mental illness has declined.[41] Patients with manic-depressive illness have a severalfold greater rate of admissions than they had before the advent of mood stabilizers.[42] Were this pattern documented elsewhere in medicine, one imagines there would be an outcry, and the system would collapse.

We have arrived on the further banks of this story, but at this point it has become a story without heroes. This is not just because it is more difficult to portray contemporaries as heroes but rather because it is not possible to be certain that any authors of any recent articles trumpeting breakthroughs have participated meaningfully in any of the work they celebrate. If there is a central figure, he is almost an antihero—Michael Shepherd, who toward the end of his life felt like the creator of an atom bomb might have felt post-Hiroshima.[43]

As its final horror, the system has begun to swallow up children in a manner that irresistibly brings forth the image of the Pied Piper of Hamelin. In the 1950s, the pharmaceutical industry expanded the range of human freedoms by helping eliminate lethal infections and disorders like malignant hypertension. Although not as impressive as that of the fabled piper, this elimination of ancient scourges was wonderfully welcome. But, as in the fairy tale, where the piper is denied his just reward and takes revenge, so also, in ways that may have seemed bewildering to many in the industry, the societal response was to restrict the piper to using his powers for the purposes of eliminating diseases only and to install physicians as the gatekeepers to profits.

Not surprisingly, companies turned to marketing diseases, and physicians have been co-opted in the process. Professors of psychiatry, even from Harvard, at a few thousand dollars per lecture are a cheaper resource than company detail men. A generation of children is now being led away, and we seem as powerless to stop this happening as Emil Kraepelin was to stop his children dying of epidemic infections.

The Once and Future Laboratory

❋ ❋ ❋

When delegates convened for the first major psychopharmacology meetings in the late 1950s and early 1960s, they came from all over the world—Christian, Hindu, Muslim and Jew, Japanese, and South American, as well as Europeans and North Americans. They came because a treatment first discovered for mania, chlorpromazine, transcended national frontiers and cultural barriers. Partly because of commonalities of social class and background training, while in the conference halls and wandering around strange cities together, they found—sometimes to their considerable surprise— there was much more that united than divided them, despite these national, religious, and ethnic differences. Many might have felt that swapping children would have made little difference as to how these children would have turned out. Yet any one of these foreigners set down outside these academic cocoons, alone in London, New York, Delhi, or Tokyo in the 1950s, would have been severely disconcerted by culture shock.

If any of these psychopharmacologists had been able to meet up with the earliest British pioneers of neuroscience in seventeenth-century Oxford, where Thomas Willis was mapping the brain, they would probably also have had much in common, and not just with the science involved. Just as Willis had to tread carefully, so also had Herman van Praag in the 1960s in supposedly liberal Holland. The new psychopharmacology of the brain was

widely perceived as intensely materialistic and van Praag, as one
of its early practitioners, was subject to death threats and protests.[1]

Psychopharmacology gave rise to yet another brain. Following
Willis, the eighteenth and nineteenth centuries had brought speculation about the location of different faculties in different brain
areas. This possibility was deeply disturbing for many concerned
about its implications for what it meant to be human. But, experimental work in the nineteenth century also led in the latter half
of the century to the view that the brain conducted its business
electrically. Curiously, this finding seemed to offer a compromise.
Many could continue to see humans as mechanical systems in
which an electrical wraith or ghost hovered in the machinery of
the brain—a ghost that might function independently of the machinery if need be— a ghost that was in some senses immaterial
or at least not particulate.

The first intimations of something different came in the years
just before the First World War, when Henry Dale and others
working in England and Germany began to demonstrate that
histamine and other agents might play a role in peripheral neurotransmission.[2] These early breakthroughs led in the 1920s and
1930s to the celebrated work of Otto Loewi on acetylcholine, and
Walter Cannon on adrenaline and noradrenaline. But despite an
accumulating body of evidence indicating that these neurohumors played a part in peripheral neurotransmission and that drug
treatments acted by modulating or blocking the effects of neurotransmitters, there was an entrenched resistance to the idea of
chemical neurotransmission.

Even the scientists who argued for chemical neurotransmission in the periphery found it almost inconceivable that the brain
might operate in a similar way. In a Moses leading his people to
the Promised Land moment, Henry Dale, along with Jack Gad-
dum, Marthe Vogt, and Wilhelm Feldberg on the one side, at
a CIBA symposium in London in 1960, found themselves faced
with Arvid Carlsson outlining the evidence that serotonin, dopamine, and noradrenaline were central neurotransmitters, but
Dale and his followers chose instead to read the evidence as indicating these chemicals, when found in the brain, functioned

as poisons.[3] The resistance to explaining the functioning of the brain in terms of chemical neurotransmission was profound.

It can be argued that chemical neurotransmission had in some sense been foreshadowed in the seventeenth century by followers of Paracelsus like van Helmont. The early chemical doctors had seen chemical interactions producing processes such as fermentation that gave rise to vapors, and it was these vapors or spirits that did the "business."[4] These vapors were in some senses not much different from the humors of Galenic medicine, or later electrical wraiths. But the emerging biochemical psychopharmacology of the 1960s was vaporless, spiritless, and particulate.

In part, the resistance displayed by the physiologists of the 1940s and 1950s unquestionably stemmed simply from the complexity of the brain, and difficulties in imagining how a chemical brain might work and the all-too-imaginable difficulties in manipulating or experimenting on this mass of neurons and their soup of fluids. But the resistance must also have been partly spiritual, where by spiritual I am referring to our ability to give some account for a human life, some understanding of why we fall in love and get gripped by causes, some truths that we pass on to our children.

Now that Prozac and Zyprexa have become such commodities, many will find it hard to credit that one of the mobilizing calls of those opposed to neuroscience in the 1960s through to the late 1980s was that neuroscience attempted to smuggle into political life social biases against ethnic groups, the poor, or others on the basis of a supposed biological taint.[5]

More generally, the new particulate brain posed questions about the continuity of the self—not just a possible continuity after death, but rather the very moment-to-moment continuity of the self in the face of shifting chemical balances. How do we emerge from our chemicals? How does the mind—or soul—fit into this new brain? If a disease like manic-depressive illness involves a chemical disorder, is there a boundary between these twisted molecules and our selves, or is the whole self in some sense diseased?

And during the 1960s when modern psychopharmacology was born, the Western world was in just as much turmoil as Willis's England in the seventeenth century. The legitimacy of poli-

tics and of an established order was thrown into question. Just as
300 years earlier a new democracy was being born, so also in the
1960s a new global democratic order was taking shape, an order
in which women, ethnic groups, and the young had a part that
they had not had previously. Just as in the 1660s, the world was
turned upside down, and it seemed as though "the people" might
subvert the established order.[6]

Willis was a clinician as well as a neuroscientist. And the problems about where to locate the human spirit he faced were faced
also by Falret and Kahlbaum. Whatever we think about other
diseases, when it comes to diseases of behavior, the capacity to
conceive of a disease like manic-depressive disorder was all but
completely constrained by our views of how humans functioned.
Once the brain emerged on the clinical stage, it became the cru-
cial backdrop to the story through to the present. Whatever view
we have of a disease like manic-depressive insanity will necessarily
be intimately tied up with how we view the self and its brain and
issues of human responsibility.

The management of mood disorders with treatments like ECT
continues to provoke the most vigorous debates in all of medicine.[7]
While the overtly spiritual aspects of these issues have gone underground since the 1960s, it is not difficult to resurrect the inner
daemons. For example, free-range versions of fashionable psychotropic brands are staples of animal husbandry aimed at reducing
stress in animals so that they can be battery farmed; can we be
certain that the point of branding is not to do the same to us?

But the story has also changed. Far from coming into wider
view, the brain of modern neuroscience risks disappearing behind
a pastiche generated in company marketing departments. And it
is here that the "spiritual" problem now lies. While the September
11th planes did not blazon their rejection of a world of chemical
imbalances, this was an attack on perceptions of Western values.

As the most profitable of corporations, pharmaceutical companies were inescapably implicated in any attack on the World
Trade Center. And while Levi jeans and other products have
frequently been held up as the fruits of the Western way of doing things, Western health care has arguably been a more central driver of Western expansion. Not only do consumers who die

young buy less, but a key reason to buy into the Western way of doing things has been because until the 1980s it came with longevity attached. Commodities like penicillin and insulin drew us together in a way that Levis and Ipods never could. The health *oikumene* has been central to Western values since Hippocrates.

No longer so. Few people on earth are likely to reject the next penicillin, insulin, or breakthrough high-tech gadget, but it is a different matter to play with our hopes and fears as the witches did with Macbeth, and this playing with our hopes and fears is the very stuff of marketing. This manipulation, rather than breakthrough products, is increasingly what sustains the share price of pharmaceutical companies.

The changing scene has been caught best by Charles Medawar. "I fear that we are heading blindly in the general direction of Pharmageddon. Pharmageddon is a gold-standard paradox: individually we benefit from some wonderful medicines while, collectively, we are losing sight and sense of health. By analogy, think of the relationship between a car journey and climate change—they are inextricably linked, but probably not remotely connected in the driver's mind. Just as climate change seems inconceivable as a journey outcome, so the notion of Pharmageddon is flatly contradicted by most personal experience of medicines."[8]

The manic-depressive story better than any other brings out a growing divide between biology on the one side and commerce and politics on the other. Developments in neuroscience have no intrinsic link with patent law arrangements and the interaction of these laws with phenomena such as branding. The links are structural and historical.

Although the rhetoric of commerce still holds that mapping our genomes will reveal the genetic causes of our diseases, we are learning in contrast to see how patterns of gene activation show the history of our interactions with our environments and what environmental agents have in fact triggered disease. Our biology is a gateway to understanding our environment. While remaining aware that the fruits of scientific progress may provide yet other means of oppression, the exploration of our biology can be a source of liberation as the roots of love lie there and probably instincts such as altruism.

There are also great discontinuities across our time frame, not least for instance in the experience of women,[9] and the almost incomprehensible difference in accessibility to material goods for those living now compared with the lot of anyone living previously. A younger scientist working in a pharmaceutical company would possibly find the journey from today's automated and computational systems to a company laboratory in the 1950s close to unimaginable or recognizable only in terms of what she might have done in high school.

This is a key and perennial problem for history: how to convey change and discontinuities when some of the most important things remain the same over millennia and these continuities need to be brought out in order make any story relevant for the present. People have always fallen in love and been driven by ideals and have needed to find words to tell their children about what it means to be human. These continuities seem uncontestable.

Other continuities can be proposed but should be contested. Thus, we can note a remarkable superficial similarity at least between the cocktails of mood stabilizers now regularly given for bipolar disorder and Galen's Theriac (chapters 1 and 6). We can also note that twenty-first-century physicians appear to practice in accord with the dictates of authorities rather than based on their own experience, just as the best Galenic physicians did (chapters 1 and 8). Physicians today who fail to adhere to guidelines run the risk of following Paracelsus and being struck off. We can point to a comparable dominance of commercial factors in medical practice in the Middle Ages and now. In chapter 1 it was suggested that the experience of parents from Hippocrates to Willis and Kraepelin in the face of untreatable epidemics might have commonalities with the experience of parents with children with manic-depressive illness today. In chapter 8, the evolution of current patent laws was noted—and this connects the experience of parents facing an untreatable AIDS epidemic in poorer parts of the globe with parents of bipolar children now.

But to set aside the almost uncontestable continuity between ancient and modern times, there is one close-to-uncontestable discontinuity between the world that emerged with Willis and our current situation. This lies in the central role of data in the world that emerged with the revolution in science that involved a new willingness to settle matters by an appeal to observable data and a growing capacity to generate data that might help settle long-standing uncertainties.

Data were also central to the emergence of democracy and modern economies. The rule of the people by the people hinged critically on knowing how many people there were, and government of ourselves by ourselves has ever since been responsive to evidence, for instance, that people living in one area may be dying faster than those living in other areas, or that particular tax arrangements yield a poorer outcome than others.

As a result, the fact that pharmaceutical companies are now sequestering data is a profound threat to our very modernity. It poses a threat to our science, our democracy, and our values and may also threaten the economy.

The common perception that drugs are made in university or company laboratories is wrong. As this history should make clear, companies may make chemicals, but we are the laboratories in which modern drugs are made. There is an immediate and less immediate sense to our role. In a very physical sense, drugs cannot come into being unless we as healthy volunteers and later as patients in clinical trials agree to take them to see what happens. Without this participation by the community, there is no drug.

Our willingness to participate in these studies was borne out of the global calamity of world war, when conditions of scarcity mandated the development of the first controlled trials. We participated on the basis that taking risks might injure us but would benefit a community that included our friends, relatives, and children. We did so for free. At first this worked and extended the compass of human freedom from the epidemics and other scourges to which our ancestors had been subject for millennia.

But now these data freely given are sequestered by corporations who market selected parts of it back to us under the banner of science. This business model has made these corporations the most profitable on the planet. The process is one that increasingly appears to jeopardize the health and well-being of our friends, relatives, and children.

In a less immediate and less physical sense companies take

our inner aspirations and fears and mold these into a strategy designed to get us to consume drugs more faithfully than we would do if we were living in a totalitarian regime and were ordered to consume.

And the same process, by which they effect this compliance, has now begun to interfere with our very conception of who we are just as much as any developments in neuroscience might do. A chemical patois that bears no relationship to the latest neuroscience is not something to hand on to children, even if the message comes in graphic form in a coloring book. The idea that the language in which we describe ourselves might be subject to change at predictable intervals coinciding with the fall of off-patent and rise of newly patented compounds is disturbing.

Companies once affected our experience by delivering us from disease, but now their capacities to control our experience seem to be escalating in inverse proportion to their ability to deliver us from new diseases, and instead their strategies appear to be infecting formerly healthy experiences.

There is no better example of this strategy than manic-depressive disorder. While there can still be some uncertainty about the ideal type or perhaps the number of ideal types there are in the family of severe affective disorders, these disorders have in all probability been continuous in all cultures across time. Our desperate need for cures for these conditions marks another point of continuity with those who have gone before us. But we now have instead a system that inhibits our abilities to find cures while encouraging companies to seek short-term profits by co-opting bipolar disorder for the purposes of increasing the sales of major tranquilizers to infants. Giving major tranquilizers to children is little different from giving children cancer chemotherapy when they have a cold. There is here an extraordinary discontinuity with the hopes we have invested in medicine.

Because our civilization appears threatened by fundamentalisms whose appeal lies in a message that we have lost sight of some of the most important things about being human, and because the creation of bipolar disorder in children is so alarming, we need to chart the currents that delivered us to this shore.

NOTES

Preface. Stories about Mania

1. Alex's story closely follows a real case history which I became aware of in 2002. Much more recently, the story of four-year-old Rebecca Riley from Boston made front-page news, as it became clear that her death may have been linked to medications for bipolar disorder, which she had been taking since the age of two. http://ahrp.blogspot.com/2007/02/4-year-old-rebecca-riley-casualty-of.html.

2. Daston L (2005). *The History of Science as European Self-Portraiture*. Praemium Erasmianum Foundation, Amsterdam.

3. This is a history that unashamedly embraces the progress of "hard" science. There is no suggestion here that science undoes itself or does not make progress in terms of things known and mastery of the world, that it is simply a reflection of a statement that Niels Bohr would have endorsed—that sometimes new ideas only triumph when the proponents of older ideas die.

4. Healy D (2004). Psychopharmacologie et histoire: Un manifeste. *Psychiatrie, Sciences Humaines et Neurosciences* 2, 3–7.

5. Cowen P (2004). Review of *The Creation of Psychopharmacology*. *Psychological Medicine* 34, 173–180.

Chapter 1. Frenzy and Stupor

1. Goodwin FK, Jamison KR (1990). *Manic Depressive Illness*. Oxford University Press, New York; Angst J, Marneros A (2001). Bipolarity from ancient to modern times: Conception, birth and rebirth. *Journal of Affective Disorders* 67, 3–19. See Nordic Psychiatry Academy, January 20, 2006. http://gdp.videoarkiv.net/janssen-cilag/20012006_JC_DK_nordic_academy/default.html, accessed March 28, 2006.

2. Kraepelin E (1899). *Psychiatrie. Ein Lehrbuch fur Studirende und Aertze*. 6th edition. JA Barth, Leipzig. Trans. Quen, JM, Watson Publishing, Canton, Mass.

3. Lloyd GER (ed.) (1950). *Hippocratic Writings*. Trans. Chadwick J, Mann WN, Penguin Books, Harmondsworth, Middlesex.

4. The various translations of Hippocrates' writings are historically uninformed and correspondingly inaccurate. The vignettes presented here are translated by the author and supplemented by Lloyd GER (ed.) (1950). *Hippocratic Writings*. Trans. Chadwick J, Mann WN, Penguin Books, Harmondsworth, Middlesex, p. 138, as well as the Greek text and French translations available on www.bium.univ-paris5.fr/histmed/medica/hipp_va.htm. From *Hippocrates,* volume 1, trans. Jones WR, Loeb Classical Library, p. 276.

5. The word *phrenitis* is translated as "brain fever" by Chadwick, for instance,

when in most cases where fever was present Hippocrates makes this clear by using πυρετός. And Hippocrates would have had no conception of a brain or of an inflammation of the brain implied by brain fever.

6. In addition to the usual difficulties translating a word, from Galen onward there have been uncertainties about whether this is δυσάνιος or δυσήνιος, which could change meaning.

7. This is rarely if ever translated as *dysthymic,* which is a word that has only recently come back into use.

8. Typically translated as *convulsions,* where the more literal spasms might be better.

9. Lloyd GER (ed.) (1950). *Hippocratic Writings.* Trans. Chadwick J, Mann WN, Penguin Books, Harmondsworth, Middlesex, pp. 134–135.

10. Lloyd GER (ed.) (1950). *Hippocratic Writings.* Trans. Chadwick J, Mann WN, Penguin Books, Harmondsworth, Middlesex, p. 215.

11. Lloyd GER (ed.) (1950). *Hippocratic Writings.* Trans. Chadwick J, Mann WN, Penguin Books, Harmondsworth, Middlesex, p. 152.

12. Lloyd GR (1979). *Magic, Reason and Experience. Studies in the Origin and Development of Greek Science.* Cambridge University Press, Cambridge.

13. Tranter R, Healy H, Cattell D, Healy D (2002). Functional variations in agents differentially selective to monoaminergic systems. *Psychological Medicine* 32, 517–524.

14. Lloyd GER (ed.) (1950). *Hippocratic Writings.* Trans. Chadwick J, Mann WN, Penguin Books, Harmondsworth, Middlesex, p. 249.

15. Lloyd GER (ed.) (1950). *Hippocratic Writings.* Trans. Chadwick J, Mann WN, Penguin Books, Harmondsworth, Middlesex, p. 248.

16. *Oxford Classical Greek Dictionary* (2002). Oxford University Press, Oxford.

17. Dysphoria here in its original sense almost certainly refers to something closer to pain than to a mood state.

18. Lloyd GER (ed.) (1950). *Hippocratic Writings.* Trans. Chadwick J, Mann WN, Penguin Books, Harmondsworth, Middlesex, pp. 128–129.

19. Brockington IF (1996). *Motherhood and Mental Illness.* Oxford University Press, Oxford; Marland H (2004). *Dangerous Motherhood. Insanity and Childbirth in Victorian Britain.* Palgrave Macmillan, New York.

20. www.perseus.tufts.edu/cgi-bin/ptextlookup=Plt.+Phaedrus+244b.

21. See Diethelm O (1971). *Medical Dissertations of Psychiatric Interest before 1750.* Karger, Basel, pp. 17–19.

22. Goodwin FK, Jamison KR (1990). *Manic Depressive Illness.* Oxford University Press, New York; Angst J, Marneros A (2001). Bipolarity from ancient to modern times: Conception, birth and rebirth. *Journal of Affective Disorders* 67, 3–19.

23. Cited in Jackson SW (1986). *Melancholia and Depression.* Yale University Press, New Haven, Conn., p. 39. See other wording in Aretaeus.

24. Diethelm O (1971). *Medical Dissertations of Psychiatric Interest before 1750.* Karger, Basel.

25. Cited in Diethelm O (1971). *Medical Dissertations of Psychiatric Interest before 1750.* Karger, Basel, pp. 72–73.

26. Fink M, Taylor MA (2003). *Catatonia*. Cambridge University Press, Cambridge.

27. Porter R (1997). *The Greatest Benefit to Mankind. A medical history of humanity from antiquity to the present*. HarperCollins, London.

28. *The Medieval Health Handbook, "Tacuinum Sanitatis"* (1976). Ed. Luisa Cogliati Arano, George Braziller, New York.

29. Paracelsus (1979). *Selected Writings*. Ed. Jolande Jacobi, Princeton University Press, Princeton, p. liii.

30. Paracelsus (1979). *Selected Writings*. Ed. Jolande Jacobi, Princeton University Press, Princeton, p. 84.

31. Pagel W (1980). *Paracelsus: An Introduction to Philosophical Medicine in the Era of the Renaissance*. Karger, Basel; Ball P (2006). *The Devil's Doctor. Paracelsus and the World of Renaissance Magic and Science*. William Heinemann, London.

32. Maehle A-H (1999). *Drugs on Trial: Experimental Pharmacology and Therapeutic Innovation in the Eighteenth Century*. Editions Rodopi, Amsterdam.

33. Porter R, Porter D (1989). The rise of the English drugs industry: The role of Thomas Corbyn. *Medical History* 33, 277–295.

34. Cited in Diethelm O (1971). *Medical Dissertations of Psychiatric Interest before 1750*. Karger, Basel, p. 32.

35. Henningus Unverzagt (1614). *De Melancholia*. Helmstadt. Cited in Diethelm O (1971). *Medical Dissertations of Psychiatric Interest before 1750*. Karge, Basel, p. 33.

36. C Vater. Cited in Diethelm O (1971). *Medical Dissertations of Psychiatric Interest before 1750*. Karger, Basel, pp. 38–39.

37. Sydenham T (1716). *The Practice of Physick*. Trans. William Salmon, London. Cited in Diethelm O (1971). *Medical Dissertations of Psychiatric Interest before 1750*. Karger, Basel, pp. 90–91.

38. Cited in Zimmer C (2004). *Soul Made Flesh*. William Heinemann, London, p. 246.

39. Healy D (1993). *Images of Trauma. From Hysteria to Post-traumatic Stress Disorder*. Faber & Faber, London, chapters 1–3.

40. Healy D (1993). *Images of Trauma. From Hysteria to Post-traumatic Stress Disorder*. Faber & Faber, London, chapter 4.

41. Fink M, Taylor MA (2003). *Catatonia*. Cambridge University Press, Cambridge; Chalassani P, Healy D, Morriss R (2005). Presentation and frequency of catatonia in new admissions to two acute psychiatric admission units in India and Wales. *Psychological Medicine* 35, 1667–1675.

42. Hare E (1981). The two manias: A study of the evolution of the modern concept of mania. *British Journal of Psychiatry* 138, 89–99.

43. Berrios GE (1981). The two manias. *British Journal of Psychiatry* 139, 258–259.

44. Kiple K (ed.) (1997). *Plagues, Pox and Pestilence. Disease in History*. Weidenfeld and Nicolson, London.

45. Cambridge only opened a clinical school in the 1970s.

Chapter 2. Circling the Brain

1. Dumit J (2004). *Picturing Personhood. Brain Scans and Biomedical Identity.* Princeton University Press, Princeton.

2. Martensen RL (2004). *The Brain Takes Shape, an Early History.* Oxford University Press, New York.

3. Descartes R (1649/1989). *The Passions of the Soul.* Hackett Publishing, Indianapolis.

4. Descartes R (1662/1972). *The Treatise on Man.* Trans. Hall TS, Harvard University Press, Cambridge, Mass. The *Treatise* was however essentially written by 1633.

5. Lloyd GER (ed.) (1950). *Hippocratic Writings.* Trans. Chadwick J, Mann WN, Penguin Books, Harmondsworth, Middlesex, p. 250.

6. Lloyd GER (ed.) (1950). *Hippocratic Writings.* Trans. Chadwick J, Mann WN, Penguin Books, Harmondsworth, Middlesex, p. 248.

7. Martensen RL (2004). *The Brain Takes Shape, an Early History.* Oxford University Press, New York; Zimmer, C. (2004). *Soul Made Flesh.* William Heinemann, London.

8. Martensen RL (2004). *The Brain Takes Shape, an Early History.* Oxford University Press, New York; Zimmer, C. (2004). *Soul Made Flesh.* William Heinemann, London.

9. Zimmer C (2004). *Soul Made Flesh.* William Heinemann, London.

10. Martensen RL (2004). *The Brain Takes Shape, an Early History.* Oxford University Press, New York.

11. Porter R (2003). *Flesh in the Age of Reason.* Allen Lane, London.

12. Koutouvidis N, Marketos SG (1995). The contribution of Thomas Sydenham (1624–1689) to the evolution of psychiatry. *History of Psychiatry* 6, 513–520.

13. Conrad LI, Neve M, Nutton V, Porter R, Wear A (1995). *The Western Medical Tradition. 800 BC to AD 1800.* Cambridge University Press, Cambridge.

14. Rational in this sense is somewhat equivalent to being logical in preference to being empirical.

15. Hill C (1972). *The World Turned Upside Down.* Penguin Books, Harmondsworth, Middlesex.

16. Febvre L (1982). *The Problem of Unbelief in the Sixteenth Century.* Harvard University Press, Cambridge, Mass.

17. Shapin S (1994). *A Social History of Truth: Science and Civility in Seventeenth Century England.* University of Chicago Press, Chicago.

18. Clark E, Jacyna LS (1987). *Nineteenth Century Origins of Neuroscientific Concepts.* University of California Press, Berkeley.

19. From Willis T (1664). Cerebri anatome: Cui accessit nervorum descriptio et usus. London. Trans. Pordage S (1681), *The Anatomy of the Brain and Nerves*; republished, Feindel W (ed), McGill University Press, Montreal, p. 124.

20. Pinero JML (1983). *Historical Origins of the Concept of Neurosis.* Trans. Berrios D, Cambridge University Press, Cambridge; French RK (1969). *Robert Whytt, the Soul and Medicine.* Wellcome Institute for the History of Medicine, London.

21. Kraepelin E (1899). *Psychiatrie. Ein Lehrbuch für Studirende und Aertze.* Barth, Leipzig, volume 1. Trans. Metoui H (1960), Science History Publications, Canton, Mass.

22. Descartes R (1639/1989). *The Passions of the Soul,* Article 16 (17).

23. French RK (1969). *Robert Whytt, the Soul and Medicine.* Wellcome Institute for the History of Medicine, London.

24. Clark E, Jacyna LS (1987). *Nineteenth Century Origins of Neuroscientific Concepts.* University of California Press, Berkeley.

25. Clark E, Jacyna LS (1987). *Nineteenth Century Origins of Neuroscientific Concepts.* University of California Press, Berkeley; Hall TS (1969). *History of General Physiology,* volume 2, University of Chicago Press, Chicago.

26. Cited in Clark E, Jacyna LS (1987). *Nineteenth Century Origins of Neuroscientific Concepts.* University of California Press, Berkeley, p. 143.

27. Laycock T (1844). *On the Reflex Functions of the Brain.* Cited in Dewhurst K (1982). *Hughlings Jackson on Psychiatry.* Sandford Publications, Oxford.

28. Scull A (2005). *Madhouse. A Tragic Tale of Megalomania and Modern Medicine.* Yale University Press, New Haven.

29. Healy D (1993). *Images of Trauma. From Hysteria to Post-traumatic Stress Disorder.* Faber & Faber, London, chapter 9.

30. Freud S (1895). In *Standard Edition of the Complete Psychological Works of Sigmund Freud,* ed. Strachey J, Hogarth Press, London, volume 1, pp. 295–391.

31. Healy D (1996). Irish psychiatry in the twentieth century: Notes towards a history. In *150 Years of British Psychiatry,* volume 2, ed. Freeman H and Berrios GE, Athlone Press, London, pp. 268–291.

32. Foucault M (1972). *Histoire de la Folie à l'âge classique.* Gallimard, Paris; Scull A (1979). *Museums of Madness.* Allen Lane, London; Scull A (1994). Somatic treatments and the historiography of psychiatry. *History of Psychiatry* 5, 1–12.

33. Shorter E (1996). *A History of Psychiatry. From the Era of the Asylum to the Age of Prozac.* J Wiley & Sons, Bristol.

34. Esquirol JED (1838). *Des maladies mentales considérées sous les rapports médical hygienique et médico-legal.* Paris, Baillière. Trans. Hunt EK (1845) as *Mental Maladies: A Treatise on Insanity,* Philadelphia, Lea and Blanchard; republished, Haffner Publishing Company, New York, 1965.

35. Esquirol JED (1838). *Des maladies mentales considérées sous les rapports médical hygienique et médico-legal.* Paris, Baillière. Trans. Hunt EK (1845) as *Mental Maladies: A Treatise on Insanity,* Philadelphia, Lea and Blanchard; republished, Haffner Publishing Company, New York, 1965, pp. 199–200.

36. Esquirol JED (1838). *Des maladies mentales considérées sous les rapports médical hygienique et médico-legal.* Paris, Baillière. Trans. Hunt EK (1845) as *Mental Maladies: A Treatise on Insanity,* Philadelphia, Lea and Blanchard; republished, Haffner Publishing Company, New York, 1965, p. 203.

37. Prichard JC (1835). *Treatise on Insanity and Other Disorders Affecting the Mind.* Sherwood, Gilbert & Piper, London. See Berrios GE (1999). J. C. Prichard and the concept of "moral insanity." *History of Psychiatry* 10, 111–116; Prichard JC (1835/1999). Moral Insanity. *History of Psychiatry* 10, 117–126.

38. Cited in Shorter ES (2005). *A Historical Dictionary of Psychiatry*. Oxford University Press, Oxford, p. 228.

39. See Jackson SW (1986). *Melancholia and Depression*. Yale University Press, New Haven, Conn., p. 257.

40. From Haslam J (1798). *Observations on Insanity*. London, Rivington. Cited in Jackson SW (1986). *Melancholia and Depression*. Yale University Press, New Haven, Conn., p. 260.

41. Crichton A (1798). *An Inquiry into the Nature and Origin of Mental Derangement*. Cadell and Davies, London. Cited in Jackson SW (1986). *Melancholia and Depression*. Yale University Press, New Haven, Conn., p. 260.

42. Esquirol JED (1838). *Des maladies mentales considérées sous les rapports médical hygienique et médico-legal*. Paris, Baillière. Trans. Hunt EK (1845) as *Mental Maladies: A Treatise on Insanity*, Philadelphia, Lea and Blanchard; republished, Haffner Publishing Company, New York, 1965.

43. Bayle A (1826). *Traité des maladies du cerveau et de ses membranes*. Paris, Gabon. See also Bayle A (1822). Researches on chronic arachnitis, published in *Anthology of French Language Psychiatric Texts*, ed. Cousin F-R, Garrabé J, Morozov D, Les Empêcheurs de Penser en Rond, Paris, pp. 148–158.

44. Falret J-P (1854). Of the non-existence of monomania. In *Leçons clinique de médecine mentale faites a l'hospice de la Salpêtrière*, Paris, Baillière; also in *Anthology of French Language Psychiatric Texts*, ed. Cousin F-R, Garrabé J, Morozov D, Les Empêcheurs de Penser en Rond, Paris, pp. 108–126.

45. Walker N (1968). *Crime and Insanity in England*. Edinburgh University Press, Edinburgh; Rosenberg C (1968). *The Trial of the Assassin Guiteau. Psychiatry and the Law in the Gilded Age*. University of Chicago Press, Chicago.

46. Hale M (1736/2003). *Historia Placitorum Coronae*, volume 1, *Lawbook Exchange*. Clark, NJ, chapter 4, p. 30.

47. Hale M (1736/2003). *Historia Placitorum Coronae*, volume 1, *Lawbook Exchange*. Clark, NJ. chapter 4, pp. 29–37.

48. Cited in Walker N (1968). *Crime and Insanity in England*. Edinburgh University Press, Edinburgh, p. 56.

49. Cited in Walker N (1968). *Crime and Insanity in England*. Edinburgh University Press, Edinburgh, pp. 77 et seq.

50. West DJ, Walk A (1977). *Daniel McNaughton. His Trial and the Aftermath*. Headley Bros, Ashford, Kent.

51. Quen JM (1983). Isaac Ray and the development of psychiatry and the law. *Psychiatric Clinics of North America* 6, 527–538; Zilboorg G (1944). Legal aspects of psychiatry. In *One Hundred Years of American Psychiatry*, American Psychiatric Association, Columbia University Press, New York, pp. 507–588.

52. Ray I (1838). *A Treatise on the Medical Jurisprudence of Insanity*. Belknap, Boston.

53. Haslam J (1817). *Medical Jurisprudence as It Relates to Insanity according to the Law of England*. Callow, London.

54. Pick D (1989). *Faces of Degeneration. A European Disorder c1848–c1918*. Cambridge University Press, Cambridge.

55. Lombroso C (1876). *L'uomo deliquente studiato in rapporto alla anthropologia, alla medicina legale ed. alla discipline carcerarie.* Milan; Lombroso C (2006). *Criminal Man.* Editions 1, 2 (1878), 3 (1884), 4 (1889), 5 (1896). Trans. Gibson M, Rafter NH, Duke University Press, Durham.

56. Rosenberg CE (1968). *The Trial of the Assassin Guiteau. Psychiatry and the Law in the Gilded Age.* University of Chicago Press, Chicago.

57. See case of Stephen Anthony Mobley. www.wadsworth.com/criminaljustice_d/templates/student_resources/0534629016_gaines/great_debates/ch2.html.

58. Healy D, Herxheimer A, Menkes D (2006). Antidepressants and violence. Problems at the interface of law and medicine. *PLoS Medicine* 3, e372, Sept, available on www.plosmedicine.org.

Chapter 3. Circular Madness

1. Wyman R (1830). Exaltation and depression. In Hunter R, MacAlpine I (eds.) (1982), *Three Hundred Years of Psychiatry. 1535–1860,* Carlisle Publishing, New York, pp. 810–811.

2. Prichard JC (1837). Moral insanity. In Hunter R, MacAlpine I (eds.) (1982), *Three Hundred Years of Psychiatry. 1535–1860,* Carlisle Publishing, New York, p. 840. In 1844, Carl Flemming outlined a similar condition and gave it a name, Dysthymia mutabilis; for details see Shorter ES (2005). *A Historical Dictionary of Psychiatry.* Oxford University Press, Oxford, pp. 165–166.

3. François-Régis C (1999). Jules Baillarger (1809–1890). In François-Régis C, Garrabé J, Morozov D (1999). *Anthology of French Language Psychiatric Texts.* Trans. Crisp J, Institute Sanofi-Synthélabo, Paris.

4. Cited in François-Régis C (1999). Jules Baillarger (1809–1890). In François-Régis C, Garrabé J, Morozov D (1999). *Anthology of French Language Psychiatric Texts.* Trans. Crisp J, Institute Sanofi-Synthélabo, Paris, pp. 181–182.

5. Pichot P (1995). The birth of the bipolar disorder. *European Psychiatry* 10, 1–10.

6. Baillarger J (1854). Notes sour un Genre de Folie dont les accés sont carecterisé par deux period régulairè, l'une de depréssion, l'autre d'excitation. *Bulletin de l'Académie de Médecine* 19, 340–352.

7. Baillarger J (1854). De la folie à double forme. *Annales médico-psychologiques* 6, 369–391.

8. Baillarger J (1854). Notes sour un Genre de Folie dont les accés sont carecterisé par deux period régulairè, l'une de depréssion, l'autre d'excitation. *Bulletin de l'Académie de Médecine* 19, 340–352.

9. From Baillarger J (1854). Dual form insanity. In François-Régis C, Garrabé J, Morozov D (1999). *Anthology of French Language Psychiatric Texts.* Trans. Crisp J, Institute Sanofi-Synthélabo, Paris, pp. 186–198 for this and subsequent quotations in text.

10. Falret JP (1854). Mémoire sur la folie circulaire. *Bulletin de l'Académie de Médecine* 19, 382–415. Also see Sedler MJ (1983). Falret's discovery: The origin of the concept of bipolar affective illness. *American Journal of Psychiatry* 140, 1127–1133.

11. Falret (1854). *Leçons clinique de médecine mentale faites à l'Hospice de Salpêtrière.*

Baillière, Paris. For this and subsequent quotations in text, see Sedler MJ (1983). Falret's discovery: The origin of the concept of bipolar affective illness. *American Journal of Psychiatry* 140, 1127–1133, especially pp. 1129–1133.

12. Baillarger J (1854). (Discussion of Falret's lecture). *Bulletin de l'Académie de Médicine* 19, 401–415.

13. Pichot P (1995). The birth of the bipolar disorder. *European Psychiatry* 10, 1–10.

14. Billod E (1856). Des diverses formes de lypemania. *Annales Médico-Psychologique* 20, 308–338.

15. Berrios GE (1996). *The History of Mental Symptoms. Descriptive Psychopathology since the Nineteenth Century.* Cambridge University Press, Cambridge.

16. Krueger S (1999). Karl Ludwig Kahlbaum, Address, American Psychiatric Association Meeting, Washington, D.C., May 15, 1999; Braunig P, Krueger S (1999). Karl Ludwig Kahlbaum. *American Journal of Psychiatry* 156, 989.

17. Krueger S, Braunig P (2000). Ewald Hecker. *American Journal of Psychiatry* 157, 1220.

18. Kahlbaum K (1863), *Die Gruppirung der psychischen Krankheiten und die Eintheilung der Seelenstorungen.* AW Kafemann, Danzig; part of which has been translated by GE Berrios (1996) as The relationships of the new groupings to old classification and to a general pathology of mental disorder. *History of Psychiatry* 7, 167–181; Hecker also put forward this argument a few years later in more readable form. Hecker E (1871/2004). On the origin of the clinical standpoint in psychiatry. *History of Psychiatry* 15, 349–360.

19. Baethge C, Salvatore P, Baldessarini RJ (2003). "On Cyclic Insanity," by Karl Ludwig Kahlbaum, MD; A translation and commentary. *Harvard Review of Psychiatry* 11, 78–90. Kahlbaum K (1882). Über cyklisches Irresein. *Der Irrenfreund-Psychiatrische Monatsschrift für praktische Aerzte* 24, 145–157. Quotation from p. 85.

20. Hecker E (1871). Die Hebephrenie. *Archiv fur pathologische Anatomie und Physiologie und fur klinische Medizin* 25, 394–429. Part of which was translated in Sedler MJ, Schoelly M-L (1985). The legacy of Ewald Hecker: A new translation of "Die Hebephrenie." *American Journal of Psychiatry* 142, 1265–1271.

21. Kahlbaum K (1874), *Katatonie oder das Spannungsirresein.* Kirschwald, Berlin. Trans. Levij Y, Pridan T, Baltimore: Johns Hopkins University Press, 1973; Lanczik M (1992). Karl Ludwig Kahlbaum and the emergence of psychopathological and nosological research in German psychiatry. *History of Psychiatry* 3, 53–58. For a contemporary American reaction to the syndrome and descriptions of cases, see Kiernan JG (1877), Katatonia: A clinical form of insanity. Reprinted in *American Journal of Psychiatry* 151, sesquicentennial supplement, 103–111.

22. Healy D (2002). *The Creation of Psychopharmacology.* Harvard University Press, Cambridge, Mass., chapter 2.

23. Baethge C, Salvatore P, Baldessarini RJ (2003). "On Cyclic Insanity," by Karl Ludwig Kahlbaum, MD; A translation and commentary. *Harvard Review of Psychiatry* 11, 78–90; Kahlbaum K (1882). Über cyklisches Irresein. *Der Irrenfreund-Psychiatrische Monatsschrift für praktische Aerzte* 24, 145–157.

24. Baethge C, Salvatore P, Baldessarini RJ (2003). Introduction: "Cyclothymia,

a Circular Mood Disorder," by Ewald Hecker. *History of Psychiatry* 14, 377–399; Hecker E (2003). Cyclothymia, a Circular Mood Disorder. Trans. Baethge C, Salvatore P, Baldessarini RJ. *History of Psychiatry* 14, 377–399; Hecker E. (1898). Die Cyklothymie, eine cirkuläre Gemüthserkrankung. *Zeitschrift für praktische Aerzte* 7, 6–15.

25. Lange CG (1886). *Om periodiske depressionstilstande.* Copenhagen, Jakob Lunds.

26. Hecker E (2003). Cyclothymia, a circular mood disorder. Trans. Baethge C, Salvatore P, Baldessarini RJ. *History of Psychiatry* 14, 394.

27. Shorter E (2005). Hypomania. In *A Historical Dictionary of Psychiatry.* Oxford University Press, Oxford, pp. 132–133.

28. Hecker E (2003). Cyclothymia, a circular mood disorder. Trans. Baethge C, Salvatore P, Baldessarini RJ. *History of Psychiatry* 14, 398.

29. Hoff P (1995). Kraepelin. In Berrios GE, Porter R, *A History of Clinical Psychiatry,* Athlone Press, London, pp. 261–279; Berrios GE, Hauser R (1995). Kraepelin. In Berrios GE, Porter R, *A History of Clinical Psychiatry,* Athlone Press, London, pp. 280–291; Engstrom EJ (1995). Kraepelin. In Berrios GE, Porter R, *A History of Clinical Psychiatry,* Athlone Press, London, pp. 292–301.

30. Kraepelin E (1892). *Ueber die Beinflussing einfacher psychischer vorgange durch einige arzneimittel.* Gustav Fischer, Jena; Healy D (1993). One hundred years of psychopharmacology. *Journal of Psychopharmacology* 7, 207–214.

31. Shorter E (1997). *A History of Psychiatry. From the Era of the Asylum to the Age of Prozac.* J Wiley & Sons, New York.

32. Kraepelin E (1987). *Memoirs.* Trans. Cheryl Wooding-Deane, Ed. Hippius H, Peters G, Ploog D, Springer Books, Berlin, pp. 60–61.

33. Kraepelin E (1987). *Memoirs.* Trans. Cheryl Wooding-Deane, Ed. Hippius H, Peters G, Ploog D, Springer Books, Berlin.

34. Kraepelin E (1899). Psychiatrie. *Ein Lehrbuch für Studirende und Aertze.* Barth, Leipzig, volume 2. Trans. Ayed S (1960), Science History Publications, Canton, Mass., p. 272.

35. Salvatore P, Baldessarini RJ, Centorrino F, Egli S, Albert M, Gerhard A, Maggini C (2002). Weygandt's "On the Mixed States of Manic-Depressive Insanity": A translation and commentary on its significance in the evolution of the concept of bipolar disorder. *Harvard Review of Psychiatry* 10, 255–275.

36. Kraepelin E (1899). *Psychiatrie. Ein Lehrbuch für Studirende und Aertze.* Barth, Leipzig, volume 2. Trans. Ayed S (1960), Science History Publications, Canton, Mass., pp. 28–33.

37. Fink M, Taylor MA (2003). *Catatonia.* Cambridge University Press, Cambridge.

38. Kraepelin E (1921). *Manic-depressive Insanity and Paranoia.* Livingstone, Edinburgh.

39. Meyer A (1896). Book review. *American Journal of Insanity* 53, 298–302.

40. Healy D (2002). Mandel Cohen and the origins of the *Diagnostic and Statistical Manual,* third edition: *DSM-III. History of Psychiatry* 13, 209–230.

41. Norman C (1904). Dementia Praecox. *British Medical Journal* 1, 972–975;

Healy D (1996). Irish psychiatry in the twentieth century: Notes towards a history. In *150 Years of British Psychiatry,* volume 2, ed. Freeman H and Berrios GE, Athlone Press, London, pp. 268–291.

42. Ion RM, Beer MD (2002). The British reaction to dementia praecox 1893–1913, part 1, *History of Psychiatry* 13, 285–304; part 2, 13, 419–432.

43. Shepherd M (1996). The two faces of Emil Kraepelin. *British Journal of Psychiatry* 167, 174–183; Shepherd M (1998). Psychopharmacology specific and non-specific. In Healy D, *The Psychopharmacologists,* volume 2, Arnold, London, pp. 237–258.

44. Pichot P (1982). The diagnosis and classification of mental disorders in French-speaking countries: Background, current views and comparison with other nomenclatures. *Psychological Medicine* 12, 475–492.

45. Kraepelin E (1987). *Memoirs.* Trans. Cheryl Wooding-Deane, Ed. Hippius H, Peters G, Ploog D, Springer Books, Berlin, pp. 55–56.

46. Robins J (1986). *Fools and Mad. A History of the Insane in Ireland.* Institute of Public Administration, Dublin; Healy D (1991). The Role of Irish members in the Medico-Psychological Association. Plus ça change. In *150 Years of British Psychiatry,* volume 1, ed. Berrios GE, Freeman HL, Gaskell, London, pp. 314–320.

47. Michael P (2003). *Care and Treatment of the Mentally Ill in North Wales. 1800–2000.* University of Wales Press, Cardiff.

48. The political situation is caught by a 1990s bumper sticker, which proclaimed that if Wales were ironed flat it would be larger than England.

49. This was the area in which JRR Tolkien set *Lord of the Rings.*

50. Berrios GE, Hauser R (1995). Kraepelin. In Berrios GE, Porter R, *A History of Clinical Psychiatry,* Athlone Press, London, pp. 280–291.

51. Harris M, Chandran S, Chakroborty N, Healy D (2005). Service utilization in bipolar disorder, 1890 and 1990 compared. *History of Psychiatry* 16, 423–434.

Chapter 4. The Stone of Madness

1. Kraepelin E (1920). Die Erscheinungsformen des Irreseins. *Zeitschrift für die gesammte Neurologie und Psychiatrie* 62, 1–29. Trans. as Patterns of mental disorder. In Hirsch S, Shepherd M (1974), *Themes and Variations in European Psychiatry,* University Press of Virginia, Charlottesville, pp. 7–30.

2. See Healy D (2002). *The Creation of Psychopharmacology.* Harvard University Press, Cambridge, Mass., chapter 2.

3. See Johnson FN (1984). *The History of Lithium Therapy.* Macmillan, London, chapter 1.

4. Bellis M (2005). *The History of 7UP.* Charles Leiper Grigg. www.inventors .about.com/library/inventors/bl7up.htm. Accessed July 11.

5. Ure A (1843). Observations and researches upon a new solvent for stone in the bladder. *Pharmaceutical Journal and Transactions* 3, 71–74.

6. Maehle A-H (1999). *Drugs on Trial: Experimental Pharmacology and Therapeutic Innovation in the 18th Century.* Cleo Medica Radopi, Amsterdam.

7. Anon (1860). Calculus in the bladder, treated by litholysis, or solution of the

stone by injections of the carbonate of Lithia, conjoined with lithotrity (under the care of Mr Ure). *Lancet* ii, 185–186.

8. Garrod AB (1859). *The Nature and Treatment of Gout and Rheumatic Gout.* Walton & Maberly, London.

9. Garrod AB (1873). Renal calculus, gravel, gout and gouty deposits, and the value of lithium salts in their treatment. *Medical Times and Gazette,* March 8, 246–247.

10. Garrod AB (1876). *A Treatise on Gout and Rheumatic Gout (Rheumatoid Arthritis).* Longmans, Green & Co, London, p. 372.

11. Trousseau A (1868). *Clinique Médicale de l'Hôtel-Dieu de Paris.* J-B Baillière et Fils, Paris.

12. Gilbrin A-A (1858). De la Diathèse Urique. Thesis for the Doctorate of Medicine presented in Paris. Quote translated from the French presented in Johnson FN (1984). *The History of Lithium Therapy.* Macmillan, London. p. 142.

13. Cited in Berrios GE (1984). Epilepsy and insanity during the early 19th century. A conceptual history. *Archives of Neurology* 41, 978–981.

14. Mitchell SW (1870). On the use of bromide of lithium. *American Journal of Medical Science* 60, 443–445.

15. Hammond WA (1871). *A Treatise on Diseases of the Nervous System.* Appleton, New York; Yeragani VK, Gerson S (1986). Hammond and lithium: Historical update. *Biological Psychiatry* 21, 1101–1102.

16. Deutsch A (1944). The history of mental hygiene. In *One Hundred Years of American Psychiatry,* American Psychiatric Association, Columbia University Press, New York, pp. 367–384.

17. Aulde J (1887). The use of lithium bromide in combination with solution of potassium citrate. *Medical Bulletin* (Philadelphia), 9, 35–39, 69–72, 228–233.

18. Aulde J (1887). The use of lithium bromide in combination with solution of potassium citrate. *Medical Bulletin* (Philadelphia), 9, 229.

19. Aulde J (1887). The use of lithium bromide in combination with solution of potassium citrate. *Medical Bulletin* (Philadelphia), 9, 230.

20. Haig A (1884). Influence of diet on headache. *Practitioner* 33, 113–118; Haig A (1892). *Uric Acid as a Factor in the Causation of Disease. A Contribution to the Pathology of High Arterial Tension, Headache, Epilepsy, Mental Depression, Gout, Rheumatism, Diabetes, Bright's and Other Disorders.* J & A Churchill, London.

21. Schioldann JA (2001). *The Lange Theory of Periodical Depression. A Landmark in the History of Lithium Therapy.* Adelaide Academic Press, Adelaide.

22. Lange C (1886). *Om Periodiske Depressionstilstande of deres Patogenese.* Copenhagen, Jacob Lunds Forlag. Trans. in Schioldann JA (2001). *The Lange Theory of Periodical Depression. A Landmark in the History of Lithium Therapy.* Adelaide Academic Press, Adelaide.

23. Schioldann JA (2001). *The Lange Theory of Periodical Depression. A Landmark in the History of Lithium Therapy.* Adelaide Academic Press, Adelaide.

24. Lange F (1894). *De vigtigste Sindssygdomsgrupper.* Gyldendalske Boghandels Forlag, Copenhagen.

25. Schou HI (1938). Lette og begyndende Sinds-sygdomme og deres Behandlung I Hjemmet. *Ugeskrift for Laeger* 9, 215–220.

26. Schou M (1998). Lithium. In Healy D, *The Psychopharmacologists,* volume 2, Arnold, London, pp. 259–284.

27. Healy D (2002). *The Creation of Psychopharmacology.* Harvard University Press, Cambridge, Mass.

28. Delay J, Deniker P (1952/2007). 38 Cas de psychoses traitées par la cure prolongée et continue de 4560 RP. *Comptes Rendus du Congrès des Médécins Alienistes et Neurologistes de Langue Française* 50, 497–502. Trans. Healy D in Deniker P (2007). *European Clinical Psychiatry. An Historical Perspective from Selected Scientific Papers by Pierre Deniker.* Pierre Deniker Association, Paris, pp. 11–22.

29. These would be termed acute and transient psychoses outside of North America.

30. Delay J, Deniker P, Ropert R (1955/2007). Etude de 300 dossiers de maladies psychotiques traits par la chlorpromazine en service fermé depuis 1952. *Encéphale* 528–535. Trans. Healy D in Deniker P (2007). *European Clinical Psychiatry. An Historical Perspective from Selected Scientific Papers by Pierre Deniker.* Pierre Deniker Association, Paris, pp. 31–40.

31. Healy D (1997). *The Antidepressant Era.* Harvard University Press, Cambridge, Mass.

32. Healy D (2004). *Let Them Eat Prozac.* New York University Press, New York.

33. Johnson FN (1984). *The History of Lithium Therapy.* Macmillan, London, chapter 3.

34. Cade JFJ (1970). The story of lithium. In Ayd FJ, Blackwell B (eds.), *Discoveries in Biological Psychiatry,* Lippincott, Philadelphia, p. 223; also in Johnson FN (1984), *The History of Lithium Therapy,* Macmillan, London, chapter 3.

35. Cade JFJ (1949). Lithium salts in the treatment of psychotic excitement. *Medical Journal of Australia* 2, 349–353. See also Cade JFJ (1967). Lithium in psychiatry: Historical origins and present positioned. *Australian and New Zealand Journal of Psychiatry* 1, 61–62.

36. Cade JFJ (1967). Lithium in psychiatry: Historical origins and present positioned. *Australian and New Zealand Journal of Psychiatry* 1, 61–62.

37. Cade JFJ (1970). The story of lithium. In Ayd FJ, Blackwell B (eds.). *Discoveries in Biological Psychiatry,* Lippincott, Philadelphia, pp. 218–229.

38. Roberts EL (1950). A case of chronic mania treated with lithium citrate and terminating fatally. *Medical Journal of Australia* 37, 251–262.

39. Ashburner JV (1950). A case of chronic mania treated with Lithium citrate and terminating fatally. *Medical Journal of Australia* 37, 386.

40. Wynn V, Simon S, Morris RJ, McDonald IR, Denton DA (1950). The clinical significance of sodium and potassium analyses of biological fluids: Their estimation by flame spectrophotometry. *Medical Journal of Australia* 37, 821–836.

41. Noack CH, Trautner EM (1951). The lithium treatment of maniacal psychosis. *Medical Journal of Australia* 38, 219–222.

42. Glesinger B (1954). Evaluation of lithium in treatment of psychotic excitement. *Medical Journal of Australia* 41, 277–283.

43. Trautner EM, Morris R, Noack CH, Gershon S (1955). The excretion and retention of ingested lithium and its effect on the ionic balance of man. *Medical Journal of Australia* 42, 280–291.

44. Cade JFJ (1970). The story of lithium. In Ayd FJ, Blackwell B (eds.), *Discoveries in Biological Psychiatry*, Philadelphia, Lippincott, pp. 218–229.

45. Johnson FN (1984). *The History of Lithium Therapy*. Macmillan, London, chapter 5.

46. Rice D (1956). The use of lithium salts in the treatment of manic states. *Journal of Mental Science* 102, 604–611.

47. Talbott JH (1950). The use of lithium salts as a substitute for sodium chloride. *Archives of Internal Medicine* 85, 1–10.

48. Gershon S, Yuwiler A (1960). Lithium ion: A specific psychopharmacological approach to the treatment of mania. *Journal of Neuropsychiatry* 1, 229–241.

49. Despinoy M, Romeuf J de (1951). Emploi des sels de lithlium en thérapeutique clinique. *Comptes Rendus du Congrès des Médécins Alienistes et Neurologistes de Langue Française*, 509–515.

50. Reyss-Brion R, Grambert J (1951). Essai de traitment des etats d'excitation psychotique par le citrate de lithium. *Journal de Médécine de Lyon* 32, 985–989.

51. Deschamps M, Denis M (1952). Premiers resultats du traitement des états d'excitation maniaque par les sels de lithium. *L'Avenir Medical* 49, 673–679.

52. Duc N, Maurel H (1953). Le traitement des états d'agitation psychomotrice par le lithium. *Le Concours Médical* 75, 1817–1820.

53. Carbère J, Pochard M (1954). Le citrate de lithium dans le traitement des syndromes d'excitation psychomotrice. *Annales Médico-Psychologiques* 112, 566–572.

54. Teulie M, Follin M, Begoin M (1955). Etude de l'action des sels de lithium dans états d'excitation psychomotrice. *Encéphale* 44, 266–285.

55. Oulès J, Soubrie R, Salles P (1955). A propos du traitement des crises de manie par les sels de lithium. *Comptes Rendus du Congrès des Médécins Alienistes et Neurologistes de Langue Française*, 570–573; Oulès J (1955). Discussion. *Annales Médico-Psychologiques* 113, 679; Sivadon P, Chanoit P (1955). L'emploi du lithium dans l'agitation psychomotrice à propos d'une experience clinique. *Annales Médico-Psychologiques* 133, 790–796.

56. Maissin CM-TLP (1955). Le traitement de la manie par le citrate de lithium. Thesis presented for the Doctorate of Medicine in the Faculty of Medicine, Paris, p. 48.

57. Maissin CM-TLP (1955). Le traitement de la manie par le citrate de lithium. Thesis presented for the Doctorate of Medicine in the Faculty of Medicine, Paris, p. 47.

58. Plichet A (1954). Le traitement des états maniaques par les sels de lithium. *Presse Médical* 62, 869–870.

59. Kingstone E (1960). The lithium treatment of hypomanic and manic states. *Comprehensive Psychiatry* 1, 317–320; Kingstone E (1998). Lithium in Canada. In Ban T, Shorter E, Healy D (eds.), *The Rise of Psychopharmacology and the Story of CINP*. Animula, Budapest, pp. 98–100.

60. Healy D (2002). *The Creation of Psychopharmacology*. Harvard University

Press, Cambridge, Mass.; Ban T, Shorter E, Healy D (eds.) (1998). *The Rise of Psychopharmacology and the Story of CINP*. Animula, Budapest.

61. Schou M (1959). Therapeutic and toxic properties of lithium. In Bradley P, Deniker P, Radouco-Thomas C (eds.), *Proceedings of the First International Congress of Neuropharmacology, Rome, September 1958,* Elsevier, Amsterdam, pp. 687–690.

62. Schou M (1962). *Proceedings of the Third CINP Congress,* Elsevier, Amsterdam, p. 600.

63. Johnson FN, Cade JFJ (1975). The historical background to lithium research and therapy. In Johnson FN (ed.), *Lithium Research and Therapy,* Academic Press, Burlington, Mass., pp. 9–21.

64. Schou M (1998). Lithium. In Healy D, *The Psychopharmacologists,* volume 2, Arnold, London, pp. 259–284.

65. Healy D (2002). *The Creation of Psychopharmacology.* Harvard University Press, Cambridge, Mass., chapter 2.

66. Jenner A (2000). Catatonia, pink spots and antipsychiatry. In Healy D, *The Psychopharmacologists,* volume 3, Arnold, London, pp. 135–156.

67. Healy D (1997). *The Antidepressant Era.* Harvard University Press, Cambridge, Mass., chapter 5.

68. Richter D, Healy D (1995). The origins of mental health oriented neuroscience in Britain. *Journal of Psychopharmacology* 4, 392–399; Richter D (1989). *Life in Research.* Stuart Phillips Publications, Kingswood, Surrey.

69. Strömgren E. Cited in Schioldann JA (2001). *The Lange Theory of Periodical Depression. A Landmark in the History of Lithium Therapy.* Adelaide Academic Press, Adelaide, p. 127.

70. Schou M (1998). Lithium. In Healy D, *The Psychopharmacologists,* volume 2, Arnold, London, pp. 259–284.

71. Cited in Johnson FN (1984). *The History of Lithium Therapy.* Macmillan, London, p. 71.

72. Baastrup PC (1964). The use of lithium in manic depressive psychosis. *Comprehensive Psychiatry* 5, 396–408.

73. Hartigan GP (1961). Experiences of treatment with lithium salts. Published in full in Johnson FN (1984). *The History of Lithium Therapy.* Macmillan, London, pp. 183–187.

74. Hartigan GP (1963). The use of lithium salts in affective disorders. *British Journal of Psychiatry* 109, 810–814.

75. Schou M (1963). Normothymotics, "mood-normalizers": Are lithium and imipramine drugs specific for affective disorders? *British Journal of Psychiatry,* 109, 803–809.

76. Schou M (1981). Address on receiving an honorary doctorate. University of Aix-Marseilles, October 29.

77. Baastrup PC, Schou M (1967). Lithium as a prophylactic agent: Its effect against recurrent depression and manic depressive psychosis. *Archives of General Psychiatry* 16, 162–172.

78. Goldberg D (1995). Michael Shepherd, 1923–1995. *Psychological Medicine* 25, 1109–1111.

79. Shepherd M (1998). Psychopharmacology: Specific and non-specific. In Healy D, *The Psychopharmacologists*, volume 2, Arnold, London, pp. 237–258.

80. Davies DL, Shepherd M (1955). Reserpine in the treatment of anxious and depressed patients. *Lancet* 2, 117–120.

81. Healy D (1997). *The Antidepressant Era.* Harvard University Press, Cambridge, Mass., chapter 3.

82. Healy D (2002). *The Creation of Psychopharmacology.* Harvard University Press, Cambridge, Mass., chapter 3.

83. Baastrup PC, Schou M (1967). Lithium as a prophylactic agent: Its effect against recurrent depression and manic depressive psychosis. *Archives of General Psychiatry* 16, 162–172.

84. Blackwell B, Shepherd M (1968). Prophylactic lithium: Another therapeutic myth? An examination of the evidence to date. *Lancet* 1, 968–970. See also Blackwell B (1969). Lithium: Prophylactic or panacea? *Medical Counterpoint,* November, 52–59.

85. Blackwell B, Shepherd M (1968). Prophylactic lithium: Another therapeutic myth? An examination of the evidence to date. *Lancet* 1, 968.

86. Blackwell B, Shepherd M (1968). Prophylactic lithium: Another therapeutic myth? An examination of the evidence to date. *Lancet* 1, 969.

87. Blackwell B (1969). Need for careful evaluation of lithium. *American Journal of Psychiatry* 125, 1131; Kline NS (1969). Dr Kline Replies. *American Journal of Psychiatry* 125, 1131–1132.

88. Shephed M (1974). Discussion. In *Psihofarmakologija 3: Proceedings of the 3rd Yugoslav Psychopharmacological Symposium, Opatija 1973, Medicinska Noklada,* pp. 329–330.

89. Grof P (1998). Fighting the recurrence of affective disorders. In Ban TA, Healy D, Shorter E, *The Rise of Psychopharmacology and the Story of CINP,* Animula Publishing, Budapest, pp. 101–105.

90. Angst J, Weis P (1967). Periodicity of depressive psychoses. In Brill AA, Cole J, Deniker P, Hippius H, Bradley PB (eds.), *Neuropsychopharmacology,* Excerpta Medical Foundation ISC 129, Amsterdam, pp. 703–710.

91. Angst J, Dittrich A, Grof P (1969). Course of endogenous affective psychoses and its modification by prophylactic administration of imipramine and lithium. *International Pharmacopsychiatry* 2, 1–11; Schou M (1968). Lithium in psychiatric therapy and prophylaxis. *Journal of Psychiatric Research* 6, 67–69; Angst J, Weiss P, Grof P, Baastrup PC, Schou M (1970). Lithium prophylaxis in recurrent affective disorder. *British Journal of Psychiatry* 116, 604–614.

92. Baastrup PC, Poulsen JC, Schou M, Thomsen K, Amdisen A (1970). Prophylactic lithium: Double-blind discontinuation in manic-depressive and recurrent depressive disorders. *Lancet* 2, 326–330.

93. Lader MH (1968). Prophylactic lithium? *Lancet* 2, 103; Saran BM (1969). Lithium. *Lancet* 2, 1208–1209.

94. Coppen A, Noguera R, Bailey J, Burns BH, Swami MS, Hare EH, Gardner R, Maggs R (1971). Prophylactic lithium in affective disorders. Controlled trial. *Lancet* 2, 275–279.

95. Mindham RS, Howland C, Shepherd M (1972). Continuation therapy with tricyclic antidepressants in depressive illness. *Lancet* 1, 854–855.

96. Glen AIM, Johnson AL, Shepherd M (1984). Continuation therapy with lithium and amitriptyline in unipolar depressive illness: A randomised double blind controlled trial. *Psychological Medicine* 14, 37–50.

97. Sheard MH (1971). Effect of lithium on human aggression. *Nature* 230, 113–114.

98. Tupin JP, Smith DB, Clanon TL, Kim LI, Nugent A, Groupe A (1973). The long-term use of lithium in aggressive prisoners. *Comprehensive Psychiatry* 14, 311–317.

99. Cole JC, Healy D (1996). The evaluation of psychotropic drugs. In Healy D, *The Psychopharmacologists*, Chapman & Hall, London, pp. 239–263.

100. Fieve RR, Platman SR, Plutchik RR (1968). The use of lithium in affective disorders. *American Journal of Psychiatry* 125, 487–498.

101. Healy D (2002). *The Creation of Psychopharmacology*. Harvard University Press, Cambridge, Mass., chapter 7.

102. Gattozzi AA (1970). *Lithium in the Treatment of Mood Disorders*, US Dept of Health, Education, and Welfare, Public Health Service, National Clearing House for Mental Health Information, Publication No. 5033.

103. Anonymous (1980). Review of Schou M, Strömgren E (1979). *Origin, Prevention and Treatment of Affective Disorders*. Academic Press, London. *Psychological Medicine* 10, 387. Written by Shepherd.

104. Grof P (1998). Fighting the recurrence of affective disorders. In Ban TA, Healy D, Shorter E, *The Rise of Psychopharmacology and the Story of CINP*, Animula Publishing, Budapest, pp. 101–105.

105. These figures are based on published studies. If unpublished studies were included, the difference between active treatment and placebo would be less.

106. Davies DL, Shepherd M (1955). Reserpine in the treatment of anxious and depressed patients. *Lancet* 2, 117–120.

107. Healy D, Savage M (1998). Reserpine exhumed. *British Journal of Psychiatry* 172, 376–378.

108. Shepherd M (1998). Psychopharmacology: Specific and non-specific. In Healy D, *The Psychopharmacologists*, volume 2, Arnold, London, pp. 237–258.

109. Smirk FH, McQueen EG (1955). Comparison of rescinamine and reserpine as hypotensive agents. *Lancet* 2, 115–116; Wallace DC (1955). Treatment of hypertension. Hypotensive drugs and mental changes. *Lancet* 2, 116–117.

110. For more on these points, see Healy D (2002). *The Creation of Psychopharmacology*. Harvard University Press, Cambridge, Mass., chapter 7.

111. Shepherd M (1993). The placebo: From specificity to the non-specific and back. *Psychological Medicine* 23, 569–578.

112. Shepherd M (1998). Psychopharmacology: Specific and non-specific. In Healy D, *The Psychopharmacologists*, volume 2, Arnold, London, pp. 237–258.

113. Shepherd M (1995). Two faces of Emil Kraepelin. *British Journal of Psychiatry* 166, 174–183.

Chapter 5. The Eclipse of Manic-Depressive Disorder

1. Kraepelin E (1987). *Memoirs.* Trans. Cheryl Wooding-Deane, Ed. Hippius H, Peters G, Ploog D, Springer Books, Berlin, p. 54.

2. Kraepelin E (1918). Hundert Jahre Psychiatrie. *Zeitschrift der Neurologie* 38, 161–275. Trans. Baskin W (1962). *One Hundred Years of Psychiatry.* Philosophical Library, New York, p. 121.

3. Kraepelin E (1920/1992). The manifestations of insanity. *History of Psychiatry* 3, 509–529.

4. Kraepelin E (1918). Hundert Jahre Psychiatrie. *Zeitschrift der Neurologie* 38, 161–275. Trans. Baskin W (1962). *One Hundred Years of Psychiatry.* Philosophical Library, New York, p. 129.

5. Neumarker K-J, Bartsch AJ (2003). Karl Kleist (1879–1960)—pioneer of neuropsychiatry. *History of Psychiatry* 14, 411–458.

6. Kleist K (1928). Ueber zykloide, paranoide und epileptoide Psychosen und uber die Frage der Degenerationspsychosen. *Schweizer Archive für Neurologie und Psychiatrie* 23, 3–37.

7. Craddock N, Owen M (2005). The beginning of the end of the Kraepelinian dichotomy. *British Journal of Psychiatry* 186, 364–366.

8. Leonhard K (1961). Cycloid psychoses—endogenous psychoses which are neither schizophrenic nor manic-depressive. *Journal of Mental Science* 107, 633–648.

9. Leonhard K (1999). *Classification of Endogenous Psychosis and their Differentiated Etiology.* Translated from German by Charles H Cahn, Springer Books, New York.

10. Gottesman I (1998). Predisposed to predispositions. In Healy D, *The Psychopharmacologists,* volume 2, London, Chapman & Hall, 377–408.

11. Angst J. (1966). *Zur Atiologie und Nosologie endogener depressiver Psychosen.* Springer, Berlin. Trans. Angst J (1973). The Etiology and nosology of endogenous depressive psychoses. A genetic, sociological and clinical study. *Foreign Psychiatry* 2, 1–94.

12. Perris C. (1966). A study of bipolar (Manic Depressive) and unipolar recurrent depressive psychoses. *Acta Psychiatrica Scandinavica* 42, supplement 194; Perris C (1968). The course of depressive psychoses. *Acta Psychiatrica Scandinavica* 44, 238–248; Perris C (1974). A study of cycloid psychoses. *Acta Psychiatrica Scandinavica,* supplement 253.

13. Rees WL, Healy D (1996). The role of clinical trials in the development of psychopharmacology. *History of Psychiatry* 8, 1–20; Coppen A (1996). Biological psychiatry in Britain. In Healy D, *The Psychopharmacologists,* volume 1, Chapman & Hall, London, pp. 265–286; Claridge G, Healy D (1994). The Psychopharmacology of Individual Differences. *Human Psychopharmacology* 9, 285–298.

14. Perris C (1966). A study of bipolar (manic depressive) and unipolar recurrent depressive psychoses. *Acta Psychiatrica Scandinavica* 42, supplement 194, p. 185.

15. Craddock N, Owen M (2005). The beginning of the end of the Kraepelinian dichotomy. *British Journal of Psychiatry* 186, 364–366.

16. Angst J, Marneros A (2001). Bipolarity from ancient to modern times: Conception, birth and rebirth. *Journal of Affective Disorders* 67, 3–19.

17. Schildkraut JJ (1965). The catecholamine hypothesis of affective disorders. A review of supporting evidence. *American Journal of Psychiatry* 122, 519–522. See Healy D (1997). *The Antidepressant Era*. Harvard University Press, Cambridge, Mass., chapter 5.

18. Katz MM, Cole JO, Barton WE (eds.) (1968). *The Role and Methodology of Classification in Psychiatry and Psychopharmacology*. Government Printing Office, Washington, D.C.; Williams TA, Katz MM, Shields JA (1972). *Recent Advances in the Psychobiology of Depressive Illness*. Superintendent of Documents, Government Printing Offices, Washington D.C., Proceedings of the Williamsburg Conference in Virginia 1969.

19. Spitzer RL, Endicott J, Robins E (1975). Research diagnostic criteria (RDC) for a selected group of functional disorders. New York State Department of Mental Hygiene, Biometrics Branch, New York.

20. Robins E, Guze SB (1972). Classification of affective disorders: The primary-secondary, the endogenous-reactive, and the neurotic-psychotic concepts. In Williams TA, Katz MM, Shields JA (1972), *Recent Advances in the Psychobiology of Depressive Illness*. Superintendent of Documents, Government Printing Offices, Washington, D.C., Proceedings of the Williamsburg Conference in Virginia 1969, pp. 283–293.

21. Guze S (2000). The Neo-Kraepelinian revolution. In Healy D, *The Psychopharmacologists*, volume 3, Arnold, London, pp. 395–414.

22. Guze S (1997). George Winokur, 1925–1996. *Archives of General Psychiatry* 54, 574–575.

23. Winokur G, Clayton PJ (1967). Family history studies: I, Two types of affective disorders separated according to genetic and clinical factors. In Wortis J (ed.), *Recent Advances in Biological Psychiatry*, volume 10, Plenum, New York, pp. 35–50.

24. Winokur G, Clayton PJ, Reich T (1969). *Manic-Depressive Illness*. Mosby, St. Louis.

25. Dunner DL (2002). After bipolar II and rapid cycling. In Ban TA, Healy D, and Shorter E, *From Psychopharmacology to Neuropsychopharmacology in the 1980s and the Story of CINP as Told in Autobiography*, Animula Publishing, Budapest, pp. 242–244.

26. Fieve RR (2000). Lithium: From introduction to public awareness. In Ban TA, Healy D, Shorter E, *The Triumph of Psychopharmacology and the Story of CINP*, Animula Publishing, Budapest, pp. 258–260.

27. Dunner DL, Fleiss JL, Fieve RR (1976). The course of development of mania in patients with recurrent depression. *American Journal of Psychiatry* 133, 905–908.

28. Akiskal HS (1983). Diagnosis and classification of affective disorders. New insights from clinical and laboratory approaches. *Psychiatric Developments* 2, 123–160; Akiskal HS (2002). The bipolar spectrum—the shaping of a new paradigm in psychiatry. *Current Psychiatry Reports* 4, 1–3.

29. Endicott J, Nee J, Andreason N, Clayton P, Keller M, Coryell W (1985). Bipolar II: Combine or keep separate? *Journal of Affective Disorders* 8, 17–28.

30. Coryell W, Endicott J, Andreasen N, Keller M (1985). Bipolar I, bipolar II, and non-bipolar major depression among the relatives of affectively ill probands. *American Journal of Psychiatry* 142, 817–821.

31. Guze S (2000). The Neo-Kraepelinian revolution. In Healy D, *The Psychopharmacologists*, volume 3, Arnold, London, pp. 395–414; Klerman GL (1977). The neo-Kraepelinian revival in American psychiatry: Its history, promise and prospect. Scientific Symposium on the retirement of Eli Robins, St. Louis, Missouri, May 27.

32. Gottesman I (1998). Predisposed to predispositions. In Healy D, *The Psychopharmacologists*, volume 2, Chapman & Hall, London, pp. 377–408.

33. Akiskal HS (2005). Bipolarity is clinically expressed as a spectrum. *Journal of Bipolar Disorders* 4, 3–5.

34. Sheehan D (2000). Angles on panic. In Healy D, *The Psychopharmacologists*, volume 3, Arnold, London, pp. 479–504; Berk M, Dodd S (2005). Bipolar II disorder: A review. *Bipolar Disorder* 7, 11–21.

35. Angst J (1990). Recurrent brief depression. A new concept of depression. *Pharmacopsychiatry* 23, 63–66.

36. Angst J (1997). Recurrent brief psychiatric syndromes: Hypomania, depression, anxiety, and neurasthenia. In Judd LL, Saletu B, Filip V (eds.), *Basic and Clinical Science of Mental and Addictive Disorders*, Karger, Basel, pp. 33–38.

37. Stoll AL, Tohen M, Baldessarini RJ, Goodwin DC, Stein S, Katz S, Geenens D, Swinson RP, Goethe JW, McGlashan T (1993). Shifts in diagnostic frequencies of schizophrenia and major affective disorders at six North American psychiatric hospitals, 1972–1988. *American Journal of Psychiatry* 150, 1668–1673.

38. Health care reforms for Americans with severe mental illnesses: Report of the National Advisory Mental Health Council (1993). *American Journal of Psychiatry* 150, 1447–1465.

39. Kessler RC, McGonagle KA, Zhao S, et al. (1994). Lifetime and 12-month prevalence of DSM-IIIR psychiatric disorders in the United States: Results from the National Comorbidity Study. *Archives of General Psychiatry* 51, 8–19.

40. Angst J (1998). The emerging epidemiology of hypomania and bipolar II disorder. *Journal of Affective Disorders* 50, 163–173.

41. Anthony JC, Folstein M, Romanoski AJ, et al. (1985). Comparison of the lay diagnostic interview schedule and a standardized psychiatric diagnosis. *Archives of General Psychiatry* 42, 667–675.

42. Regier DA, Kaelber CT, Rae DS, Farmer ME, Knauper B, Kessler RC, Norquist GS (1998). Limitations of diagnostic criteria and assessment instruments for mental disorders. *Archives of General Psychiatry* 55, 109–115.

43. Spitzer RL (1998). Diagnosis and need for treatment are not the same thing. *Archives of General Psychiatry* 55, 116.

44. Horwitz AV, Wakefield JC (2006). The epidemic in mental illness: Clinical fact or survey artifact? *Contexts* 5, 19–23.

45. In Carey B (2005). Most will be mentally ill at some point, study says. *New York Times*, June 7.

46. Jamison KR (1993). *Touched by Fire. Manic-Depressive Illness and the Artistic Temperament*. Simon & Schuster, New York.

47. Jamison KR (1995). *An Unquiet Mind. A Memoir of Moods and Madness*. A. Knopf, New York.

48. Ellis HA (1926). *A Study of British Genius*. New York, Houghton Mifflin.

49. Storr A (1976). *The Dynamics of Creation*. Penguin, Harmondsworth, Middlesex.

50. Porter R (1987). *Social History of Madness*. Weidenfeld & Nicolson, London.

51. Andreasen NJC (1987). Creativity and mental illness: Prevalence rates in writers and their first degree relatives. *American Journal of Psychiatry* 144, 1288–1292; Claridge G, Pryor R, Watkins G (1990). *Sounds from the Bell Jar. Ten Psychotic Authors*. Macmillan Press, London.

52. Hayden D (2003). *Pox. Genius, Madness, and the Mysteries of Syphilis*. Basic Books, New York.

53. Goodwin FK, Jamison KR (1990). *Manic Depressive Illness*. Oxford University Press, New York.

54. Perris C (1974). A study of cycloid psychoses. *Acta Psychiatrica Scandinavica*, supplementum 253, pp. 1–77; Perris C (1990). The importance of Karl Leonhard's classification of endogenous psychoses. *Psychopathology* 23, 282–290; Brockington IF, Perris C, Meltzer HY (1982). Cycloid psychoses. Diagnosis and heuristic value. *Journal of Nervous and Mental Disease* 170, 651–656; Brockington IF, Perris C, Kendell RE, Hillier VE, Wainwright S (1982). The course and outcome of cycloid psychosis. *Psychological Medicine* 12, 97–105.

55. Perris C (1988). The concept of cycloid psychotic disorder. *Psychiatric Developments* 1, 37–56.

56. Brockington IF (1996). *Motherhood and Mental Illness*. Oxford University Press, Oxford.

57. Kraepelin E (1899). *Psychiatrie. Ein Lehrbuch für Studirende und Aertze*. Barth, Leipzig, volume II. Trans. Ayed S (1960), Science History Publications, Canton, Mass., p. 28.

58. Kraepelin E (1899). *Psychiatrie. Ein Lehrbuch für Studirende und Aertze*. Barth, Leipzig, volume 2. Trans. Ayed S (1960), Science History Publications, Canton, Mass., p. 33.

59. Gentile S (2005). The role of estrogen therapy in postpartum psychiatric disorders: An update. *CNS Spectrums* 10, 944–952.

60. Robertson E, Jones I, Haque S, Holder R, Craddock N (2005). Risk of puerperal and non-puerperal recurrence of illness following bipolar affective (postpartum) psychosis. *British Journal of Psychiatry* 186, 258–259; Chaudron LH, Pies RW (2003). The relationship between postpartum psychosis and bipolar disorder: A review. *Journal of Clinical Psychiatry* 64, 1284–1292.

61. Fink M, Taylor MA (2003). *Catatonia*. Cambridge University Press, Cambridge.

62. Jones M (2000). Cure it with drugs. *New York Times Magazine*, October 15, pp. 88–89.

63. Moynihan R, Cassels A (2005). *Selling Sickness*. Nation Books, New York.

64. Nager A, Johansson L-M, Sundquist K (2005). Are sociodemographic factors and year of delivery associated with hospital admission for postpartum psy-

chosis? A study of 500,000 first-time mothers. *Acta Psychiatrica Scandinavica* 112, 47–53.

65. Healy D, Savage M, Michael P, Harris M, Hirst D, Carter M, Cattell D, McMonagle T, Sohler N, Susser E (2001). Psychiatric bed utilisation: 1896 and 1996 compared. *Psychological Medicine* 31, 779–790.

66. Tschinkel S, Harris M, Le Noury J, Healy D (2007). Postpartum psychosis: Two cohorts compared, 1875–1924 and 1994–2005. *Psychological Medicine* 37, 529–536.

67. Taylor MA, Fink M (2006). *Melancholia Defined.* Cambridge University Press, Cambridge.

68. Perris C (1992). A cognitive-behavioral treatment program for patients with a schizophrenic disorder. *New Directions for Mental Health Services* 53, 21–32.

69. Perris C (1986). *Kognitiv terapi I teori och praktik.* Natur och kultur, Stockholm.

70. Herlofson J (2000). Obituary. Carlo Perris. *Scandinavian Journal of Behaviour Therapy* 29, 97–99. Some of the material cited also depends on information from Hjördis Perris and Jan-Otto Ottosson.

71. Chalassani P, Healy D, Morriss R (2005). Presentation and frequency of catatonia in new admissions to two acute psychiatric admission units in India and Wales. *Psychological Medicine* 35, 1667–1675.

72. Craddock N, Owen M (2005). The beginning of the end of the Kraepelinian dichotomy. *British Journal of Psychiatry* 186, 364–366.

73. Bentall RP (2003). *Madness Explained.* Allen Lane, London.

74. Marshall BL, Katz S (2002). Forever functional. Sexual fitness and the aging male body. *Body & Society* 8, 43–70; Katz S, Marshall BL (2004). Is the functional "normal"? Age, sex and the biomarking of successful living. *History of the Human Sciences* 17, 53–75.

75. Elliot C (2003). *Better than Well. American Medicine Meets the American Dream.* WW Norton & Co, New York; Rothman SM, Rothman DJ (2003). *The Pursuit of Perfection. The Promise and Perils of Medical Enhancement.* Pantheon Books, New York.

76. Fish F (1962). *Fish's Schizophrenia.* John Wright & Sons, Bristol; Fish F (1964). *An Outline of Psychiatry.* John Wright & Sons, Bristol.

77. Fish F (1964). The influence of the tranquilizers on the Leonhard schizophrenic syndromes. *Encephale* 53, 245–249.

78. See Ban T (2004). Neuropsychopharmacology and the history of pharmacotherapy. In Ban T, Shorter E, Healy D (eds.), *Reflections on Twentieth Century Psychopharmacology,* Animula, Budapest, pp. 697–721; Ban TA (2006). The neurotransmitter era in neuropsychopharmacology. In Ban TA, Ucha Udabe R (eds.). *The Neurotransmitter Era in Neuropsychopharmacology,* Editorial Polemos, Buenos Aires, pp. 265–274.

79. Ban TA (1987). Prolegomenon to the clinical prerequisite. Psychopharmacology and the classification of mental disorders. *Progress in Neuro-Psychopharmacology & Biological Psychiatry* 11, 527–580; Ban T (1996). They used to call it psychiatry. In Healy D, *The Psychopharmacologists,* volume 1, Chapman & Hall, London, pp. 540–580.

80. Kraepelin's tombstone reads: Dein Name mag vergeben, Bleibt nur dein Werk bestehen. In Kraepelin E (1987). *Memoirs.* Trans. Cheryl Wooding-Deane, Ed. Hippius H, Peters G, Ploog D, Springer Books, Berlin, p. 270.

Chapter 6. Branded in the USA

1. Chouinard G, Steinberg S, Steiner W (1985). Estrogen-progesterone combination: Another mood stabilizer? *American Journal of Psychiatry* 144, 826.

2. Sachs GS (1996). Bipolar mood disorder: Practical strategies for acute and maintenance phase treatment. *Journal of Clinical Psychopharmacology* 16, supp. 1, 32s–47s; Bowden CL (1998). New concepts in mood stabilization: Evidence for the effectiveness of Valproate and Lamotrigine. *Neuropsychopharmacology* 19, 194–199; Ghaemi SN (2001). On defining "mood stabilizer." *Bipolar Disorder* 3, 154–158.

3. Burton BS (1882). On the propyl derivatives and decomposition products of ethyl acetoacetate. *American Chemical Journal* 3, 385–395. Quote from p. 389.

4. Meijer JW, Meinardi H, Binnie CD (1983). The development of antiepileptic drugs. In Parnham MJ, Bruinvels J (eds.), *Discoveries in Pharmacology*, volume 1, Elsevier, Amsterdam, pp. 447–477.

5. Meunier G, Carraz G, Meunier Y, Eymard P, Aimard M (1963). Propriétés pharmaco-dynamiques de l'acide n-dipropylacétique. *Thérapie* 18, 435–438.

6. Carraz G, Lebreton S, Boitard M, Borselli S, Bonnin J (1965). A propos de deux nouveaux anti-epileptiques de la serie n-dipropylacetique. *Encephale,* 458–465.

7. Carraz G, Boucherle A, Lebreton S, Benoit-Guyon JL, Boitard M (1964). Le neurotropisme de la structure n-dipropylacétique. *Thérapie* 19, 917–920.

8. Comite Lyonnais de Recherches Thérapeutiques en Psychiatrie (2000). The birth of psychopharmacotherapy: Explorations in a new world—1952–1968. In Healy D, *The Psychopharmacologists,* volume 3, Arnold, London, pp. 1–54.

9. Revol L, Achaintre A, Balvet P, Beaujard M, Berthier C, Broussolle P, Lambert P, Perrin J, Requet A (1956). *La thérapeutique par la chlorpromazine en pratique psychiatrique.* Masson & Cie, Paris; Achaintre E (1985). Histoire du Comité Lyonnais de Recherches Thérapeutiques en Psychiatrie (CLRTP). Docteur en Medicine Thèse, L'université Claude Bernard, Lyon.

10. Lambert PA, Revol L (1960). Classification psychopharmacologique et clinique des différents neuroleptiques. Indications thérapeutiques générales dans les psychoses. *Presse Médicale* 68, 1509–1511. See also Lambert PA, Revol L (1969). Classification of neuroleptics. *Comprehensive Psychiatry* 10, 50–58.

11. Lambert PA, Guyotat J (1961). Un nouvel antidépresseur sédatif derive de l'iminobenzyle; le 7162RP-Essais thérapeutiques. *Presse Médicale* 69, 1425–1428.

12. Guyotat J, Marin A, Dubor P, Bonhomme P, Rozier P (1960). L'Imipramine en dehors des états dépressifs. *Le Journal de Médicine de Lyon,* April, 367–375.

13. Carraz G, Lebreton S, Boitard M, Borselli S, Bonnin J (1965). A propos de deux nouveaux anti-epileptiques de la serie n-dipropylacetique. *Encephale,* 458–465; Lambert P-A, Borselli S, Midenet J, Baudrand C, Marcou G, Bouchardy M (1968). L'action favorable du Depamide sur l'evolution a long terme des psychoses maniaco-depressives. *Comptes Rendus Congrès de Psychiatrie et de Neurologie de Langue Française,* Masson, Paris, pp. 489–495.

14. Lambert P-A, Borselli S, Marcou G, Bouchardy M, Carraz G (1966). Proprietes neuro-psychotropes du Depamide: Action psychique chez les epileptiques et les malades presentant des troubles caracteriels. *Comptes Rendus Congrès de Psychiatrie et de Neurologie de Langue Française,* Masson, Paris, pp. 1034–1039.

15. Lambert P in Comite Lyonnais de Recherches Thérapeutiques en Psychiatrie (2000). The birth of psychopharmacotherapy: Explorations in a new world—1952–1968. In Healy D, *The Psychopharmacologists,* volume 3, Arnold, London, pp. 1–54, citation from p. 47.

16. Lambert P-A, Carraz G, Borselli S, Bouchardy M (1975). Le dipropylacetamide dans le traitement de la psychose maniaco-depressive. *Encephale,* 25–31.

17. Lambert P-A (1984). Acute and prophylactic therapies of patients with affective disorders using valpromide. In Emrich HM, Okuma T, Muller AA (eds.), *Anticonvulsants in Affective Disorders,* Elsevier, Amsterdam, pp. 33–44.

18. Ruffat M (1996). *175 Years of French Pharmaceutical Industry. History of Synthélabo.* Editions la Découverte, Paris.

19. Emrich HM, von Zerssen D, Kissling W, Moller H-J, Windorfer A (1980). Effect of sodium valproate on mania: GABA-hypothesis of affective disorders. *Archiv für Psychiatrie und Nervenkrankheiten* 229, 1–16.

20. United States Patent 4,988,731. Date of Patent Jan 29th 1991.

21. United States Patent 5,212,326. Date of Patent May 18th 1993.

22. Pope HG, McElroy SL, Keck PE, Hudson JI (1991). Valproate in the treatment of acute mania. *Archives of General Psychiatry* 48, 62–68.

23. Bowden CL, Brugger AM, Swann AC, Calabrese JR, Janicak DG, Petty F, Dilsaver SC, Davis JM, Rush AJ, Small JG, Garza-Trevino ES, Risch SC, Goodnick PJ, Morris DD (1994). Efficacy of divalproex, lithium and placebo in the treatment of mania. *Journal of American Medical Association* 271, 918–924.

24. Forty-fourth Psychopharmacologic Drugs Advisory Committee Meeting (1995). NDA 20-320: Depakote. Transcript of Proceedings. Department of Health and Human Services. Washington, D.C., February 6.

25. Comite Lyonnais de Recherches Thérapeutiques en Psychiatrie (2000). The birth of psychopharmacotherapy: Explorations in a new world—1952–1968. In Healy D, *The Psychopharmacologists,* volume 3, Arnold, London, pp. 1–54.

26. Harris M, Chandran S, Chakroborty N, Healy D (2003). Mood stabilizers: The archaeology of the concept. *Bipolar Disorders* 5, 446–452.

27. Healy D (1997). *The Antidepressant Era.* Harvard University Press, Cambridge, Mass., chapter 2.

28. Domenjoz R (2000). From DDT to imipramine. In Healy D, *The Psychopharmacologists,* volume 3, Arnold, London, pp. 357–370.

29. Maxwell RA, Eckhardt SB (1990). *Drug Discovery. A Casebook and Analysis. Carbamazepine.* Humana Press, Clifton, N.J., pp. 193–206.

30. Schindler W (1961). 5-H-dibenzazepines. US patent 2,948,718. Chemical Abstracts 55, 1671; Maxwell RA, Eckhardt SB (1990). *Drug Discovery. A Casebook and Analysis. Carbamazepine.* Humana Press, Clifton, N.J., pp. 193–206.

31. Theobald W, Kunz HA. Zur pharmacologie des antiepilepticums 5-carbamoyl–5H-dibenz(b,f)azepine. *Arzneimittelforschung* 13, 122–125.

32. Hernandez-Peon R (1964). Anticonvulsant action of G 32885. In Bradley P, Flugel F, Hoch P (eds.), *Neuropsychopharmacology*. Proceedings of the 3rd CINP Congress, Elsevier, Amsterdam, pp. 303–311.

33. Bonduelle M, Bouygues P, Sallou C, Chemaly R (1964). Bilan de l'experimentation clinique de l'anti-epileptique G 32883. In Bradley P, Flugel F, Hoch P (eds.), *Neuropsychopharmacology*. Proceedings of the 3rd CINP Congress, Elsevier, Amsterdam, pp. 312–316.

34. Bonduelle M, Bouygues P, Sallou C, Groebius S(1964). Experimentation clinique de l'antiepileptique G 32883 (Tegretol); Resultants portant sur 100 cas observes en trois ans. *Revue Neurologie* 110, 209–215.

35. Lorge M (1964). Uber ein neuartiges Antiepilepticum der Iminostilbenreihe (G 32883). In Bradley P, Flugel F, Hoch P (eds.), *Neuropsychopharmacology*. Proceedings of the 3rd CINP Congress, Elsevier, Amsterdam, pp. 299–302.

36. Cereghino JJ, Brock JT, Van Meter JC, Perry JK, Smith LD, White BG (1974). Carbamazepine for epilepsy. A controlled prospective evaluation. *Neurology* 24, 401–410.

37. Healy D (2002). *The Creation of Psychopharmacology*. Harvard University Press, Cambridge, Mass.

38. Okuma T (2000). The discovery of the psychotropic effects of carbamazepine. In Healy D, *The Psychopharmacologists*, volume 3, Arnold, London, pp. 259–280.

39. Takezaki H, Hanaoka M (1971). The use of carbamazepine (Tegretol) in the control of manic-depressive psychosis and other manic-depressive states. *Seishin Igaku* 13, 173–183.

40. Okuma T, Kishimoto A, Inoue K, Matsumoto H, Ogura A, Matsushita T, Nakao T, Ogura C (1973). Anti-manic and prophylactic effects of carbamazepine (Tegretol) on manic-depressive psychosis—A preliminary report. *Folia Psychiatrie und Neurologie Japonica* 27, 283–297; Okuma T, Kishimoto A, Inoue K, et al. (1975). Anti-manic and prophylactic effects of carbamazepine (Tegretol) on manic depressive psychosis. *Seishin Igaku* 17, 617–630.

41. Okuma T, Kishimoto A (1977). Anti-manic and prophylactic effects of Tegretol. In *Abstracts of the 6th World Congress of Psychiatry Honolulu*, Ciba-Geigy, Summit, N.J.

42. Okuma T, Inanaga K, Otsuki S (1979). Comparison of the antimanic efficacy of carbamazepine and chlorpromazine: A double blind controlled study. *Psychopharmacology* 66, 211–217.

43. Okuma T (2000). The discovery of the psychotropic effects of carbamazepine. In Healy D, *The Psychopharmacologists*, volume 3, Arnold, London, pp. 259–280.

44. Takahashi R, Sakuma A, Itoh H (1975). Comparison of the antimanic efficacy of lithium carbonate and chlorpromazine in mania. Report of collaborative study group on treatment of mania in Japan. *Archives of General Psychiatry* 32, 1310–1318.

45. Okuma T, Yamashita I, Takahashi R (1990). Comparison of the antimanic efficacy of carbamazepine and lithium carbonate by double-blind controlled study. *Pharmacopsychiatry* 23, 143–150.

46. Ballenger JC, Post RM (1980). Carbamazepine in manic-depressive illness: A new treatment. *American Journal of Psychiatry* 137, 782–790.

47. Lewin J, Sumners D (1992). Successful treatment of episodic dyscontrol with carbamazepine. *British Journal of Psychiatry* 161, 261–262.

48. Post RM (2000). Three decades of research on bipolar illness. In Ban TA, Healy D, Shorter E, *The Triumph of Psychopharmacology and the Story of CINP,* Animula Publishing, Budapest, pp. 296–299.

49. Silberman EK, Post RM, Nurnberger J, Theodore W, Boulenger AP (1985). Transient sensory, cognitive and affective phenomena in affective illness. *British Journal of Psychiatry* 146, 81–89; Post RM, Rubinow D, Ballenger JC (1986). Conditioning and sensitization in the longitudinal course of affective illness. *British Journal of Psychiatry* 149, 191–201; Post RM, Weiss SRB (1989). Kindling and manic-depressive illness. In Bolwig TG, Trimble MR (eds.), *The Clinical Relevance of Kindling.* J Wiley & Sons, London, pp. 209–230.

50. See chapter 3; Falret JP (1860 and 1861). Sur l'état mental des épileptiques. *Archives of General Medicine* (December 1860 and 1861).

51. Shorter E, Healy D. (2007). *Shock Therapy. A History of Electroconvulsive Therapy in Mental Illness.* Rutgers University Press, New Brunswick, N.J., chapter 11.

52. Satzinger G (1993). A provocative reminiscence. *Drug News Perspective* 6, 623–627. Satzinger G (2001). Drug discovery and commercial exploitation. *Drug News Perspective* 14, 197–207.

53. Melody Petersen (2002). Madison Avenue plays growing role in drug research. *New York Times,* November 22.

54. Pandey AC, Crockatt JG, Janney CA, Werth JL, Tsarouchag G. (2000). Gabapentin in bipolar disorder: A placebo-controlled trial of adjunctive therapy. *Bipolar Disorder* 2, 249–255.

55. K Applbaum has pointed out that recent editions of the psychotropics *Physicians' Desk Reference* sponsored by GlaxoSmithKline that American residents are given as a gift have exactly one ad in it. It is the only color page in the book, and it is thick, card-like, so that the book automatically opens to that page every time you touch it. The ad is for Lamictal (lamotrigine). It shows the picture of an attractive woman busy with kids, and reads roughly: She is stable for now. But how long will that last?

56. Post RM (2000). Three decades of research on bipolar illness. In Ban T, Shorter E, Healy D (eds.), *The Triumph of Psychopharmacology,* Animula, Budapest, pp. 296–302.

57. Findling RL, Kowatch RA, Post RM (2003). *Pediatric Bipolar Disorder. A Handbook for Clinicians.* Martin Dunitz, London; Post RM (2002). Treatment resistance in bipolar disorder. Royal College of Psychiatrists Meeting, Newcastle, England. October 17. From abstract book available from author.

58. Shorter E (2002). Looking backwards: A possible new path for drug discovery in psychopharmacology. Nature reviews. *Drug Discovery,* Perspective 1, 1003–1006.

59. The term hypnotic in the 1950s, though, primarily referred to agents that might be useful in the induction of hypnosis rather than agents that would put someone to sleep.

60. Litchfield H (1960). Aminophenylpyridone, A new mood stabilizing drug. *Archives of Pediatrics* 77, 133–137.

61. Cantelmo AL 1960. Clinical evaluation of aminophenylpyridone (dornwal): A new drug for stabilizing emotional behavior. *Current Therapeutic Research, Clinical and Experimental* 2, 72–75.

62. Cass LJ, Frederik WS, Teodoro J (1960). Evaluation of calmative agents. *American Practitioner and Digest of Treatment*, April, 285–288.

63. Janssen P (1998). From Haloperidol to Risperidone. In Healy D, *The Psychopharmacologists*, volume 2, Arnold, London, pp. 39–70.

64. Berger FM (1970). Anxiety and the discovery of the tranquilizers. In Ayd F, Blackwell B (eds.), *Discoveries in Biological Psychiatry*, Lippincott, Philadelphia, 115–129.

65. Berger FM, Bradley W (1946). The pharmacological properties of alpha, beta-dihydroxy-gamma-(2-methylphenoxy)-propane (myanesin). *British Journal of Pharmacology* 1, 265–272.

66. Thuillier J (1981). *Les dix ans qui ont changé la folie*. Editions Robert Laffont, Paris, pp. 299–301. Trans. Hickish G, Healy D (1999). *Ten Years that Changed the Face of Mental Illness*. Dunitz, London.

67. Berger FM, Schwartz RP (1948). Oral myanesin in the treatment of spastic and hyperkinetic disorders. *Journal of the American Medical Association* 137, 772–774.

68. Berger FM. Interview with DH. January 15, 2006.

69. Berger FM. Interview with DH. January 1, 2006.

70. Berger FM (1955). Miltown, a long-acting mephenesin-like drug. *Federation Proceedings* 14, 318–319.

71. Bein HJ (1970). Biological research in the pharmaceutical industry with reserpine. In Ayd FJ, Blackwell B (eds.), *Discoveries in Biological Psychiatry*, Lippincott, Philadelphia, 142–152.

72. SmithKline Beecham, as a late entrant into the serotonin reuptake inhibiting class, did just this with extraordinary success thirty years later when it christened paroxetine, the selective serotonin reuptake inhibitor or SSRI.

73. Ironically quite unaware of this, the advocates of mood stabilizers now argue against using antidepressants in people with a bipolar disorder.

74. Advertisement for nortriptyline in *British Journal of Psychiatry*, 1964.

75. Morton Mintz (1967). *By Prescription Only*. Houghton Mifflin, Boston.

76. Azima H, Arthurs D, Silver A (1961). The effect of aminophenidone in anxiety states, a multi-blind study. *American Journal of Psychiatry* 118, 159–160.

77. Azima H, Arthurs D (1961). A controlled trial of thalidomide, a new hypnotic agent. *American Journal of Psychiatry* 118, 554–555.

78. Chouinard G, Steinberg S, Steiner W (1987). Estrogen-progesterone combination: Another mood stabilizer? *American Journal of Psychiatry* 144, 826–827.

79. Chouinard G, Beauclair L, Geiser R, Etienne P (1990). A pilot study of magnesium aspartate hydrochloride (Magnesiocard) as a mood stabilizer for rapid cycling bipolar affective disorder patients. *Progress in Neuro-Psychopharmacology & Biological Psychiatry* 14, 171–180.

80. Hollister L (1987). Strategies for research in clinical psychopharmacology. In Meltzer HY, et al. (eds.), *Neuropsychopharmacology. The Third Generation of Progress*, Raven Press, New York, p. 35.

81. Leonard BE (1992). *Fundamentals of Psychopharmacology*. J Wiley & Sons, Bristol; Ayd FJ Jr (1996). *Lexicon for Psychiatry, Neurology and the Neurosciences*. Williams and Wilkins, Baltimore.

82. Gorman J (1992). *The Essential Guide to Psychiatric Drugs*. St Martin's Press, New York.

83. Gruber AJ, Cole JO (1991). Antidepressant effects of flupenthixol. *Pharmacotherapy* 11, 450–459.

84. Healy D (1990). The psychopharmacological era: Notes toward a history. *Journal of Psychopharmacology* 4, 152–167.

85. Zarate CA, Tohen M, Banov MD, Weiss MK, Cole JO (1995). Is clozapine a mood stabilizer? *Journal of Clinical Psychiatry* 56, 108–112.

86. Grinspoon L, Bakalar JB (1995). The use of cannabis as a mood stabilizer in bipolar disorder: Anecdotal evidence and the need for clinical research. *Journal of Psychoactive Drugs* 30, 171–177.

87. Bowden C, Brugger A, Swann A (1994). Efficacy of divalproex vs lithium and placebo in the treatment of mania. *Journal of the American Medical Association* 271, 918–924; Bowden CL (1998). New concepts in mood stabilization: Evidence for the effectiveness of valproate and lamotrigine. *Neuropsycho-pharmacology* 19, 194–199.

88. Harris M, Chandran S, Chakroborty N, Healy D (2003). Mood stabilizers: The archaeology of the concept. *Bipolar Disorders* 5, 446–452; commentary by P Grof.

89. Tollefson GD (1997). Zyprexa Product Team: 4 Column Summary. Zyprexa MultiDistrict Litigation 1596, Document ZY200270343.

90. Allan Young, Newcastle, Lecture at Yorkshire.

91. Berk M, Dodd S (2005). Bipolar II disorder: A review. *Bipolar Disorder* 7, 11–24.

92. Healy D (2004). *Let Them Eat Prozac*. New York University Press, New York, chapter 5.

93. American Psychiatric Association (2003). Meeting Program.

94. Oepen G, Baldessarini RJ, Salvatore P (2004). "On the periodicity of manic-depressive insanity," by Eliot Slater (1938); translated excerpts and commentary. *Journal of Affective Disorders* 78, 1–9.

95. Healy D (2006). Neuroleptics and mortality: A 50-year cycle. *British Journal of Psychiatry* 188, 128.

96. Torrey EF (2002). The going rate on shrinks. Big pharma and the buying of psychiatry. *The American Prospect*, July 15, pp. 15–16.

97. Heath J, Potter A (2005). *The Rebel Sell. How the Counterculture Became Consumer Culture*. Capstone, Chichester.

98. Applbaum puts it like this: "Considering the role of psychiatric congresses . . . we can observe that drug companies are uninterested in sponsoring congresses whose core scientific program is not corroborative of a pharmacological approach to treatment. The relationship between a drug company's interests and the organization

of a psychiatric congress is never a blunt one . . . However, the influences [can be] interpreted as having "structural force" [rather] than being directly persuasive. This effect . . . can be seen more or less directly when we consider the organization of the conference itself." Applbaum K (2004). How to organize a psychiatric congress. *Anthropological Quarterly* 77, 306.

99. My excuse for participating is for fieldwork purposes. Perhaps we're all doing the same thing.

100. Exactly this criticism was offered of this argument by an anonymous reviewer of Healy D (2006). The latest mania. Selling bipolar disorder. *PLoS Medicine.* http://dx.doi.org/10.1371/journal.pmed.0030185.

101. Post RM (2000). Three decades of research on bipolar illness. In Ban T, Shorter E, Healy D (eds.), *The Triumph of Psychopharmacology*, Animula, Budapest, pp. 296–302.

102. There was ferocious pressure on Post and others within NIMH, for instance, to take out patents on possible new treatments like TMS. Shorter E, Healy D. (2007). *Shock Therapy. A History of Electroconvulsive Therapy in Mental Illness.* Rutgers University Press, New Brunswick, N.J., chapter 11.

103. www.bipolarhelpcenter.com/resources/mdq.jsp.

104. Moynihan R, Cassels A (2005). *Selling Sickness.* Nation Books, New York.

105. Tollefson GD (1997). Zyprexa Product Team: 4 Column Summary. Zyprexa MultiDistrict Litigation 1596, Document ZY200270343.

106. Healy D (2002). *The Creation of Psychopharmacology.* Harvard University Press, Cambridge, Mass., chapter 3.

107. Warawa E (2000). From neuroleptics to antipsychotics. In D Healy, *The Psychopharmacologists*, volume 3, London, Arnold, pp. 505–521.

108. US Patent No. 5,229,382, filed on May 22, 1992 (a continuation of an application filed on April 23, 1991). European patent, EP0,454,436, filed on April 24, 1991.

109. Details from Wyden P (1997). *Conquering Schizophrenia.* Alfred A Knopf, New York.

110. Tohen M, Calabrese JR, Sachs G, Banov MD, Detke HC, Risser R, Baker RW, Chou JC-Y, Bowden CL (2006). Randomized, placebo-controlled trial of olanzapine as maintenance therapy in patients with bipolar I disorder responding to acute treatment with olanzapine. *American Journal of Psychiatry* 163, 247–256.

111. www.prnewswire.com/cgi-bin/micro_stories.pl?ACCT=916306&TICK=LLY.

112. *Staying Well . . . with Bipolar Disorder.* Relapse Prevention Booklet. Produced in Association with the Manic-Depressive Fellowship Sponsored by Eli Lilly and Company, p. 17.

113. De Hert M, Thys E, Magiels G, Wyckaert S (2005). *Anything or Nothing.* Self-guide for people with Bipolar Disorder. Uitgeverij Houtekiet, Antwerp, p. 35.

114. Healy D (2006). The latest mania. Selling bipolar disorder. *PLoS Medicine.* http://dx.doi.org/10.1371/journal.pmed.0030185.

115. Colton CW, Manderscheid RW (2006). Congruencies in increased mortality rates, years of potential life lost, and causes of death among public mental health clients in eight states. *Prevention of Chronic Disease.* www.cdc.gov/pcd/issues/2006/apr/05_0180.htm.

116. Tondo L, Baldessarini RJ, Hennen J, Floris G, Silvetti F, Tohen M (1998). Lithium treatment and risk of suicidal behavior. *Journal of Clinical Psychiatry* 59, 405–414.

117. Healy D (2006). The latest mania. Selling bipolar disorder. *PLoS Medicine.* http://dx.doi.org/10.1371/journal.pmed.0030185.

118. Zyprexa Primary Care Sales Force Resource Guide. Zyprexa MDL 1596. ZY20006 1996.

119. Drahos P, Braithwaite J (2002). *Information Feudalism. Who Owns the Knowledge Economy.* Earthscan, London.

120. See Lieberman JA, Stroop TS, McEvoy JP, Swartz MS, et al. (2005). Effectiveness of antipsychotic drugs in patients with chronic schizophrenia. *New England Journal of Medicine* 353, 1209–1223. Having researched this issue, the author is not aware of any other drug capable of inducing comparable increases in lipid levels with the possible exception of cyclosporine.

121. Marson A, Jacoby A, Johnson A, Kim L, Gamble C, Chadwick D (2005). Immediate versus deferred antiepileptic drug treatment for early epilepsy and single seizures: A randomized controlled trial. *Lancet* 365, 2007–2013.

Chapter 7. The Latest Mania

1. Brooks K (2000). No small burden. Families with mentally ill children confront health care shortcomings, undeserved stigma of "bad parenting." *Star-Telegram,* July 19.

2. Kluger J, Song S (2002). Young and bipolar. Once called manic depression, the disorder afflicted adults. Now it's striking kids. Why? *Time,* August 19, 30–41.

3. Volkmar FR (2002). Changing perspectives on mood disorders in children. *American Journal of Psychiatry* 159, 893–894.

4. Papolos D, Papolos J (2000). *The Bipolar Child.* Random House, New York.

5. Isaac G (2001). Bipolar not ADHD. Unrecognized epidemic of manic-depressive illness in children. Writers' Club Press, Lincoln, Neb.

6. Findling RL, Kowatch RA, Post RM (2003). *Pediatric Bipolar Disorder. A Handbook for Clinicians.* Martin Dunitz, London.

7. Anglada T (2004). *Brandon and the Bipolar Bear.* Trafford Publishing, Victoria, B.C.

8. Hebert B (2005). *My Bipolar Roller Coaster Feeling Book.* Trafford Publishing, Victoria, B.C.

9. www.jbrf.org/cbq/cbq_survey.cfm. Accessed December 1, 2005.

10. www.jbrf.org/juv_bipolar/faq.html. Accessed December 1, 2005.

11. Papolos D, Papolos J (2000). *The Bipolar Child.* Random House, New York, p. 14.

12. Harris J (2005). The increased diagnosis of juvenile "bipolar disorder," what are we treating? *Psychiatric Services* 56, 529–531.

13. Baethge C, Glovinsky R, Baldessarini RJ (2004). Manic-depressive illness in children: An early twentieth century view by Theodore Ziehen (1862–1950). *History of Psychiatry* 15, 201–226. See also Homburger A (1926). *Vorlesungen über Psycho-*

pathologie des Kindesalters. Reprint, Wissenschaftliche Buchgesellschaft, Darmstadt, 1967, chapter 30, pp. 462–483.

14. Mick E, Biederman J, Dougherty M, Aleardi M (2004a). Comparative efficacy of atypical antipsychotics for pediatric bipolar disorder. *Acta Psychiatrica Scandinavica* 1110, 50, 29; Mick E, Biederman J, Aleardi M, Dougherty M (2004b). Open trial of atypical antipsychotics in pre-schoolers with bipolar disorder. *Acta Psychiatrica Scandinavica* 1110, 51, 29.

15. Carlson G (1990). Child and adolescent mania: Diagnostic considerations. *Journal of Child Psychology and Psychiatry* 31, 331–342; Werry JS, McClellan JM, Chard L (1991). Childhood and adolescent schizophrenic, bipolar and schizoaffective disorders: A clinical and outcome study. *Journal of the American Academy of Child and Adolescent Psychiatry* 30, 457–465.

16. Geller B, Williams M, Zimmerman B, Frazier J (1996). Washington University in St Louis Kiddie Schedule for Affective Disorders and Schizophrenia (Wash-U-KSADS). St. Louis, Washington University.

17. Geller B, Craney J, Bolhoffer K, DelBello MP, Axelson D, Luby J, Williams M, Zimerman B, Nickelsburg MJ, Frazier J, Beringer L (2003). Phenomenology and longitudinal course of children with a prepubertal and early adolescent bipolar disorder phenotype. In Geller B, DelBello MP (eds.), *Bipolar Disorder in Childhood and Early Adolescence*, Guilford Press, New York, pp. 25–50.

18. Biederman J, Faraone S, Mick E, Wozniak J, Chen L, Ouellette C, Marrs A, Moore P, Garcia J, Mennin D, Lelon E (1996). Attention-deficit hyperactivity disorder and juvenile mania: An overlooked co-morbidity? *Journal of the American Academy of Child and Adolescent Psychiatry* 35, 997–1008; Faraone SV, Biederman J, Mennin D, Wozniak J, Spencer T (1997). Attention-deficit hyperactivity disorder with bipolar disorder: A familial subtype? *Journal of the American Academy of Child and Adolescent Psychiatry* 36, 1378–1387.

19. Lewinsohn P, Klein D, Seeley J (2000). Bipolar disorder during adolescence and young adulthood in a community sample. *Bipolar Disorder* 2, 281–293.

20. National Institute of Mental Health Research Roundtable on Prepubertal Bipolar Disorder (2001). *Journal of the American Academy of Child and Adolescent Psychiatry* 40, 871–878.

21. Healy D, Le Noury J (2007). Paediatric bipolar disorder. An object of study in the creation of an illness. *Int J Risk & Safety in Medicine* 19, 209–221.

22. Kowatch RA, Fristad M, Birmaher B, Wagner KD, Findling RL, Hellander M, and the Child Psychiatric Workgroup on Bipolar Disorder (2005). Treatment guidelines for children and adolescents with bipolar disorder. *Journal of the American Academy of Child and Adolescent Psychiatry* 44, 213–235.

23. Groopman J (2007). What's Normal?—The difficulty of diagnosing bipolar disorder in children. *New Yorker,* April 9, pp. 28–33.

24. Cooper W, Arbogast PG, Ding H, Hickson GB, Fuchs C, Ray WA (2006). Trends in prescribing of antipsychotic medications for U.S. children. *Ambulatory Pediatrics* 6, 79–83.

25. Blader JC, Carlson GA (2006). Increased rates of bipolar disorder diagnoses among U.S. child, adolescent and adult inpatients, 1996–2004. *Biological Psychiatry* 62, 107–114.

26. Harpaz-Rotem I, Rosenheck R (2004). Changes in outpatient psychiatric diagnosis in privately insured children and adolescents from 1995 to 2000. *Child Psychiatry and Human Development* 34, 329–340; Moreno C, Laje G, Blanco C, Jiang H, Schmidt AB, Olfson M (2007). National trends in outpatient diagnosis and treatment of bipolar disorder in youth. *Archives of General Psychiatry* 64, 1032–1039.

27. Harris J (2005). The increased diagnosis of juvenile "bipolar disorder," what are we treating? *Psychiatric Services* 56, 529–531.

28. Dilsaver S (2005). Review of Harris J. The increased diagnosis of juvenile bipolar disorder: What are we treating? *Journal of Bipolar Disorders* 4, 8.

29. Tollefson GD (1997). Zyprexa Product Team: 4 Column Summary. Zyprexa MultiDistrict Litigation 1596, Document ZY200270343.

30. Krishnamoorthy J, King BH (1998). Open-label olanzapine treatment in five preadolescent children. *Journal of Child and Adolescent Psychopharmacology* 8, 107–113.

31. National Institute for Health and Clinical Excellence (NICE) (2006). *Bipolar Disorder*. Clinical Guideline 38. Available on www.nice.org.uk.

32. Klein R (2000). Children and psychopharmacology. In Healy D, *The Psychopharmacologists*, volume 3, Arnold, London, pp. 309–332; Rapoport J (2000). Phenomenology, psychopharmacotherapy and child psychiatry. In Healy D, *The Psychopharmacologists*, volume 3, Arnold, London, pp. 333–356. There were, however, psychiatrists prescribing drugs to children such as Barbara Fish, Magda Campbell, Joveon Simeon, and John Werry.

33. Jung CG (1923). *Psychological Types*. Harcourt, Brace, New York.

34. IP Pavlov (1928). *Lectures on Conditioned Reflexes*. Trans. Gantt WH, International Publishers, New York.

35. Eysenck HJ (1947). *Dimensions of Personality*. Routledge and Kegan Paul, London; Eysenck HJ (1990). *Rebel with a Cause*. WH Allen, London.

36. Sulser F (2000). From the presynaptic neuron to the receptor to the nucleus. In Healy D, *The Psychopharmacologists*, volume 3, Arnold, London, pp. 239–258.

37. Kretschmer EA (1934). *Textbook of Medical Psychology*. Trans. Strauss EB, Oxford University Press.

38. Sheldon WH (1942). *The Varieties of Temperament*. Harper, New York. See Gottesman I (1998). Predisposed to predispositions. In Healy D, *The Psychopharmacologists*, volume 2, Arnold, London, pp. 377–408.

39. Rees WL, Healy D (1997). The place of clinical trials in the evolution of psychopharmacology. *History of Psychiatry* 8, 1–20.

40. Claridge G, Healy D (1994). The psychopharmacology of individual differences. *Human Psychopharmacology* 9, 285–298.

41. Temkin O (1963). The scientific approach to disease: Specific entity and individual sickness. In Crombie AC (ed.), *Scientific Change*, Heinemann, London, pp. 629–647; Rosenberg CE (2002). The tyranny of diagnosis: Specific entities and individual experience. *Milbank Quarterly* 80, 237–260; Rosenberg CE (2003). What is disease? In memory of Owsei Temkin. *Bulletin of the History of Medicine* 77, 491–505.

42. See introduction and Goldberg C (2007). Bipolar labels for children stir concern. *Boston Globe*, February 15.

43. Healy D (2006). Manufacturing consensus. *Culture, Medicine & Psychiatry* 30, 135–156; Rosenheck R (2005). The growth of psychopharmacology in the 1990s: Evidence-based practice or irrational exuberance? *International Journal of Law & Psychiatry* 28, 467–483.

44. Healy D, Nutt D (1997). British Association for Psychopharmacology consensus on statement on childhood and learning disabilities psychopharmacology. *Journal of Psychopharmacology* 11, 291–294.

45. Sharav VH (2003). The impact of FDA modernization act on the recruitment of children for research. *Ethical Human Sciences and Services* 5, 83–108.

46. *Newsweek* (2002). Depression. 3 million kids suffer from it. What you can do? October 7, 52–61.

47. Healy D (2004). *Let Them Eat Prozac*. New York University Press, New York.

48. Emslie G, Mann JJ, Beardslee W, Fawcett J, Leon A, Meltzer H, Goodwin F, Shaffer D, Wagner K, Ryan N (2004). *ACNP*. Preliminary report of the task force on SSRIs and suicidal behavior in youth. January 21.

49. There are good grounds to argue that all fifteen studies failed to show efficacy. See Healy D (2006). Manufacturing consensus. *Culture, Medicine & Psychiatry* 30, 135–156.

50. www.fda.gov/ohrms/dockets/ac/04/transcripts/4006T1.htm.

51. Cited in Healy D (2006). Manufacturing Consensus. *Culture, Medicine & Psychiatry* 30, 135–156.

52. Keller MD, Ryan ND, Strober M, Klein RG, Kutcher SP, Birmaher B, Hagino OR, Koplewicz H, Carlsson GA, Clarke GN, Emslie GJ, Feinberg D, Geller B, Kusumakar V, Papatheodorou G, Sack WH, Sweeney M, Wagner KD, Weller E, Winters NC, Oakes R, McCafferty JP (2001). Efficacy of paroxetine in the treatment of adolescent major depression: A randomized, controlled trial. *Journal of the American Academy of Child and Adolescent Psychiatry* 40, 762–772.

53. Central Medical Affairs Team. Seroxat/Paxil. Adolescent Depression. Position Piece on the Phase III studies. October 1998. SmithKline Beecham Confidential Document, available from the author. This is also available on the *Canadian Medical Association Journal* Web site.

Chapter 8. The Engineers of Human Souls

1. Mol AM (2006). *De logica van het zorgen*. Van Gennep, Amsterdam. Trans. (2008). *The Logic of Care*. Routledge, London.

2. Coyle JT, Pine DS, Charney DS, Lewis L, Nemeroff CB, Carlson GA, Joshi PT, Reiss D, Todd RD, Hellander M, and the Depression & Bipolar Support Alliance Consensus Development Panel (2003). Depression & Bipolar Support Alliance Consensus Statement on the unmet needs in the diagnosis and treatment of mood disorders in children and adolescents. *Journal of the American Academy of Child and Adolescent Psychiatry* 42, 1494–1503.

3. This isn't the only article that includes this phrase. In addition to Harvard and Yale, Oxford seems to have been folded into the loop: Chengappa KR, Goodwin GM (2005). Characterizing barriers, challenges and unmet needs in the management of bipolar disorder. *Bipolar Disorders* 7, supp. 1, 5–7.

4. Drahos P, Braithwaite J (2002). *Information Feudalism. Who Owns the Knowledge Economy.* Earthscan, London.

5. Swann JP (1988). *Academic Scientists and the Pharmaceutical Industry. Cooperative Research in Twentieth Century America.* Johns Hopkins University Press, Baltimore.

6. Liebenau J (1987). *Medical Science and Medical Industry.* Macmillan Press, Basingstoke.

7. This happened in different countries in different years; in Germany in 1967 but in Canada not till 1993.

8. Applbaum K (2006). Personal communication.

9. Applbaum K (2004). *The Marketing Era.* Routledge, New York. Applbaum "found unmet needs to be the overarching model [that] drives the organization forward." These were "self-serving suppositions that work simultaneously as market research constructs." "In their putative effort to fulfil consumer wishes, corporations see needs and desires, the valuable constituents of which marketers regard as latent or unmet until they have tapped them, as the quarry from which to extract their sustenance. The profession's modus vivendi is to ascertain what [unmet] needs exist and should be marketed to; marketing science is the system of practices devoted to determining these as objective categories into which designated products and services can be launched and directed."

10. Applbaum K (2004). *The Marketing Era.* Routledge, New York. See also Applbaum K (2006). Pharmaceutical marketing and the invention of the medical consumer. *PLoS Medicine* 3, issue 4, e189, publicly available on plosmedicine.org, April 2006.

11. Pedersen V, Bogeso K (1998). Drug hunting. In D Healy, *The Psychopharmacologists,* volume 2, Arnold, London, pp. 561–580.

12. This paragraph is heavily dependent on inputs from Tom Ban and Kal Applbaum.

13. Healy D (1997). *The Antidepressant Era.* Harvard University Press, Cambridge, Mass., chapter 5.

14. Healy D (1997). *The Antidepressant Era.* Harvard University Press, Cambridge, Mass., chapter 6.

15. Healy D (1997). *The Antidepressant Era.* Harvard University Press, Cambridge, Mass., chapter 6.

16. Ellenberger H (1955). A comparison on European and American psychiatry. *Bulletin of the Menninger Clinic* 19, 43–52.

17. Goodwin F, Ghaemi SN (1997). Prospects for a scientific psychiatry. *Acta Neuropsychiatrica* 9, 49–51.

18. Coyle JT, Pine DS, Charney DS, Lewis L, Nemeroff CB, et al. (2003). Depression & Bipolar Support Alliance Consensus Statement on the unmet needs in the diagnosis and treatment of mood disorders in children and adolescence. *Journal of the American Academy of Child and Adolescent Psychiatry* 42, 1494–1503.

19. Sheldon TA, Smith GD (1993). Consensus conferences as drug promotion. *Lancet* 341, 100–102.

20. Gilbert DA, Altshuler KZ, Rego WV, Shon SP, Crismon ML, Toprac MG,

Rush AJ (1998). Texas Medication Algorithm Project: Definitions, rationale, and methods to develop medication algorithms. *Journal of Clinical Psychiatry* 59, 345–351.

21. Hughes CW (1999). The Texas children's Medication Algorithm Project: Report of the Texas consensus conference panel on medication treatment of childhood major depressive disorder. *Journal of the American Academy of Child and Adolescent Psychiatry* 38, 1442–1454.

22. As of 2004, these guidelines had been adopted at some point by Pennsylvania, California, Colorado, Nevada, Illinois, Kentucky, New Mexico, New York, Ohio, South Carolina, Maryland, Missouri, and Washington, D.C., or by jurisdictions within those states.

23. Healy D (2006). Manufacturing Consensus. *Culture, Medicine & Psychiatry* 30, 135–156.

24. Healy D (2008). Trussed in evidence: Guidelines, tramlines and faultlines. *Transcultural Psychiatry*, in press.

25. See Healy D (2002). *The Creation of Psychopharmacology*. Harvard University Press, Cambridge, Mass.

26. Davies H (2001). The role of the private sector in protecting human subjects. Talk to Institute of Medicine, August 21, www.acrohealth.org/policy/pdfs/testimony_082101.pdf; Getz K, De Bruin A (2000). Breaking the development speed barrier. *Drug Information Journal* 34, 725–736.

27. See Stecklow S, Johannes L (1997). Questions arise on new drug testing. Drug makers relied on clinical researchers who now await trial. *Wall Street Journal*, August 15; Eichenwald K, Kolata G (1999). Drug trials hide conflict for doctors. *New York Times*, May 16, pp. 1, 28, 29; A doctor's drug studies turn into fraud. *New York Times*, May 17, pp. 1, 16, 17; Boseley S (1999). Trial and error puts patients at risk. *Guardian Newspaper*, July 27, p. 8.

28. Lemmens T, Freedman B (2000). Ethics review for sale? Conflict of interest and commercial research review boards. *Milbank Quarterly* 78, 547–584.

29. Petryna A (2006). Globalizing human subjects research. In Petryna A, Lakoff A, Kleinman A (eds.), *Global pharmaceuticals. Ethics, markets, practices*. Duke University Press, Durham, pp. 33–60.

30. Drahos P, Braithwaite J (2002). *Information Feudalism. Who Owns the Knowledge Economy*. Earthscan, London.

31. Angell M (2004). *The Truth about the Drug Companies*. Random House, New York; Kassirer JP (2004). *On the Take*. Oxford University Press, New York; Krimsky S (2003). *Science in the Private Interest*. Rowman & Littlefield, Lanham, Md.

32. Kraepelin E (1987). *Memoirs*. Trans. Cheryl Wooding-Deane, Ed. Hippius H, Peters G, Ploog D, Springer Books, New York.

33. Healy D (2004). Shaping the intimate. Influences on the experience of everyday nerves. *Social Studies of Science* 34, 219–245.

34. Heath I (2006). Combating disease mongering: Daunting but nonetheless essential. *PLoS Medicine* 3, e146. April. Available on www.plosmedicine.org.

35. Healy D (2006). The Antidepressant Tale: Figures signifying nothing? *Advances in Psychiatric Treatment* 12, 320–328.

36. Bittker TE (1985). The industrialization of American psychiatry. *American Journal of Psychiatry* 142, 149–154.

37. Sinaikin PM (2003). Categorical diagnosis and a poetics of obligation: An ethical commentary on psychiatric diagnosis and treatment. *Ethical Human Sciences and Services* 5, 141–148; Sinaikin PM (2004). Coping with the medical model in clinical practice or "How I learned to stop worrying and love DSM." *Journal of Critical Psychology, Counselling and Psychotherapy,* 204–213.

38. Shorter E, Healy D (2007). *Shock Therapy. A History of Electroconvulsive Therapy in Mental Illness.* Rutgers University Press, New Brunswick, N.J., chapter 11.

39. Healy D, Savage M, Michael P, Harris M, Hirst D, Carter M, Cattell D, McMonagle T, Sohler N, Susser E (2001). Psychiatric bed utilisation: 1896 and 1996 compared. *Psychological Medicine* 31, 779–790.

40. Healy D, Harris M, Tranter R, Gutting P, Austin R, Jones-Edwards G, Roberts AP (2006). Lifetime suicide rates in treated schizophrenia: 1875–1924 and 1994–1998 cohorts compared. *British Journal of Psychiatry* 188, 223–228.

41. Colton CW, Manderscheid RW (2006). Congruencies in increased mortality rates, years of potential life lost, and causes of death among public mental health clients in eight states. *Prevention of Chronic Disease.* www.cdc.gov/pcd/issues/2006/apr/05_0180.htm.

42. Harris M, Chandran S, Chakroborty N, Healy D (2005). Service utilization in bipolar disorder, 1890 and 1990 compared. *History of Psychiatry* 16, 423–434.

43. Shepherd M (1998). Psychopharmacology: Specific and non-specific. In Healy D, *The Psychopharmacologists,* volume 2, Arnold, London, pp. 237–258.

Coda. The Once and Future Laboratory

1. Healy D (1997). *The Antidepressant Era.* Harvard University Press, Cambridge, Mass., chapter 5.

2. Valenstein ES (2005). *The War of the Soups and the Sparks.* Columbia University Press, New York.

3. Vane JR, Wolstenholme GE, O'Connor M (1960). *Adrenergic Mechanisms.* Ciba Foundation Symposium, J & A Churchill Ltd, London; Carlsson A (1996). The rise of neuropsychopharmacology: Impact on basic and clinical neuroscience. In Healy D, *The Psychopharmacologists,* volume 1, Chapman & Hall, London, pp. 51–80.

4. Debus AG (1991). *The French Paracelsians.* Cambridge University Press, Cambridge.

5. Gottesman I (1998). Predisposed towards predispositions. In Healy D, *The Psychopharmacologists,* volume 2, Arnold, London, pp. 377–408.

6. Healy D (2002). *The Creation of Psychopharmacology.* Harvard University Press, Cambridge, Mass., chapters 4 and 8.

7. Shorter E, Healy D. (2007). *Shock Therapy. A History of Electroconvulsive Therapy in Mental Illness.* Rutgers University Press, New Brunswick, N.J., chapter 11.

8. www.socialaudit.org.uk/6070225.htm.

9. Shorter E (1982). *A History of Women's Bodies.* Penguin, Harmondsworth, Middlesex.

INDEX

Page numbers in *italics* refer to figures.

Abbott Laboratories, 168–69, 185–86, 204
academics: childhood diagnosis and,
202–8; co-optation of, 244; pharmaceutical industry and, 188–89; sidelin-
ing of, 235–36; statistics and, 240
ADHD. *See* Attention Deficit Hyperactivity Disorder
admissions per annum, 243
adolescence and marketing, 227
age at diagnosis, 198–202, 205, 207–8
Akimoto, Haruo, 114
Akiskal, Hagop, 148
alienists: American, 48; asylums and, 37;
forensic issues and, 49; German, 34;
hope of, 51; lithium compounds and,
93–94; manic-depressive illness and,
54; view of insanity by, 88. *See also*
Falret, Jean-Pierre; Kraepelin, Emil;
Pinel, Philippe; Wernicke, Karl
American Psychiatric Association, 187–88,
206
aminophenidone/aminophenylpyridine,
179, 183–84
amitriptyline, 227
Anatomy (Vesalius), 14
Anatomy of the Brain (Willis), 28–29
Angst, Jules, 121–22, 127, 142, 144–45, 149
anthropometry, 211
anticonvulsants: for behavioral purposes,
208; carbamazepine, 168, 169–73, 174;
epilepsy and, 196; gabapentin, 168,
175–76; as mood stabilizers, 174–76,
196–97; studies of, 165–68; suicide and,
195; valproate, 164, 168, 175
antidepressants, *130*, 170, 183–84, 213–18.
See also selective serotonin reuptake
inhibitors (SSRIs)
antipsychotics: Baldessarini and, 188; bipolar disorder and, 193; life expectancy
and, 194; major tranquilizers as, 182;
mania, depression, and, 185, 191; side

effects of, 165. *See also* mood
stabilizers
anxiolytics, 182, 185
Aretaeus of Cappadocia, 8, 10–11
Arfwedson, Johann August, 91
Aristotle, 12
Arnold, Ned, 45–46
artists and mental illness, 75, 150
Ashburner, Val, 103
Astra-Zeneca, 192, 193, 204
asylums: brain and, 37–43; in Britain,
78–79; carbamazepine in, 171; epileptics
in, 165–66, 172–73; lithium compounds
and, 93. *See also* North Wales, asylum at
Attention Deficit Hyperactivity Disorder
(ADHD), 187, 199, 202, 203, 208, 213,
227, 230
Aulde, John, 94
Australia, 100–105
Aventyl. *See* nortriptyline
Ayd, Frank, 227
Azima, Hazim, 184

Baastrup, Poul, 113–14, 115, 118, 122
Baillarger, Jules, 43, 54–59, 63
Bakalar, Jim, 185
Baldessarini, Ross, 188
Ballenger, Jim, 172, 174
Ban, Tom, 160, 224
Bayle, Auguste, 42
Bell, Charles, 34
benzodiazepines, 167, 182, 183, 184
Berger, Frank, 180–82, 206
Berrios, German, 19
Berzelius, Jon Jacobs, 91
Biederman, Joseph, 203
biological psychiatry, 211
The Bipolar Child (Papolos and Papolos),
198, 200, 202
bipolar disorder: across time, 19–23; birth
of, 142–45; DSM-III and, 18; global

---

bipolar disorder (cont'd.)
character of, 187–88; Kraepelin and, 135; landscape of, xv–xvi; marketing of, 190–91; pediatric, 198–208; prevalence of, 149–50, 187; as social entity, xiii; substance abuse and, 70, 148; terminology for, 151; types I and II, 125, 147–48
bipolar spectrum, 148
Bittker, Thomas, 240–41
Blackwell, Barry, 118–20
Bleuler, Eugen, 75
Bleuler, Manfred, 145
borderline personality disorder, 17, 148, 149
Borselli, Sergio, 164–66
Bowden, Charles, 168–69, 186
brain: asylums and, 37–43; Hippocrates and, 6–7; model of functioning of, 136–37; "nerves" and, 31–37; science of, 25–31, 246–48
branding, 76, 223–26
Breuer, Josef, 71–72
Britain, 75, 77–80, 207, 232, 233. See also North Wales, asylum at
Broca, Paul, 136
Brockington, Ian, 152
Brooks, Karen, 198–99, 205
Broussolle, Paul, 165
Bunney, William (Biff), 123, 124, 173
Burton, Beverly, 163

Cade, John, 100–103, 112
Cameron, Ewen, 108
Canada, 108
carbamazepine, 168, 169–73, 174–76, 208
care, dynamics and logic of, 220–21
Carlsson, Arvid, 99, 246
Carraz, George, xviii, 163–64, 169
cartels, 222
Carter-Wallace, 181–82
cases, discussion of, 15–17, 101–3, 131
catalepsy, 11, 17–18
catatonia: benzodiazepines and, 184; disease and, 157; in Germany, 67–68; Gjessing and, 111; Kahlbaum and, 11; Kraepelin and, 73–74; prevalence of, 19
catecholamine hypothesis of depression, 111, 145–47, 226
Celexa. See citalopram
Charpentier, Paul, 98
chemical imbalance, 226
Child and Adolescent Bipolar Foundation, 204

children: antidepressants and, 214–18; diagnosis of, 198–202, 212–13; marketing and, 227; mental health system and, 243–44; suicide in, and SSRIs, 213–14, 217–18, 235, 238; treatment of, 177–78, 195, 208, 252; unmet need concept and, 221–22
chlordiazepoxide, 179, 181, 182
chlorpromazine: carbamazepine and, 172; effects of, 98–99, 166–67, 172, 182; lithium and, 108, 172; as mood stabilizer, 179; tardive dyskinesia and, 191; and tranquilizer idea, 179
cholera, xii
Chouinard, Guy, 161, 185
circular insanity, 68, 84
citalopram, 214, 215
classification of disorders: Kraepelin and, 74, 89, 135; Leonhard and, 141–42; Sydenham and, 30; unipolar-bipolar distinction, 147–48. See also Diagnostic and Statistical Manual of Mental Disorders
clinical judgment, 201–2
Clinical Research Organizations (CROs), 233–35
clinical trials, 101–3, 112, 160, 177. See also randomized controlled trials (RCTs)
clozapine, 185, 191, 192, 195
cocaine, 173–74
Cole, Jonathan, 117, 185
Collegium Internationale Neuropsychopharmacologium, 108–10, 114, 117
Comité Lyonnaise pour Recherches et Thérapeutiques en Psychiatrie, 164–65
commerce and science, 13–19, 21–22
community, benefit to, and patents, 224, 242
consensus conferences, 231–33
constitutional types, 211
consumer input into medicine, 229–30
Cotton, Henry, 35
course of disorders: Kahlbaum, Hecker, and, 65; Kraepelin and, 72, 74; manic-depression, 122, 127
Covance, 234
creativity and mental illness, 75, 150
Crichton, Alexander, 41, 46
Cullen, William, 32–33, 38–39
cycloid psychoses, 139, 140, 151–57
cyclothymia, 68–71

Darwin, Charles, 36
data, lack of access to, 239–42, 250–52